Management of Inpatient Inflammatory Bowel Disease

Joseph D. Feuerstein
Adam S. Cheifetz
Editors

Management of Inpatient Inflammatory Bowel Disease

A Comprehensive Handbook

Springer

Editors
Joseph D. Feuerstein
Harvard Medical School
Beth Israel Deaconess
Medical Center
Boston, MA, USA

Adam S. Cheifetz
Harvard Medical School
Beth Israel Deaconess
Medical Center
Boston, MA, USA

ISBN 978-1-0716-1986-5 ISBN 978-1-0716-1987-2 (eBook)
https://doi.org/10.1007/978-1-0716-1987-2

This Springer imprint is published by the registered company Springer Science+Business Media, LLC part of Springer Nature
The registered company address is: 1 New York Plaza, New York, NY 10004, U.S.A.

Introduction

The management of patients hospitalized with acute severe ulcerative colitis and Crohn's disease often requires complex multidisciplinary management with hospitalists, gastroenterologists, inflammatory bowel disease (IBD) specialists, and surgeons. Over the last decade, the pharmacologic armamentarium and surgical techniques for managing IBD has evolved dramatically providing additional new options for managing patients hospitalized with IBD. We are excited that this book, *Management of Inpatient IBD: A Comprehensive Handbook*, provides the readers with expert reviews on critical topics pertaining to the management of hospitalized patients with IBD.

The book includes chapters focused on both Crohn's disease and ulcerative colitis. Each author was carefully selected for their clinical and research expertise in the management of hospitalized patients with IBD and their ability to succinctly summarize the latest evidence-based medicine approach.

The first four chapters focus on the pharmacologic management and surgical management of acute severe ulcerative colitis. These chapters are authored by Dr. Schwartz, Dr. Farraye, Dr. Maser, and Dr. Messaris.

Chapters 5, 6 and 7 review the management of hospitalized patients with Crohn's disease, with a focus on the pharmacologic and surgical management of inflammatory, stricturing, and fistulizing Crohn's disease. These chapters are authored by Drs. Weizman, Flier, and Remzi.

The remaining chapters (Chaps. 8, 9, 10, 11, 12 and 13) focus on the management of co-infection with cytomegalovirus (CMV) and clostridium difficile, nutritional management, quality of care, pediatric IBD, and pregnancy. These chapters are authored by Dr. Achkar, Dr. Grossman, Dr. Barnes, Dr. Bousevaros, Dr. Israel, and Dr. Friedman.

We believe this book will provide the reader with a thorough review of the latest evidence on managing a challenging group of patients, those hospitalized patients with inflammatory bowel disease.

Boston, MA, USA

Joseph D. Feuerstein
Adam S. Cheifetz

Contents

Editors and Contributors

Editors

Joseph D. Feuerstein Division of Gastroenterology, Center for Inflammatory Bowel Disease, Beth Israel Deaconess Medical Center, Department of Medicine, Harvard Medical School, Boston, MA, USA

Adam S. Cheifetz Center for Inflammatory Bowel Disease, Beth Israel Deaconess Medical Center, Department of Medicine, Harvard Medical School, Boston, MA, USA

Contributors

Jean-Paul Achkar, MD Department of Gastroenterology, Hepatology and Nutrition, Cleveland Clinic, Cleveland, OH, USA

Edward L. Barnes Division of Gastroenterology and Hepatology, University of North Carolina at Chapel Hill, Chapel Hill, NC, USA

Multidisciplinary Center for Inflammatory Bowel Diseases, University of North Carolina at Chapel Hill, Chapel Hill, NC, USA

Center for Gastrointestinal Biology and Disease, University of North Carolina at Chapel Hill, Chapel Hill, NC, USA

Athos Bousvaros Professor of Pediatrics, Harvard Medical School, Inflammatory Bowel Disease Center, Boston Children's Hospital, Boston, MA, USA

R. Chibbar Division of Gastroenterology, Department of Medicine, University of Alberta, Edmonton, AB, Canada

Rahul S. Dalal Division of Gastroenterology, Hepatology, and Endoscopy, Department of Medicine, Brigham and Women's Hospital, Harvard Medical School, Boston, MA, USA

Robin Dalal Vanderbilt University Medical Center, Nashville, TN, USA

Francis A. Farraye Gastroenterology and Hepatology, Mayo Clinic Arizona, Scottsdale, AZ, USA

S. N. Flier Division of Gastroenterology, Beth Israel Deaconess Medical Center, Boston, MA, USA

Sonia Friedman Division of Gastroenterology, Hepatology, and Endoscopy, Department of Medicine, Brigham and Women's Hospital, Harvard Medical School, Boston, MA, USA

Center for Clinical Epidemiology, Odense University Hospital, Odense, Denmark

Research Unit of Clinical Epidemiology, Department of Clinical Research, University of Southern Denmark, Odense, Denmark

Harvard Medical School, Brigham and Women's Hospital, Center for Crohn's and Colitis, Chestnut Hill, MA, USA

Stephanie Lauren Gold The Rogosin Institute, Inc, New York, NY, USA

Michael J. Grieco NYU Langone Health, NYU Grossman School of Medicine, New York, NY, USA

Andrew B. Grossman Department of Pediatrics, Division of Gastroenterology, Hepatology and Nutrition, Children's Hospital of Philadelphia, Philadelphia, PA, USA

Joshua L. Hudson Department of Medicine, University of North Carolina School of Medicine, Chapel Hill, NC, USA

Esther Israel Department of Pediatrics, Harvard Medical School, Boston, MA, USA

Talha A. Malik Gastroenterology and Hepatology, Mayo Clinic Arizona, Scottsdale, AZ, USA

Elana A. Maser Gastroenterology, Mount Sinai Hospital, New York, NY, USA

Evan Messaris Division of Colon and Rectal Surgery, Beth Israel Deaconess Medical Center, Boston, MA, USA

Christopher J. Moran Pediatric Gastroenterology, MassGeneral Hospital for Children, Boston, MA, USA

Sara El Ouali, MD Digestive Disease Institute, Cleveland Clinic, Abu Dhabi, UAE

Trusha Patel Department of Pediatrics, Division of Gastroenterology, Hepatology and Nutrition, Children's Hospital of Philadelphia, Philadelphia, PA, USA

Loren Galler Rabinowitz Department of Medicine, Mount Sinai Hospital, New York, NY, USA

Feza H. Remzi NYU Langone Health, NYU Grossman School of Medicine, New York, NY, USA

David Schwartz Vanderbilt University Medical Center, Nashville, TN, USA

Punyanganie de Silva Division of Gastroenterology, Hepatology, and Endoscopy, Department of Medicine, Brigham and Women's Hospital, Harvard Medical School, Boston, MA, USA

Harvard Medical School, Brigham and Women's Hospital, Center for Crohn's and Colitis, Chestnut Hill, MA, USA

Natalie L. Stoner Center for Pediatric Inflammatory Bowel Disease, Children's Hospital of Philadelphia, Philadelphia, PA, USA

Parul Tandon Division of Gastroenterology and Hepatology, Mount Sinai Hospital, Department of Medicine, University of Toronto, Toronto, ON, Canada

Adam V. Weizman Division of Gastroenterology and Hepatology, Mount Sinai Hospital, Department of Medicine, University of Toronto, Toronto, ON, Canada

Daniel Wong Division of Colon and Rectal Surgery, Beth Israel Deaconess Medical Center, Boston, MA, USA

Epidemiology and Risk Factors for Hospitalization in Patients with Ulcerative Colitis and Crohn's Disease

1

Robin Dalal and David Schwartz

The inflammatory bowel diseases encompass both ulcerative colitis (UC) and Crohn's disease (CD). The incidence and prevalence of inflammatory bowel disease (IBD) have increased with time throughout the world with the highest annual incidence and reported prevalence of both UC and CD occurring in Europe and North America [1]. Between 1970 and 2010, incidence rates for UC and CD have increased, and it is estimated that there are approximately 1.6 million persons in the United States (US) with inflammatory bowel disease (IBD) [2].

Due to the chronic nature of IBD, patients can develop flares or worsening disease which can result in hospitalizations and need for surgery. Since the discovery of these entities, trends in hospitalizations have changed with time. The most recent interpretation of widespread data for all IBD admissions worldwide (34 coun-

R. Dalal (✉) · D. Schwartz
Vanderbilt University Medical Center, Nashville, TN, USA
e-mail: robin.dalal@vumc.org; david.a.schwartz@Vanderbilt.Edu

J. D. Feuerstein, A. S. Cheifetz (eds.), *Management of Inpatient Inflammatory Bowel Disease*,
https://doi.org/10.1007/978-1-0716-1987-2_1

tries) showed hospitalization rates were highest in North America and Europe but that the rates had stabilized or decreased over time and that rates may be increasing in Asia [3].

Specifically for UC, hospitalization rates increased since the discovery of the disease but have stabilized recently. Early data regarding hospitalizations dates back to the 1930s. Edwards and Truelove prospectively followed a series of 624 patients from 1938 to 1962, and during this time, 38% required hospitalization [4]. Annual incidence rates of hospitalization in UC began to be more widely reported in the late 1960s and 1970s with rates ranging from 4.6 to 4.8 per 100,000 in Europe and the USA [5, 6]. In one series, 20.8% of patients required hospitalization within the first year of diagnosis [7]. Since that time, hospitalization rates have increased for UC throughout the world but have stabilized recently.

In the USA, reports using data from the Nationwide Inpatient Sample showed there was a 3% annual relative increase in the hospitalization rate for UC with an overall rate reported at 10.8 per 100,000 [8]. When using the National Hospital Discharge Survey Data in the USA, hospitalization rates for UC were reported as stable during this time at 8.1–12.4 per 100,000 [9]. In California, the Kaiser Permanente system reported a 29% decrease in UC hospitalizations from 1998 to 2005 [10]. Data from Olmstead County, Minnesota, noted that from 1970 to 2004, the cumulative probability of a first hospitalization for UC was 29.4% at 5 years (95% confidence interval [CI], 24.5–34.1%), 38.7% at 10 years (33.1–43.8%), 49.2% at 20 years (42.7–55.2%), and 52.3% at 30 years (45.1–59.7%) [11]. In Canada, age-adjusted hospitalization rates remained stable from 12.6 to 13.3 per 100,000 [12]. European data from Italy and Portugal also note stable rates of hospitalization in the 2000s with rates of 4.4–4.9 per 100,000 [13, 14].

For CD, hospitalization rates have increased over time throughout the world. The annual incidence rate of hospitalization from Baltimore, Maryland, in the 1960s was reported at 1.8 per 100,000 [5]. Between 1962 and 1987, one series in Denmark reported an 83% overall admission rate within the first year of diagnosis and then 20% per year over the next 5 years [15]. In Italy, incidence of first hospitalizations of CD was 2.7 per 100,000 in the late 1980s [16]. Between 1998 and 2004, using the US Nationwide Inpatient Sample data, rates of hospitalizations increased for CD in the USA with a 4.3% annual relative increase in hospitalization rate ($P < 0.0001$) [8]. Data from the National Hospital Discharge Survey showed hospitalization rates ranging from 9.3 to 17.1 per 100,000 with a significant trend for increasing hospital rates from the 1990s to 2000s [9]. In Canada, when comparing CD patients in 2000–2001 to 1990–1991, patients were more likely in 2000–2001 to have an overnight hospital stay (RR 2.32; 95% CI 2.16–2.49) [17].

While rates have certainly increased since the first descriptions of CD, more recently, reports indicate that hospital rates for CD may be decreasing. In Canada, from 1994 to 2001, age-adjusted hospitalization rates declined from 29.2 per 100,000 to 26.9 per 100,000, and from 2003 to 2014, CD-related hospitalizations declined 32.4% [12, 18]. Hospitalization costs have also declined in CD patients over this time significantly [19]. In the USA, hospitalization rates from emergency room visits decreased 12.1% for IBD in 2014 compared to 2006 (64.7% rate of hospitalization in 2006 to 52.6% in 2014) [20].

For both UC and CD, intensive care unit (ICU) admissions are less common. In a retrospective study looking at 5 years of data from 2003 to 2008 of all IBD patients to one tertiary care center in the USA, ICU admissions accounted for only 1.43% of IBD admissions [21]. In this study, over the 5-year period, annual incidence of ICU hospitalizations increased from 0.1% in 2003 to 2.6% in 2008, and the 30-day mortality was calculated at 18.9%. In Europe, an 18-year prospective study showed that IBD-ICU admissions accounted for only 0.46% of total ICU admissions during this time period [22]. The IBD-ICU admissions were due to either IBD-specific complications, sepsis, or thromboembolic complications.

Data regarding readmission rates in IBD varies between studies. For UC, readmission rates have been reported between 14.6% and 33.7% within 90 days [12, 23–25]. For CD, readmission rates have been reported between 12.6% and 39.4% within 90 days [12, 24]. In a study of US veterans looking at readmission rates between 2007 and 2013, the 30-day readmission rate was 17.3%, and the 90-day readmission rate was 29.2%. Patients with CD had a higher risk of readmission than UC patients (OR 3.90, 95% CI 1.82–8.90) [26]. For IBD readmissions, predictors that have been reported include opioid use disorder, younger age, mood disorder (depression and/or anxiety), and lack of follow-up visit after hospitalization [26–29].

Specific risks for hospitalization in IBD have been evaluated including demographic factors, environmental exposures, and disease characteristics. The sex, age, race, and socioeconomic status of patients have variable impact on a patient's risk of hospitalization for IBD. In CD, women have been shown to have a higher risk of hospitalization than males, especially during the childbearing period [30–33]. For UC, there is conflicting data with some studies reporting risk of hospitalization being higher in females and some with a slight male predominance [32, 33]. As with the onset of IBD, there appears to be a bimodal risk of age for hospitalizations in IBD. In the USA, hospitalization rates for UC are highest in the 20–29-year-old and 70–79-year-old age groups and for CD are highest in the 20–29-year-old, 50–59-year-old, and 70–79-year-old age groups [30–32]. Within these peaks, younger patients are higher risk. Elderly patients only account for 25% of total IBD hospitalizations and overall have less hospitalization rates when compared with younger adults for both CD and UC (CD IRR 0.62, 95% CI 0.59–0.65 and UC IRR 0.64, 95% CI 0.57–0.71) [34, 35].

Data on patient's race and risk of hospitalization is not consistent overall. Earlier studies noted a twofold higher risk of hospitalization for whites than blacks (RR 2.18, 95% CI 2.18–2.19) and higher rates in both white patients and black patients when compared to Hispanics [31, 36]. A more recent evaluation of over 5000 IBD patients did not note any difference in hospitalization rates between black and white patients [37]. Other studies have shown that since the 2000s, hospitalization rates have decreased for non-Hispanic whites but not for black patients and the ratio of IBD hospitalizations to prevalence of disease was disproportionately higher among non-Hispanic blacks (7.3% compared to 3% for non-Hispanic whites and 2% for Hispanics) [38, 39]. Lower-income levels were associated with higher hospitalization rate. In a retrospective analysis of CD patients, the incidence rate for hospitalization for lowest-income group was 118 per 100-person years (CI 91.4–152.3) and for the highest-income group was 29 (CI 21.7–38.9) [40]. In CD, smoking has also been shown to increase the risk of hospitalization [41].

Geographical variation in hospitalization has also been noted in IBD. Urban areas have higher rates of hospitalization than non-urban areas [6, 36, 42]. Two studies have shown that within the USA, northern states have higher rates of hospitalizations than southern states establishing a "North to South" gradient for hospitalizations in IBD similar to the known gradient that exists with IBD incidence in general [36, 43]. The first study, in 1991, evaluated Medicare discharges, and the second study used data from the Nationwide Inpatient Sample. Seasonality has not been found to be associated with any difference in hospitalization rates [43, 44]. UV exposure has also been examined, and hospitalization rates were increased for both CD and UC in lower UV exposure areas [45].

Disease characteristics in CD have been shown to factor into a patient's risk of hospitalization as well. An analysis of a cohort of CD patients showed that patients with structuring or fistulizing phenotype of disease had a higher risk (58% vs. 41%) of hospitalization within the first year of diagnosis [46]. Over 10 years, admission rate was 2.4% per year (95% CI, 1.4–3.8%) in patients with inflammatory disease and 13% per year (95% CI, 11.5–14.6%) in the patients with structuring or fistulizing phenotypes [46]. An additional analysis from Asia showed that patients with upper GI location of CD had an 86.9% risk of hospitalization over 3 years (95% CI 73.8–100%) compared to non-upper GI location of disease (49.3% risk of hospitalization, 95% CI 39.3–59.3%) [47].

Similar to the general incidence and prevalence of IBD, the hospitalization rates for IBD have overall increased since description and discovery of these diseases. In UC, rates have stabilized in recent years, while in CD, rates have started to decrease according to some studies. The risk factors for hospitalization in IBD vary, akin to the heterogeneity of IBD itself.

References

1. Molodecky NA, Soon IS, Rabi DM, et al. Increasing incidence and prevalence of the inflammatory bowel diseases with time, based on systematic review. Gastroenterology. 2012;142(1):46–54.e42. https://doi.org/10.1053/j.gastro.2011.10.001.
2. Shivashankar R, Tremaine WJ, Harmsen WS, Loftus EVJ. Incidence and prevalence of Crohn's disease and ulcerative colitis in Olmsted County, Minnesota from 1970 through 2010. Clin Gastroenterol Hepatol. 2017;15(6):857–63. https://doi.org/10.1016/j.cgh.2016.10.039.
3. King JA, Underwood FE, Panaccione N, et al. Trends in hospitalisation rates for inflammatory bowel disease in western versus newly industrialised countries: a population-based study of countries in the Organisation for Economic Co-operation and Development. Lancet. 2019;4(4):287–95. https://doi.org/10.1016/S2468-1253(19)30013-5.
4. Edwards FC, Truelove SC. The course and prognosis of ulcerative colitis: part II Long-term prognosis. Gut. 1963;4(4):309–15. https://doi.org/10.1136/gut.4.4.309.
5. Monk M, Mendeloff AI, Siegel CI, Lilienfeld A. An epidemiological study of ulcerative colitis and regional enteritis among adults in Baltimore. I. Hospital incidence and prevalence, 1960 to 1963. Gastroenterology. 1968;54(4):198–210. https://doi.org/10.1016/S0016-5085(19)34227-1.
6. Linden G, Moller C. Ulcerative colitis in Finland: one-year incidence in all hospitals. Dis Colon Rectum. 1971;14(4):264–6. https://doi.org/10.1016/S0031-3955(05)70404-1.
7. Ritchie JK, Powell-Tuck J, Lennard-Jones J. Clinical outcome of the first ten years of ulcerative colitis and proctitis. Lancet. 1978;1:1140–3.
8. Nguyen GC, Tuskey A, Dassopoulos T, Harris ML, Brant SR. Rising hospitalization rates for inflammatory bowel disease in the United States between 1998 and 2004. Inflamm Bowel Dis. 2007;13:1529–35. https://doi.org/10.1002/ibd.20250.
9. Bewtra M, Su C, Lewis JD. Trends in hospitalization rates for inflammatory bowel disease in the United States. Clin Gastroenterol Hepatol. 2007;5:597–601. https://doi.org/10.1016/j.cgh.2007.01.015.
10. Herrinton LJ, Liu L, Fireman B, et al. Time trends in therapies and outcomes for adult inflammatory bowel disease, northern California, 1998–2005. Gastroenterology. 2009;137(2):502–11. https://doi.org/10.1053/j.gastro.2009.04.063.
11. Samuel S, Ingle S, Dhillon S, et al. Cumulative incidence and risk factors for hospitalization and surgery in a population-based cohort of ulcerative colitis. Inflamm Bowel Dis. 2013;19(9):1858–66. https://doi.org/10.1097/MIB.0b013e31828c84c5.CUMULATIVE.
12. Bernstein CN, Nabalamba A. Hospitalization, surgery, and readmission rates of IBD in Canada: a population-based study. Am J Gastroenterol. 2006;101:110–9. https://doi.org/10.1111/j.1572-0241.2006.00330.x.

13. Dias CC, Santiago M, Correia L, et al. Hospitalization trends of the inflammatory bowel disease landscape: a nationwide overview of 16 years. Dig Liver Dis. 2019;51(7):952–60. https://doi.org/10.1016/j.dld.2019.01.016.
14. Kohn A, Fano V, Monterubbianesi R, et al. Surgical and nonsurgical hospitalization rates and charges for patients with ulcerative colitis in Italy: a 10-year cohort study. Dig Liver Dis. 2012;44(5):369–74. https://doi.org/10.1016/j.dld.2011.11.009.
15. Munkholm P, Langholz E, Davidsen M, Binder V. Disease activity courses in a regional cohort of Crohn's disease patients. Scand J Gastroenterol. 1995;30(7):699–706. https://doi.org/10.3109/00365529509096316.
16. Cottone M, Cipolla C, Orlando A, Oliva L, Aiala R, Puleo A. Epidemiology of Crohn's disease in Sicily: a hospital incidence study from 1987–1989. Eur J Epidemiol. 1991;7(6):636–40.
17. Longobardi T, Bernstein CN. Health care resource utilization in inflammatory bowel disease. Clin Gastroenterol Hepatol. 2006;4(6):731–43. https://doi.org/10.1016/j.cgh.2006.02.013.
18. Rahman A, Jairath V, Feagan BG, et al. Declining hospitalisation and surgical intervention rates in patients with Crohn's disease: a population – based cohort. Aliment Pharmacol Ther. 2019;50:1086–93. https://doi.org/10.1111/apt.15511.
19. Targownik LE, Kaplan GG, Witt J, et al. Longitudinal trends in the direct costs and health care utilization ascribable to inflammatory bowel disease in the biologic era: results from a Canadian population-based analysis. Am J Gastroenterol. 2020;115(1):128–37. https://doi.org/10.14309/ajg.0000000000000503.
20. Ballou S, Hirsch W, Singh P, et al. Emergency department utilisation for inflammatory bowel disease in the United States from 2006 to 2014. Aliment Pharmacol Ther. 2018;47:913–21. https://doi.org/10.1111/apt.14551.
21. Ha C, Maser EA, Kornbluth A. Clinical presentation and outcomes of inflammatory bowel disease patients admitted to the intensive care unit. J Clin Gastroenterol. 2013;47:485–90.
22. Huber W, Herrmann G, Schuster T, et al. Life-threatening complications of Crohn's disease and ulcerative colitis: a systematic analysis of admissions to an ICU during 18 years. Dtsch Med Wochenschr. 2010;135(14):668–74. https://doi.org/10.1055/s-0030-1251915.
23. Jalan KN, Smcus W, Card WI, et al. An experience of ulcerative colitis III. Long term outcome. Gastroenterology. 1970;59(4):598–609. https://doi.org/10.1016/S0016-5085(19)33714-X.
24. Frolkis A, Kaplan GG, Patel A, et al. Postoperative complications and emergent readmission in children and adults with inflammatory bowel disease who undergo intestinal resection: a population-based study. Inflamm Bowel Dis. 2014;20:1316–23. https://doi.org/10.1097/MIB.0000000000000099.

25. Poojary P, Saha A, Chauhan K, et al. Predictors of hospital readmissions for ulcerative colitis in the United States: a National Database Study. Inflamm Bowel Dis. 2017;23(3):347–56. https://doi.org/10.1097/MIB.0000000000001041.Predictors.
26. Malhotra A, Phatharacharukul P, Thongprayoon C. Risk factors for 90-day readmission in veterans with inflammatory bowel disease – does post-discharge follow-up. Mil Med Res. 2018;5(5):1–6. https://doi.org/10.1186/s40779-018-0153-x.
27. Charilaou P, Mohapatra S, Joshi T, et al. Opioid use disorder increases 30-day readmission risk in inflammatory bowel disease hospitalizations: a nationwide matched analysis. J Crohns Colitis. 2020;14(5):636–45. https://doi.org/10.1093/ecco-jcc/jjz198.
28. Cohen-Mekelburg S, Rosenblatt R, Gold S, Shen N, Fortune B. Fragmented care is prevalent among inflammatory bowel disease readmissions and is associated with worse outcomes. Am J Gastroenterol. 2019;114:276–90.
29. Barnes EL, Kochar B, Long MD, et al. Modifiable risk factors for hospital readmission among patients with inflammatory bowel disease in a nationwide database. Inflamm Bowel Dis. 2017;23(6):875–81. https://doi.org/10.1097/MIB.0000000000001121.Modifiable.
30. Garland CF, Lilienfeld AM, Mendeloff AI, et al. Incidence rates of ulcerative colitis and Crohn's disease in fifteen areas of the United States. Gastroenterology. 1981;81(6):1115–24. https://doi.org/10.1016/S0016-5085(81)80021-2.
31. Kurata JH, Kantor-fish S, Frankl H, Godby P, Vadheim C. Crohn' s disease among ethnic groups in a large health maintenance organization. Gastroenterology. 1992;102:1940–8.
32. Primatesta P, Goldacre MJ. Crohn's disease and ulcerative colitis in England and the Oxford record linkage study area: a profile of hospitalized morbidity. Int J Epidemiol. 1995;24(5):922–8.
33. Sonnenberg A. Demographic characteristics of hospitalized IBD patients. Dig Dis Sci. 2009;54:2449–55. https://doi.org/10.1007/s10620-009-0973-3.
34. Ananthakrishnan AN, Mcginley EL, Binion DG. Inflammatory bowel disease in the elderly is associated with worse outcomes: a national study of hospitalizations. Inflamm Bowel Dis. 2009;15(2):182–9. https://doi.org/10.1002/ibd.20628.
35. Nguyen GC, Sheng L, Benchimol EI. Health care utilization in elderly onset inflammatory bowel disease a population-based study. Inflamm Bowel Dis. 2015;21:777–82. https://doi.org/10.1097/MIB.0000000000000306.
36. Sonnenberg A, Mccarty DJ, Jacobsen SJ. Geographic variation of inflammatory bowel disease within the United States. Gastroenterology. 1991;100:143–9.

37. Barnes EL, Kochar B, Long MD. Lack of difference in treatment patterns and clinical outcomes between black and white patients with inflammatory bowel disease. Inflamm Bowel Dis. 2018;24(12):2634–40. https://doi.org/10.1093/ibd/izy179.
38. Xu F, Wheaton AG, Liu Y, Lu H, Greenlund KJ. Hospitalizations for inflammatory bowel disease among medicare fee-for-service beneficiaries – United States, 1999–2017. Morb Mortal Wkly Rep. 2019;68(49):1134–8.
39. Nguyen GC, Chong CA, Chong RY. National estimates of the burden of inflammatory bowel disease among racial and ethnic groups in the United States. J Crohns Colitis. 2014;8(4):288–95. https://doi.org/10.1016/j.crohns.2013.09.001.
40. Walker C, Allamneni C, Orr J, et al. Socioeconomic status and race are both independently associated with increased hospitalization rate among Crohn' s disease patients. Sci Rep. 2018;8:1–6. https://doi.org/10.1038/s41598-018-22429-z.
41. Seksik P, Nion-Larmurier I, Sokol H, Beaugerie L, Cosnes J. Effects of light smoking consumption on the clinical course of Crohn's disease. Inflamm Bowel Dis. 2009;15(5):734–41. https://doi.org/10.1002/ibd.20828.
42. de Boer Visser N, Bryant HE, Hershfield NB. Predictors of hospitalization early in the course of Crohn's disease. A pilot study. Gastroenterology. 1990;99(2):380–5. https://doi.org/10.1016/0016-5085(90)91019-3.
43. Stein AC, Gaetano JN, Jacobs J, Kunnavakkam R, Bissonnette M, Pekow J. Northern latitude but not season is associated with increased rates of hospitalizations related to inflammatory bowel disease: results of a multi-year analysis of a National cohort. PLoS One. 2016;11(8):1–12. https://doi.org/10.1371/journal.pone.0161523.
44. Don BAC, Goldacre MJ. Absence of seasonality in emergency hospital admissions for inflammatory bowel disease. Lancet. 1984;2:1156–7.
45. Limketkai BN, Bayless TM, Brant SR, Hut SM. Lower regional and temporal ultraviolet exposure is associated with increased rates and severity of inflammatory bowel disease hospitalisation. Aliment Pharmacol Ther. 2014;40:508–17. https://doi.org/10.1111/apt.12845.
46. Veloso FT, Ferreira JT, Barros L, Almeida S. Clinical outcome of Crohn's disease: analysis according to the Vienna classification and clinical activity. Inflamm Bowel Dis. 2001;7(4):306–13.
47. Chow D, Sung J, Wu J, Tsoi K, Leong R, Chan FKL. Upper gastrointestinal tract phenotype of Crohn's disease is associated with early surgery and further hospitalization. Inflamm Bowel Dis. 2009;15(4):551–7. https://doi.org/10.1002/ibd.20804.

Routine Management of Hospitalized Patients with Ulcerative Colitis

2

Talha A. Malik and Francis A. Farraye

Background

All patients seen with ulcerative colitis (UC) in the ER or in the outpatient setting should have their disease activity graded and based on the findings, management options discussed and treatment undertaken. Acute severe ulcerative colitis (ASUC) is a term used to describe patients with UC with severely active disease whose symptoms progress rapidly. Patients with ASUC are hospitalized for inpatient management. UC is classified as ulcerative proctitis, ulcerative proctosigmoiditis, left-sided ulcerative colitis, or pancolitis based on its extent. Disease activity is graded as mild, moderate, or severe based on several clinical scores including the Mayo clinical score that includes only clinical parameters such as number of additional bowel movements per day, amount of blood, and physician assessment (Table 2.1). Another clinical

T. A. Malik (✉) · F. A. Farraye
Gastroenterology and Hepatology, Mayo Clinic Arizona, Scottsdale, AZ, USA
e-mail: Malik.Talha@mayo.edu; Farraye.Francis@mayo.edu

J. D. Feuerstein, A. S. Cheifetz (eds.), *Management of Inpatient Inflammatory Bowel Disease*,
https://doi.org/10.1007/978-1-0716-1987-2_2

Table 2.1 Mayo UC score

Composite Mayo score
A. Stool frequency
0, Normal number of stools for this patient
1, 1–2 stools more than normal
2, 3–4 stools more than normal
3, 5 or more stools more than normal
B. Rectal bleeding
0, No blood found
1, Streaks of blood with stool less than half the time
2, Obvious blood with stool most of the time
3, Blood alone passed
C. Sigmoidoscopic findings
0, Normal or inactive disease
1, Mild disease (erythema, decreased vascular pattern, mild friability)
2, Moderate disease (marked erythema, absent vascular pattern, friability, erosions)
3, Severe disease (spontaneous bleeding, ulceration)
D. Physician's global assessment
0, Normal
1, Mild disease
2, Moderate disease
3, Severe disease
Total
0 = Remission
1–4 = Mild
5–8 = Moderate
9–12 = Severe

score widely used in ulcerative colitis is the Truelove and Witts clinical score that includes both clinical and biochemical parameters (Table 2.2).

The decision to hospitalize a patient for inpatient management should be based on clinical evaluation and biochemical assessment. In 2019, the American College of Gastroenterology (ACG) proposed a disease severity scoring system that included clinical, biochemical, and endoscopic metrics (Table 2.3) [1].

Table 2.2 Truelove and Witts UC score

Truelove and Witts score	Mild	Moderate	Severe
Bowel movements per day	<4	4–6	>6
Blood in stool	Intermittent	Frequent	Continuous
Temperature greater than 37.5 °C	No	No	Yes
Heart rate > 90	No	No	Yes
Anemia No (Hb)	>11 g/dL	10.5–11 g/dL	<10.5 g/dL
ESR (mm/h) or C-reactive protein (mg/L)	Normal	<30	>30

Table 2.3 2019 ACG UC activity index

2019 ACG UC activity index	Remission	Mild	Moderate-severe	Fulminant
Stools	Formed	<4	6–10	>10
Blood in stool	None	Intermittent	Frequent	Continuous
Urgency	None	Mild, occasional	Often	Continuous
Hemoglobin	Normal	Normal	<75% of normal	Transfusion required
ESR (mm/h)	<30	<30	>30	>30
CRP (mg/L)	Normal	Elevated	Elevated	Elevated
Fecal calprotectin (ug/g)	<150–200	>150–200	>150–200	>150–200
Mayo endoscopy subscore	0–1	1	2–3	3
UC endoscopic index of severity	0–1	2–4	5–6	7–8

Epidemiology

Based on a 2010 systematic review of a cohort of 750 UC patients followed for a median of 12 years, the risk of developing at least one episode of acute severe ulcerative colitis (ASUC) in these patients was approximately 25% [2].

Before the routine use of steroids, reports suggested that a quarter of patients with fulminant UC died but in recent studies, mortality has been reduced to 1% [3–5]. In regard to rates of colectomy, the risk is 20% among patients with UC admitted for ASUC during the same admission [2].

Based on a multicenter retrospective study published in 2020, of patients with ASUC who responded to intravenous steroids, their colectomy-free survival was 96% at 1 year and 92% at approximately 5 years. Relapse-free survival in these patients was 58% at 1 year and 40% at 5 years. Those with ASUC who had <6 loose stools per day at day 3 and a clinical Mayo score of <2 at day 5 and those who were placed on anti-TNF maintenance therapy were less likely to relapse [6].

Characterizing UC Patients with ASUC

In 2019 the ACG proposed a comprehensive classification for disease severity in UC though the most common classification used to characterize patients with acute severe ulcerative colitis (ASUC) as of the writing of this chapter is the Truelove and Witts classification of severity of UC. As opposed to the Montreal and the Mayo classification of disease severity, Truelove and Witts criteria further distinguish between severe disease and fulminant disease including biochemical parameters as well as objective vital sign parameters. Based on Truelove and Witts criteria, ASUC is defined by more than six bloody bowel movements per day and at least one of the following clinical features: fever (>37.8 °C), tachycardia (>90 bpm), anemia (hemoglobin <10.5 g/dl), or elevated inflammatory markers (traditionally, erythrocyte sedimentation rate greater than 30 mm/h or, more recently, C-reactive protein (CRP) greater than 30 mg/L (ULN 10 mg/L)). It further classifies those within the ASUC category as having acute severe fulminant colitis as defined by having more than ten stools per day, continuous rectal bleeding, abdominal pain, colonic dilatation on abdominal X-ray film, and toxic symptoms that include fever and anorexia. While the initial management regimen for both these categories is the same, those with severe fulminant acute colitis are considered to be at a much higher risk of progressing to toxic megacolon and bowel perforation and therefore warrant close monitoring including surgical consultation [1, 3, 7].

Approach to Inpatient Management of ASUC

General Principles

All patients with ASUC are admitted for inpatient management. Colorectal surgery is consulted. A history and physical examination is performed and vital signs monitored. Diagnostic tests including biochemical, radiological, and endoscopic evaluation should follow promptly. Patients without absolute contraindications receive DVT prophylaxis with subcutaneous unfractionated or low molecular weight heparin or fondaparinux. All patients are allowed to eat a low-fiber diet based on their tolerance, and whenever possible, parental nutrition must be avoided. A summary of the approach to management of ASUC is outlined in Table 2.4.

Table 2.4 Approach to inpatient management of ASUC

History	History of the use of NSAIDs, antibiotics, opioid medications, and recreational drugs. Travel history and history of exposure to others with infections. Comorbid illnesses
Physical exam	Physical examination including abdominal exam, rectal exam, and vital signs
Labs	CBC, CMP, CRP, fecal calprotectin, stool for *C. diff*
Radiological testing	KUB in all patients, consider CT abdomen/pelvis with contrast if abdominal tenderness
Endoscopic testing	Flexible sigmoidoscopy with biopsy to assess disease activity and rule out CMV colitis
VTE prophylaxis	Subcutaneous unfractionated or low molecular weight heparin or fondaparinux
Diet	Oral low-fiber diet as tolerated; parenteral nutrition only if severe malnutrition and unable to eat
Hydration	Crystalloids, preferably normal saline
Medication	Methylprednisolone 60 mg IV daily for 3–5 days
Colorectal surgery consult	Surgery for toxic megacolon, perforation, severe hemorrhage, failure of inpatient medical therapy

History, Physical Examination, and Vital Signs

Medication history for the use of NSAIDs, antibiotics, opioid medications, and recreational drugs is sought. Travel history and history of exposure to others with infections is obtained. Inquiry into potential triggers for disease exacerbation is made and comorbid illnesses are assessed. Physical examination is completed promptly and should include abdominal and rectal exam. Vital signs should be monitored.

Diagnostic Work-Up

Blood and stool studies to assess electrolytes, blood counts, inflammatory markers, and comorbid illnesses including infection with *C. difficile* and other enteric pathogens are obtained on admission. All patients should undergo flexible sigmoidoscopy to assess severity of endoscopic inflammation, and biopsies should be taken to r/o CMV. Imaging to assess for toxic megacolon and perforation is performed. The entire diagnostic work should be systematic in order to identify and grade UC severity and rule out other causes of the patients' symptoms.

Initial Treatment

Once the diagnosis of ASUC is established, intravenous corticosteroids at a dose of 60 mg of methylprednisolone daily for 3–5 days should be instituted. There is no benefit of a dose higher than 60 mg daily. There is no benefit of continuous infusion over interval IV dosing [8].

If there is evidence of toxic megacolon, perforation, or severe hemorrhage, the patient should undergo surgery. If improvement on 3–5 days of IV steroids occurs, transition to any number of maintenance therapies should be initiated. If no response to IV steroids at 3–5 days albeit without significant worsening, one should consider induction with infliximab or cyclosporine. If cyclosporine is chosen, concomitant induction with vedolizumab can be considered. Tacrolimus may be used when cyclosporine is not an option or not available. Alternatives include considering ustekinumab or tofacitinib, but evidence for these medications is limited and evolving.

Monitoring Response

Patients' response to intravenous steroids should be assessed with repeat labs including CBC, electrolytes, and CRP daily along with an assessment of the total number of bowel movements over a 24-h period, with special attention to their overall response after 3 days of treatment [33–36]. The Oxford index is a traditional index used to assess and monitor response to therapy. Based on the Oxford index, ASUC patients with eight or more loose bowel movements or between three and eight loose bowel movements and a serum CRP of 45 mg/L or greater (ULN 10 mg/L) at the end of 3 days of intravenous steroids had an 85% likelihood of colectomy. By end of days 3–5 of intravenous steroid therapy, patients who have not had a response should be considered for therapy with infliximab or cyclosporine. If medical therapy with these agents is not an option, then colectomy should be considered. Delay in institution of medical therapy and/or surgery has been associated with poorer outcomes. Figure 2.1 provides a simplified algorithm for the overall approach to UC management.

Evidence for Recommended Approach to Inpatient Management of UC

Evidence for Intravenous Steroids

The efficacy of intravenous steroids in severe UC was first demonstrated by Truelove and Jewell in their 1974 case series published in the Lancet [9]. In this study, 49 patients hospitalized with severe colitis were administered prednisolone intravenously at a dose of 60 mg per day in divided doses along with topical

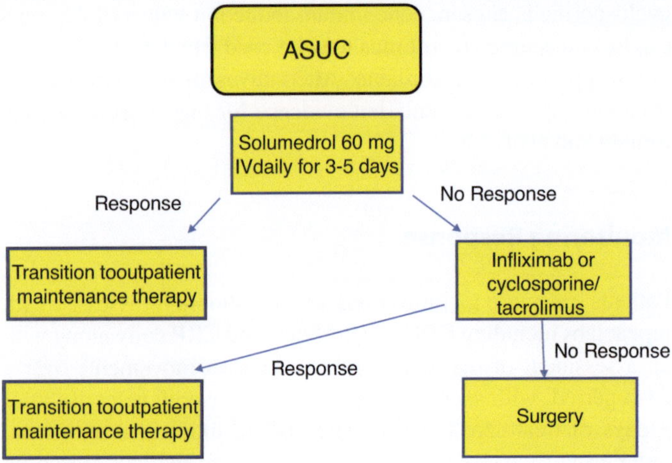

Fig. 2.1 Flow chart for therapy

hydrocortisone enemas. At day 5, 73% of these patients were in remission. Colectomy rate in these patients was reported as 18% [9]. Since then, not a single dose-ranging clinical trial for intravenous corticosteroids has been published. Based on a 2007 systematic review of 32 trials by Turner et al., among patients who failed oral steroids, up to two thirds responded to intravenous corticosteroids [10]. Their meta-regression failed to demonstrate a steroid dose-colectomy association [10]. They did note that there was no evidence of benefit at a dose higher than methylprednisolone 60 mg IV per day [10].

Evidence for Intravenous Fluids

Many UC patients admitted with ASUC have significant volume depletion and intravenous fluids (IVF) should be administered. There are no studies comparing one type of IVF to another in this group, and there are no specific guidelines pertaining to the rate and amount of IVF.

Evidence for VTE Risk and Prevention

The risk of venous thromboembolism (VTE) in hospitalized patients with IBD (both Crohn's and UC) is higher than for inpatients without IBD. VTE in hospitalized patients with IBD is associated with a 2.5-fold increased mortality [11]. Rectal bleeding is expected in ASUC and, unless life threatening, is not a contraindication to chemical VTE prophylaxis. Based on current research, beyond the need for inpatient VTE prophylaxis in ASUC, there is no clear guidance regarding the type, amount, or duration.

Evidence Against Anti-motility Agents

Anti-motility agents such as loperamide and diphenoxylate/atropine should generally be avoided as they may provoke toxic megacolon as anticholinergic agents may lead to worsening gastric and small bowel distension in UC patients, thus furthering the risk of toxic megacolon and perforation [12].

Evidence Against Use of Opiates

In addition to their undesirable anti-motility effect, the use of opiates has been associated with poor outcomes among inpatients and outpatients with IBD, including increased morbidity and mortality. Pain severe enough to require opiates should raise suspicion for toxic megacolon, perforation, or a non-inflammatory etiology. If opiates are utilized, they should be ordered as one-time doses and the patient should be reassessed for each dose. Gan and colleagues also suggested higher risk of toxic megacolon and complications in ASUC patients who received opiates [12]. A more recent study noted an association between heavy use of any opiate and premature mortality in patients with UC [13].

Evidence Against Use of NSAIDs

Similarly, data against the use of NSAIDs during ASUC is also extrapolated from outpatient IBD studies in which there is evidence of increased inflammatory bowel disease activity with NSAID use [14]. Therefore, NSAIDs should generally be avoided in hospitalized UC patients.

Evidence in Regard to Nutrition

There is no evidence that bowel rest with parenteral nutrition improves outcomes in ASUC, and therefore oral intake among those who can tolerate it is not contraindicated and in fact encouraged. Among those with toxic megacolon or fulminant colitis, oral intake should be avoided due to high risk of imminent surgery.

Evidence for Use of Mesalamine Agents

In general, there is no evidence that suggests an advantage of the continued use of mesalamine agents in patients hospitalized and being treated for ASUC, and therefore they should be discontinued. In fact, an idiosyncratic reaction of worsening of colitis can occur in 1–2% of patients treated with mesalamine.

Evidence for Antibiotics

There is no role for the routine use of antibiotics in patients hospitalized with ASUC. As use of antibiotics raises the risk of *C. difficile* infection and antibiotic resistance, they should generally be avoided in these patients other than in those with suspected toxic megacolon or perforation. Regarding using antibiotic prophylaxis against *Pneumocystis jiroveci* pneumonia (PJP) in ASUC patients treated with triple immunosuppression (i.e., steroids plus two other agents, e.g., cyclosporine or infliximab and a thiopurine), it may be advisable despite an overall very low absolute incidence of PJP in IBD patients.

Evidence for Infliximab Standard Regimen

Evidence for use of infliximab in ASUC is based on several clinical trials and case series.

The initial trial for infliximab use in ASUC was published by Sands and colleagues in 2001 in which four of eight patients with steroid-refractory ASUC who received one infusion of infliximab vs. zero of three patients who received placebo experienced response at 2 weeks [15]. In 2005, another randomized controlled trial was published by Jarnerot et al. in which a single infusion of infliximab 5 mg/kg IV given to 24 steroid-refractory ASUC patients was associated with a significantly lower colectomy rate (29%) at 3 months compared to 21 patients who received placebo (66%), and this benefit was maintained at 3 years of follow-up (50% vs. 76%) [16, 17]. In a Swedish single-arm retrospective study published in 2013, colectomy-free survivals at 3, 12, 36, and 60 months among 211 patients with steroid-refractory active UC who received infliximab were 71%, 64%, 59%, and 53%, respectively, with 50% of these patients in steroid-free remission at 12 months [18].

Evidence for Accelerated Infliximab Regimen

To date, there are no clinical trials examining the efficacy of accelerated or dose-optimized infliximab regimens in ASUC. It is however established that in severely active UC, there is significant fecal infliximab loss and therefore accelerated infliximab regimens have been employed. A 2015 retrospective study by Gibson et al. examined 50 patients who received accelerated infliximab induction, defined as 3 induction doses within a median period of 24 days. They noted a lower rate of colectomy with the accelerated regimen (7%) compared with standard dosing (40%). At a median 2.4 years' follow-up, the colectomy rate was 27% in the dose-intensified group versus 51.4% in the cohort that received the standard regimen [19]. A 2017 qualitative review of all cohort and case-control studies looking at the benefit of accelerated infliximab regimens in ASUC suggested a benefit of dose-optimized/accelerated infliximab induction regimens in at least 50% of patients with ASUC with an 80% reduction in 3-month colectomy rates among those who received one or two additional infliximab infusions in the first 3 weeks [20].

Evidence for Cyclosporine

The first clinical trial suggesting efficacy of cyclosporine in severe ulcerative colitis refractory to steroid therapy was published by Lichtiger in 1994. In their study, cyclosporine at a dose of 4 mg/kg IV daily or placebo was given to 20 patients with severe ulcerative colitis refractory to 7 days of intravenous corticosteroids. They found that 9 of the 11 patients (82%) treated with cyclosporine responded at 7 days vs. 0 of the 9 patients who got placebo [21]. Van Assche et al. published a clinical trial in 2003 in which they found that intravenous cyclosporine was equally efficacious when used as a 2 mg/kg IV infusion versus for mg/kg IV infusion albeit with less side effects [22].

Evidence Comparing Infliximab vs. Cyclosporine

Three clinical trials published between 2012 and 2016 sought to compare cyclosporine and infliximab in ASUC but did not find any statistically significant differences in rates of treatment failure, mucosal healing, colectomy, long-term colectomy-free survival, serious adverse events, or death [23–25]. A meta-analysis published in 2016 by Narula et al. did not demonstrate any statistically significant difference in response to infliximab vs. cyclosporine in ASUC [26].

In 2017, Ordas et al. published a long-term cohort study of 740 patients with steroid-refractory ASUC with median follow-up of

71 months. They did not find any difference in colectomy rates between patients treated with infliximab versus cyclosporine (26.2% vs. 25.4%). They however did note a lower rate of serious adverse events in the cyclosporine group versus those who received infliximab (15.4% vs. 26.5%) ($p = 0.001$) [27]. Of note, these studies compared standard regimens of both agents. Also, in the CONSTRUCT trial published by Williams et al. in 2016, there was higher patient and physician satisfaction with the use of infliximab. Finally, a 2014 European study reported a lower length of hospital stay in ASUC patients who received infliximab (median of 4 days (IQR 4.0–5.75)) vs. those who received cyclosporine (median of 11 days) [28].

Evidence for Infliximab-Cyclosporine Sequential Use

There have been several studies published examining the use of cyclosporine or infliximab as sequential therapy to induction with the other agent, and while the response rates have been encouraging, limiting factors have been higher rates of serious adverse events [29–31].

Narula and colleagues published a systematic review examining sequential therapy and noted short-term treatment response in 62.4%, remission in 38.9%, colectomy at 3 months in 28.3%, and colectomy at 12 months in 42.3%. Adverse event rate was 23.0%, serious infections were noted in 6.7%, and the mortality rate was 1% [32]. Based on this research, sequential infliximab/cyclosporine therapy in patients with ASUC may be cautiously considered at specialized tertiary care centers on a case-by-case basis and after risks are discussed with the patient.

Evidence for Tacrolimus Use

Evidence for the use of oral tacrolimus in acute severe ulcerative colitis emanates from two randomized controlled trials published in 2006 and 2012, respectively, both by Ogata et al.

In the 2006 trial, patients with refractory active UC were randomized to oral tacrolimus based on high versus low trough concentrations with the third group receiving placebo. The responses rate was noted to be 68.4% in the oral tacrolimus high trough concentration group compared to 10.0% in the placebo group ($p < 0.001$). There were no serious adverse events of concern and no deaths attributed to the agent [33].

In 2012, they published a placebo-controlled, double-blind study of 62 patients with steroid-refractory, moderate-to-severe UC. Patients were randomized into either an oral tacrolimus or placebo group. At week 2, clinical response rate was 50.0% in the tacrolimus vs. 13.3% in the placebo group. The rate of mucosal healing observed was 43.8% vs. 13.3%, respectively, and clinical remission in 9.4% vs. 0.0%. There were no serious adverse events reported in either group [34]. Based on these two relatively small trials, tacrolimus may be used as an alternative to cyclosporine and infliximab in steroid-refractory acute severe ulcerative colitis.

Evidence for Vedolizumab

To date, there are no clinical trials published examining the efficacy of vedolizumab in ASUC.

In 2018, Pellet and colleagues published results of a retrospective observational study in which they collected data from 12 referral centers in France. In the study, they examined 39 patients who had active steroid-refractory severely active UC that received a calcineurin inhibitor as induction therapy along with vedolizumab as maintenance therapy. At 12 months, colectomy-free survival was 68% in the group with 44% still on vedolizumab. There were no deaths and there were four severe adverse events [35]. In 2019, Feagan and colleagues published results of a post hoc analysis of the GEMINI vedolizumab trials. They found that in patients with active UC, who received vedolizumab, 19.1% (overall) and 22.3% (those that were TNF antagonist naive) achieved a composite score of rectal bleeding of 0 and stool frequency ≤1 based on the Mayo score at week 2 compared to 10% (overall) and 6.6% (TNF antagonist naive) in the placebo group [36].

In 2019, Christensen and colleagues published results of a subanalysis of patients who received vedolizumab and concomitant calcineurin inhibitors in the treatment of both active UC and Crohn's in their prospective database. Among the 11 active UC patients who received concomitant vedolizumab induction and a calcineurin inhibitor (cyclosporine or tacrolimus), clinical response was achieved in 73%, 82%, and 64% and clinical remission in 55%, 45%, and 45% at weeks 14, 30, and 52, respectively [37].

Evidence for Tofacitinib

To date, there are no clinical trials published examining the efficacy of tofacitinib in ASUC.

In 2019, Berinstein et al. published a case series of four patients with ASUC who received induction with tofacitinib at an off-label dosing regimen of 10 mg oral three times daily for 3 days. They all had rapid improvement in clinical symptoms and CRP. One of these three patients was not on concurrent IV steroids [38]. Also in 2019, Hanauer et al. published results of a post hoc analysis of the OCTAVE I, two trials of tofacitinib in UC. They noted that compared with placebo, 3 days of tofacitinib therapy at a dose of 10 mg oral twice daily induced significantly greater reductions from baseline in patient-reported stool frequency and rectal bleeding (P less than 0.01 for each measure). This effect was independent of prior treatment or baseline levels of CRP [39].

Evidence for Ustekinumab

To date, there are no clinical trials published examining the efficacy of ustekinumab in ASUC.

In a retrospective study published in 2020, Ochsenkuhn et al. examined the effectiveness of ustekinumab as rescue therapy in active UC patients refractory or intolerant to steroids and all approved therapies except tofacitinib. Of the 19 patients who received induction with ustekinumab, 53% (10/19) were in clinical remission at 1 year. Of note, 5 of the 19 patients did not continue therapy after induction due to ongoing active disease or side effects [40].

Surgery in ASUC

Colorectal surgery should be consulted on all patients admitted with ASUC. If there is evidence of toxic megacolon, perforation, or severe hemorrhage on admission or at any point during the hospital stay, the patient should undergo surgery instead of medical therapy. Those with ASUC without toxic megacolon, perforation, or severe hemorrhage should be initiated on intravenous corticosteroids. By end of days 3–5 of intravenous steroid therapy, those who have not had a response should be considered for therapy with infliximab or cyclosporine. If medical therapy with these agents is not an option, then colectomy should be considered. Delay in institution of medical therapy and/or surgery has been associated with poorer outcomes. Those who fail rescue medical therapy should undergo surgery to avoid further complications [41, 42].

Based on a 2016 systematic review, the risk of early (<30 days post-op) complications in patients with ASUC who underwent colectomy ranged between 9% and 65%, whereas late (>30 days post-op) complications ranged between 17% and 55%. The overall postoperative mortality associated with colectomy for UC was 1% [43]. At the time of writing of this chapter, the three-stage restorative proctocolectomy with ileal pouch-anal anastomosis (IPAA) was the surgical procedure of choice for patients with ASUC who failed medical therapy.

Summary

In summary, all patients with ASUC should be hospitalized for inpatient management. A thorough and systematic diagnostic work-up should be undertaken. This includes history, physical examination, and diagnostic studies. Once the diagnosis of ASUC is established, intravenous (IV) steroids should be initiated for 3–5 days. Unless contraindicated, all should receive DVT prophylaxis and be fed orally. If improvement on 3–5 days of IV steroids occurs, transition to any number of outpatient maintenance therapies is initiated. If there is no response to IV steroids at 3–5 days, infliximab or cyclosporine as rescue therapy should be considered. Patients that fail to respond to intravenous steroids or rescue therapy should undergo surgery.

Disclosures

- Relevant disclosures: Dr. Farraye is a consultant for Janssen and Pfizer.
- Relevant disclosures: Dr. Malik has no disclosures relevant to this publication.

References

1. Rubin DT, Ananthakrishnan AN, Siegel CA, Sauer BG, Long MD. ACG clinical guideline: ulcerative colitis in adults. Am J Gastroenterol. 2019;114(3):384–413.
2. Dinesen LC, Walsh AJ, Protic MN, Heap G, Cummings F, Warren BF, et al. The pattern and outcome of acute severe colitis. J Crohns Colitis. 2010;4(4):431–7.
3. Truelove SC, Witts LJ. Cortisone in ulcerative colitis; final report on a therapeutic trial. Br Med J. 1955;2(4947):1041–8.
4. Jakobovits SL, Travis SP. Management of acute severe colitis. Br Med Bull. 2005;75-76:131–44.
5. Lynch RW, Lowe D, Protheroe A, Driscoll R, Rhodes JM, Arnott ID. Outcomes of rescue therapy in acute severe ulcerative colitis: data from the United Kingdom inflammatory bowel disease audit. Aliment Pharmacol Ther. 2013;38(8):935–45.
6. Salameh R, Kirchgesner J, Allez M, Carbonnel F, Meyer A, Gornet JM, et al. Long-term outcome of patients with acute severe ulcerative colitis responding to intravenous steroids. Aliment Pharmacol Ther. 2020;51(11):1096–104.
7. Fudman DI, Sattler L, Feuerstein JD. Inpatient management of acute severe ulcerative colitis. J Hosp Med. 2019;14(12):766–73.
8. Bossa F, Fiorella S, Caruso N, Accadia L, Napolitano G, Valvano MR, et al. Continuous infusion versus bolus administration of steroids in severe attacks of ulcerative colitis: a randomized, double-blind trial. Am J Gastroenterol. 2007;102(3):601–8.

9. Truelove SC, Jewell DP. Intensive intravenous regimen for severe attacks of ulcerative colitis. Lancet. 1974;1(7866):1067–70.
10. Turner D, Walsh CM, Steinhart AH, Griffiths AM. Response to corticosteroids in severe ulcerative colitis: a systematic review of the literature and a meta-regression. Clin Gastroenterol Hepatol. 2007;5(1):103–10.
11. Grainge MJ, West J, Card TR. Venous thromboembolism during active disease and remission in inflammatory bowel disease: a cohort study. Lancet. 2010;375(9715):657–63.
12. Gan SI, Beck PL. A new look at toxic megacolon: an update and review of incidence, etiology, pathogenesis, and management. Am J Gastroenterol. 2003;98(11):2363–71.
13. Burr NE, Smith C, West R, Hull MA, Subramanian V. Increasing prescription of opiates and mortality in patients with inflammatory bowel diseases in England. Clin Gastroenterol Hepatol. 2018;16(4):534–41.e6
14. Takeuchi K, Smale S, Premchand P, Maiden L, Sherwood R, Thjodleifsson B, et al. Prevalence and mechanism of nonsteroidal anti-inflammatory drug-induced clinical relapse in patients with inflammatory bowel disease. Clin Gastroenterol Hepatol. 2006;4(2):196–202.
15. Sands BE, Tremaine WJ, Sandborn WJ, Rutgeerts PJ, Hanauer SB, Mayer L, et al. Infliximab in the treatment of severe, steroid-refractory ulcerative colitis: a pilot study. Inflamm Bowel Dis. 2001;7(2):83–8.
16. Jarnerot G, Hertervig E, Friis-Liby I, Blomquist L, Karlen P, Granno C, et al. Infliximab as rescue therapy in severe to moderately severe ulcerative colitis: a randomized, placebo-controlled study. Gastroenterology. 2005;128(7):1805–11.
17. Gustavsson A, Jarnerot G, Hertervig E, Friis-Liby I, Blomquist L, Karlen P, et al. Clinical trial: colectomy after rescue therapy in ulcerative colitis – 3-year follow-up of the Swedish-Danish controlled infliximab study. Aliment Pharmacol Ther. 2010;32(8):984–9.
18. Sjoberg M, Magnuson A, Bjork J, Benoni C, Almer S, Friis-Liby I, et al. Infliximab as rescue therapy in hospitalised patients with steroid-refractory acute ulcerative colitis: a long-term follow-up of 211 Swedish patients. Aliment Pharmacol Ther. 2013;38(4):377–87.
19. Gibson DJ, Heetun ZS, Redmond CE, Nanda KS, Keegan D, Byrne K, et al. An accelerated infliximab induction regimen reduces the need for early colectomy in patients with acute severe ulcerative colitis. Clin Gastroenterol Hepatol. 2015;13(2):330–5.e1
20. Hindryckx P, Novak G, Vande Casteele N, Laukens D, Parker C, Shackelton LM, et al. Review article: dose optimisation of infliximab for acute severe ulcerative colitis. Aliment Pharmacol Ther. 2017;45(5):617–30.
21. Lichtiger S, Present DH, Kornbluth A, Gelernt I, Bauer J, Galler G, et al. Cyclosporine in severe ulcerative colitis refractory to steroid therapy. N Engl J Med. 1994;330(26):1841–5.

22. Van Assche G, D'Haens G, Noman M, Vermeire S, Hiele M, Asnong K, et al. Randomized, double-blind comparison of 4 mg/kg versus 2 mg/kg intravenous cyclosporine in severe ulcerative colitis. Gastroenterology. 2003;125(4):1025–31.
23. Laharie D, Bourreille A, Branche J, Allez M, Bouhnik Y, Filippi J, et al. Ciclosporin versus infliximab in patients with severe ulcerative colitis refractory to intravenous steroids: a parallel, open-label randomised controlled trial. Lancet. 2012;380(9857):1909–15.
24. Croft A, Walsh A, Doecke J, Cooley R, Howlett M, Radford-Smith G. Outcomes of salvage therapy for steroid-refractory acute severe ulcerative colitis: ciclosporin vs. infliximab. Aliment Pharmacol Ther. 2013;38(3):294–302.
25. Williams JG, Alam MF, Alrubaiy L, Arnott I, Clement C, Cohen D, et al. Infliximab versus ciclosporin for steroid-resistant acute severe ulcerative colitis (CONSTRUCT): a mixed methods, open-label, pragmatic randomised trial. Lancet Gastroenterol Hepatol. 2016;1(1):15–24.
26. Narula N, Marshall JK, Colombel JF, Leontiadis GI, Williams JG, Muqtadir Z, et al. Systematic review and meta-analysis: infliximab or cyclosporine as rescue therapy in patients with severe ulcerative colitis refractory to steroids. Am J Gastroenterol. 2016;111(4):477–91.
27. Ordas I, Domenech E, Manosa M, Garcia-Sanchez V, Iglesias-Flores E, Penalva M, et al. Long-term efficacy and safety of cyclosporine in a cohort of steroid-refractory acute severe ulcerative colitis patients from the ENEIDA registry (1989–2013): a nationwide multicenter study. Am J Gastroenterol. 2017;112(11):1709–18.
28. Lowenberg M, Duijvis NW, Ponsioen C, van den Brink GR, Fockens P, D'Haens GR. Length of hospital stay and associated hospital costs with infliximab versus cyclosporine in severe ulcerative colitis. Eur J Gastroenterol Hepatol. 2014;26(11):1240–6.
29. Maser EA, Deconda D, Lichtiger S, Ullman T, Present DH, Kornbluth A. Cyclosporine and infliximab as rescue therapy for each other in patients with steroid-refractory ulcerative colitis. Clin Gastroenterol Hepatol. 2008;6(10):1112–6.
30. Chaparro M, Burgueno P, Iglesias E, Panes J, Munoz F, Bastida G, et al. Infliximab salvage therapy after failure of ciclosporin in corticosteroid-refractory ulcerative colitis: a multicentre study. Aliment Pharmacol Ther. 2012;35(2):275–83.
31. Leblanc S, Allez M, Seksik P, Flourie B, Peeters H, Dupas JL, et al. Successive treatment with cyclosporine and infliximab in steroid-refractory ulcerative colitis. Am J Gastroenterol. 2011;106(4):771–7.
32. Narula N, Fine M, Colombel JF, Marshall JK, Reinisch W. Systematic review: sequential rescue therapy in severe ulcerative colitis: do the benefits outweigh the risks? Inflamm Bowel Dis. 2015;21(7):1683–94.

33. Ogata H, Matsui T, Nakamura M, Iida M, Takazoe M, Suzuki Y, et al. A randomised dose finding study of oral tacrolimus (FK506) therapy in refractory ulcerative colitis. Gut. 2006;55(9):1255–62.
34. Ogata H, Kato J, Hirai F, Hida N, Matsui T, Matsumoto T, et al. Double-blind, placebo-controlled trial of oral tacrolimus (FK506) in the management of hospitalized patients with steroid-refractory ulcerative colitis. Inflamm Bowel Dis. 2012;18(5):803–8.
35. Pellet G, Stefanescu C, Carbonnel F, Peyrin-Biroulet L, Roblin X, Allimant C, et al. Efficacy and safety of induction therapy with calcineurin inhibitors in combination with vedolizumab in patients with refractory ulcerative colitis. Clin Gastroenterol Hepatol. 2019;17(3):494–501.
36. Feagan BG, Lasch K, Lissoos T, Cao C, Wojtowicz AM, Khalid JM, et al. Rapid response to vedolizumab therapy in biologic-naive patients with inflammatory bowel diseases. Clin Gastroenterol Hepatol. 2019;17(1):130–8.e7
37. Christensen B, Gibson PR, Micic D, Colman RJ, Goeppinger SR, Kassim O, et al. Safety and efficacy of combination treatment with calcineurin inhibitors and vedolizumab in patients with refractory inflammatory bowel disease. Clin Gastroenterol Hepatol. 2019;17(3):486–93.
38. Berinstein JA, Steiner CA, Regal RE, Allen JI, Kinnucan JAR, Stidham RW, et al. Efficacy of induction therapy with high-intensity tofacitinib in 4 patients with acute severe ulcerative colitis. Clin Gastroenterol Hepatol. 2019;17(5):988–90.e1
39. Hanauer S, Panaccione R, Danese S, Cheifetz A, Reinisch W, Higgins PDR, et al. Tofacitinib induction therapy reduces symptoms within 3 days for patients with ulcerative colitis. Clin Gastroenterol Hepatol. 2019;17(1):139–47.
40. Ochsenkuhn T, Tillack C, Szokodi D, Janelidze S, Schnitzler F. Clinical outcomes with ustekinumab as rescue treatment in therapy-refractory or therapy-intolerant ulcerative colitis. United European Gastroenterol J. 2020;8(1):91–8.
41. Gallo G, Kotze PG, Spinelli A. Surgery in ulcerative colitis: when? How? Best Pract Res Clin Gastroenterol. 2018;32-33:71–8.
42. Randall J, Singh B, Warren BF, Travis SP, Mortensen NJ, George BD. Delayed surgery for acute severe colitis is associated with increased risk of postoperative complications. Br J Surg. 2010;97(3):404–9.
43. Peyrin-Biroulet L, Germain A, Patel AS, Lindsay JO. Systematic review: outcomes and post-operative complications following colectomy for ulcerative colitis. Aliment Pharmacol Ther. 2016;44(8):807–16.

3 Management of Hospitalized Patient with Ulcerative Colitis Refractory to Corticosteroids

Loren Galler Rabinowitz,
Stephanie Lauren Gold, and Elana A. Maser

Introduction

Patients with acute severe ulcerative colitis (ASUC) are at increased morbidity and mortality risk and represent a particular challenge for physicians and health systems due to their clinical complexity and high cost of care. By Truelove-Witts criteria, patients with at least six bowel movements per day, continuously bloody stools, pyrexia, tachycardia, erythrocyte sedimentation rate (ESR) >30, and hemoglobin less than 75% that of baseline are considered to have severe ulcerative colitis [1]. Any patient

L. G. Rabinowitz
Department of Medicine, Mount Sinai Hospital, New York, NY, USA

S. L. Gold
The Rogosin Institute, Inc, New York, NY, USA

E. A. Maser (✉)
Gastroenterology, Mount Sinai Hospital, New York, NY, USA
e-mail: elana.maser@mountsinai.org

J. D. Feuerstein, A. S. Cheifetz (eds.), *Management of Inpatient Inflammatory Bowel Disease*,
https://doi.org/10.1007/978-1-0716-1987-2_3

requiring inpatient hospitalization for management of ulcerative colitis is considered to be at high risk for poor outcomes, including emergent colectomy and mortality [2].

Early recognition initiation of steroid therapy has been shown to decrease mortality rates in these patients [3, 4]. However, approximately 30% of ASUC patients will fail to clinically improve with steroid exposure [5, 6]. In the past, urgent colectomy was the only therapeutic option available in steroid-refractory disease. However, the past decade has seen a rise in the number of available rescue and maintenance biologic options, requiring careful consideration of cost and efficacy in each patient's individual context.

In this chapter, we review management options for patients with ASUC that is refractory to steroid monotherapy. We discuss the initial selection of a biologic agent, reviewing both mechanisms of action and clinical effectiveness, as well as appropriate dosing and administration. The decision of when, whether, and how to switch from one biologic agent to another will also be addressed. Finally, we review indications for colectomy and the economics and of caring for patients with acute severe ulcerative colitis.

Defining Nonresponse

Typically, patients remain on intravenous steroids for 72 hours prior to initiation of additional rescue therapy, administered at not more than 60 mg methylprednisolone in a 24-hour period [7, 8]. Travis et al. published a study in 1997, which followed 49 patients with severe ulcerative colitis; frequent stools (> 8/day) or raised CRP (> 45 mg/l) were found to have 85% positive predictive value for colectomy during admission [9]. In 1998, Lindgren et al. identified elevated body temperature, persistently bloody stools, and rising or persistently elevated CRP on day 3 of IV steroids as predictors of steroid resistance and poor outcomes in a cohort of 97 patients, who were followed prospectively for 30 days following hospitalization and initiation of IV steroids [10]. Other studies have suggested that some patients may exhibit slower steroid response, with clinical improvement on longer courses of intravenous steroids [11, 12]. However, evaluation for and the initiation of additional medical or surgical therapies at the 3-day point remains a cornerstone of clinical practice.

Biologics: Choosing a Rescue Therapy

Historically, patients with acute severe UC who failed to respond to intravenous steroids were recommended for surgical intervention. Maintenance therapy with 5ASA and oral steroids following an intravenous course has not been found to be an effective long-term management strategy. Given the significant risks associated with high-dose, long-term steroids, a steroid-sparing agent should be considered almost immediately once a severe flare has begun.

With the advent of biologic agents, salvage therapy has become an alternative for steroid-refractory patients in order to induce remission and reduce the need for colectomy [13]. To date, research on salvage medical therapy has centered on infliximab and cyclosporine; however, novel therapies, including small molecules and immunomodulators, may provide additional options for patients with refractory disease.

Infliximab and Cyclosporine

Infliximab (IFX) is often considered the first-line medical therapy for patients with steroid-refractory ASUC given its efficacy, safety profile, and wide availability. In patients who have failed to improve despite 3 days of intravenous steroids, IFX can be used to both induce and maintain clinical and endoscopic remission, potentially obviating the need for colectomy [14–16]. In a randomized, placebo-controlled trial comparing IFX (5 mg/kg) to placebo, 29% of patients in the IFX group compared to 67% of patients in the placebo group required colectomy within 3 months ($p = 0.017$, OR4.9, 95%CI 1.4–17) [15]. Similarly, a trial performed in Sweden found that 69% of patients treated with IFX for 3 months avoided colectomy compared to 33% of those who received a placebo [17]. At 3-year follow-up, the rate of colectomy remained significantly lower in those who received IFX (50%) compared to those on placebo (76%) ($p = 0.012$) [17]. Another study reported remission rates at 2 weeks, 6 weeks, and 1 year of 46%, 58%, and 45%, respectively, with a 1-, 3-, and 5-year cumulative colectomy avoidance rate of 80%, 78%, and 75%, respectively [18]. These studies suggest that IFX is effective at inducing clinical remission in ASUC, thereby reducing the rate of colectomy.

Despite the data to support the efficacy of IFX in ASUC patients, the optimal dosing remains unclear. Given the high inflammatory burden associated with ASUC, traditional induction dosing with IFX 5 mg/kg may prove to be insufficient. Studies have shown that in patients with ASUC and hypoalbuminemia, there is increased drug clearance due to fecal losses and therefore lower IFX trough levels [19]. In one study from 2016, IFX levels at day 14 following a single dose of 5 mg/kg in patients were lower in patients hospitalized with ASUC, compared to those with moderate disease being treated in the clinic [20]. Furthermore, numerous studies have demonstrated that higher serum IFX concentrations are associated with higher rates of clinical and endoscopic remission as well as lower rates of colectomy [19, 21] and, inversely, with low IFX levels predicting need for colectomy [19, 22], underscoring the need for likely higher initial dosing regimens and a treat-to-target approach.

Evaluating 50 patients with steroid-refractory ASUC, Gibson et al. showed significantly lower colectomy rates (6.7%) in patients who received an "intensified" IFX dosing regimen, which included three doses of IFX 5 mg/kg within 24 days compared to the rate of 40% in those who received traditional induction dosing at 0, 2, and 6 weeks [19, 23]. Conversely, a recent systematic review with meta-analysis evaluated the impact of higher-dosage IFX and more frequent dose intervals of IFX on colectomy-free survival in patients with ASUC. This study showed that dose intensification did not significantly reduce colectomy-free survival at 3 months (OR 0.7, p 0.24) or 12 months (OR 0.83, p = 0.31), compared to standard dosage [24]. In addition, there was no statistically significant difference in colectomy rates in those who received traditionally spaced induction doses compared to those who received accelerated induction [24].

Although not yet evidence based, given the importance of maintaining sufficient levels and the known fecal loss across the mucosal barrier in high inflammatory states, our practice is to begin with IFX 10 mg/kg in IFX-naïve, ASUC patients with albumin <3.0. If patients have a partial response to the high-dose infusion with improvement in CRP but continued clinical symptoms, we often give a second dose of 10 mg/kg 3–5 days after the initial infusion. That said, there is variability in best practice, even among providers in a single IBD center [25]. Looking forward, data from prospective RCTs, such as the PREDICT UC trial, will help determine optimal IFX dosing for patients with severe refractory disease.

Cyclosporine (CyA), a calcineurin inhibitor, which blocks T cell activation, has also been for use as a rescue medical therapy in patients with steroid-refractory ASUC. Multiple randomized controlled trials as well as prospective and retrospective studies have demonstrated CyA's efficacy in inducing clinical remission and avoiding colectomy. In 1994, Lichtiger et al. [26] published one of the first RTCs comparing the use of CyA with placebo in patients with severe UC. In this study, 82% of those who received CyA responded and 0% of those who received placebo responded. When five of those who initially received placebo were subsequently given CyA, 100% had clinical response [26]. Given these results, the study was stopped early due to ethical reasons [26, 27].

In a subsequent retrospective study, 42 steroid-refractory patients with ASUC were treated with intravenous CyA (4 mg/kg/day); 86% of patients responded, 31 (74%) continued on oral CyA after discharge, and only 20% required colectomy. Six patients had complications requiring cessation of the drug [28]. Furthermore, in a large study in the UK, only 26% of steroid-refractory patients treated with CyA required colectomy prior to discharge [13, 27, 29]. Van Assche et al. [30] evaluated the optimal dose of CyA in patients with ASUC, demonstrating that patients who received

4 mg/kg/day did not have a higher clinical response rate (84%) compared to those who received 2 mg/kg/day (85.7%) after 4 days. Similarly, in this study, patients who received higher-dose CyA did not have a lower colectomy rate at day 14 (13.1%) compared to those who received lower-dose CyA (8.6%) [30].

The use of CyA for ASUC has been limited, however, largely due to safety concerns, complicated dosing regimens that require frequent laboratory monitoring, and potentially higher long-term relapse rates. Patients treated with CyA require frequent serum CyA level monitoring (target 100–200 ng/mL) as well as monitoring of serum creatinine, liver function tests, lipids, and blood pressure every 2–4 days in the initial period. Short-term side effects include hypertension, nausea/vomiting, renal injury, headaches, infection, and seizures [13, 27]. While the majority of these side effects improve with dose reduction, mortality rates associated with CyA use in patients with inflammatory bowel disease have ranged from 1.8 to 3.5% [27, 31]. Some studies have suggested that reducing the dose from 4 mg/kg/day IV to 2 mg/kg/day IV reduces the risks of major side effects including seizures, infections, renal insufficiency, and even death [27, 30, 32, 33]. Intravenous CyA should be avoided in patients with low cholesterol, hypomagnesemia, and decreased renal function and in those recently immunosuppressed with another agent such as IFX [13]. Notably, oral formulations of CyA are associated with less neurotoxicity compared to IV formulations [27].

Infectious complications are most prevalent in patients with concomitant immunosuppression with another agent. In a univariate analysis, concomitant use of corticosteroids (OR 3.4), azathioprine (OR 3.1), or IFX (OR 4.4) was associated with significantly higher rates of infection [34]. In the multivariate analysis, the use of two or more of these agents in addition to CyA was associated with a significantly higher rate of opportunistic infection (OR 14.5, 95% CI 4.9–43) compared to only one additional agent (OR 2.9, 95% CI 1.5–5.3) [27, 34]. Furthermore, total cholesterol should be greater than 170 to avoid 3% risk of seizures with drug administration [6, 35]. Given these side effects, CyA needs to be used with caution, carefully monitoring serum CyA levels and renal function as well as for potentially life-threatening infectious complications.

While CyA has demonstrated excellent short-term efficacy, the data on long-term, sustained remission is less striking. In a study looking at long-term success with CyA use as rescue therapy for steroid-refractory ASUC, 74% of patients achieved initial remission. However, 65% of those patients had relapsed after 1 year and 90% after 3 years. In this study, after 7 years, 58% of those who initially responded to CyA required colectomy [36]. In a 2009 retrospective study looking at long-term efficacy of CyA for patients with ASUC, among those who had an incomplete initial response to CyA, 50% had a colectomy within 1 year and 70% within 5 years [37]. Similarly, investigators from Belgium published a study evaluating long-term efficacy of CyA; 83% of the reported patients had an initial response to CyA and avoided colectomy during the acute hospitalization; however, 33% of patients had a colectomy at 1 year and 88% required colectomy by 7 years [13, 27, 38].

Interestingly, Cohen et al. [28] showed that 66% of patients treated with combination therapy, CyA and a thiopurine, were able to avoid colectomy compared to 40% treated with CyA alone. However, Moskowtiz et al. [38] showed that co-administration of a thiopurine was only beneficial in those who were naïve to the medication prior to treatment with CyA, as 77% of those who were taking azathioprine on admission required colectomy despite combination therapy (CyA and a thiopurine) compared to 35% of those who were started on azathioprine within the first year of CyA. Therefore, these studies suggest the initiation of a thiopurine in combination with CyA could improve durable, long-term response [13, 27].

Given efficacy of both IFX and CyA as salvage therapy for patients with ASUC, head-to-head trials have been completed to compare the two drugs. The first head-to-head comparison was done in an open-label randomized trial (GETAID), evaluating the use of CyA and IFX in patients hospitalized with steroid-refractory UC. In this study, treatment failure was seen in 60% (OR 1.4) of those treated with CyA compared to 54% (OR 1.3) of those treated with IFX, with no significant difference in colectomy or serious adverse event rates [39]. In a very recent meta-analysis comparing long-term outcomes with CyA and IFX in patients with steroid-refractory ASUC, pooled odds ratio for colectomy-free survival was higher with IFX compared to CyA at 1-, 2-, and 3-year follow-up [40]. However, at the fourth year, this difference was no longer detectible. In addition, no difference in adverse events or mortality was noted between the groups [40]. Similarly, another systematic review demonstrated that among three randomized controlled trials, no difference in remission rate or colectomy rate was seen comparing IFX and CyA use at 3 and 12 months [41]. However, in this study, among nonrandomized studies, IFX was found to be associated with significantly higher rates of treatment response and lower 12-month colectomy rates [41]. Importantly, no significant difference was seen in adverse, drug-related events, postoperative complications, or mortality [41].

In terms of cost, one study demonstrated that IFX was associated with significantly higher healthcare costs compared with CyA [42]. Therefore, to date, the consensus appears to be that both drugs have similar efficacy, with IFX requiring less monitoring (though overall higher costs), while CyA requires more monitoring, but is less expensive despite increased length of stay for intravenous therapy. IFX is the appropriate first-line salvage therapy for most patients. However, CyA should be considered in patients with prior IFX failure or known antibodies to IFX, those who strongly prefer oral maintenance therapy, or those patients presenting significant hypoalbuminemia.

Other TNF Inhibitors

While there is an abundance of literature on the use of other TNF inhibitors including adalimumab and golimumab in patients with moderate to severe ulcerative colitis, there are few studies looking at the use of these agents in patients with steroid-refractory, acute, severe disease [43]. In a retrospective study evaluating the use of adalimumab as salvage therapy in patients who were refractory to steroids as well as calcineurin inhibitors, 41% of patients required colectomy despite salvage therapy [44]. Similar conclusions were seen in a subsequent study looking at the efficacy of Exemptia, suggesting that salvage therapy with a TNF inhibitor after failing cyclosporine therapy is associated with a high colectomy rate [45]. Of note, other anti-TNF agents, such as golimumab, have been shown to be effective at inducing and maintaining remission in patients with moderate to severe UC; however, these studies did not include patients with severe disease refractory to intravenous steroids [2, 46]. Further studies are needed to evaluate the efficacy of these TNF inhibitors in hospitalized patients with acute, severe, steroid-refractory disease.

Vedolizumab and Ustekinumab

Utilizing a different mechanism of action, vedolizumab (VDZ) targets the $\alpha 4\beta 7$ integrin, reducing the trafficking of leukocytes to the gastrointestinal tract. VDZ has been shown to induce and maintain remission in patients with moderate to severe UC, but there is limited data on its use as salvage therapy for ASUC. In patients with severe disease refractory to steroids, VDZ can be considered in those who are older in age or who have significant comorbidities, including underlying malignancies, given its safety profile and decreased risk for systemic immunosuppression compared to other biologic classes. In a small pediatric study, four patients with ASUC refractory to steroids and TNF inhibitors were treated with VDZ. By the fourth dose, two (50%) showed a clinical response and avoided colectomy [47].

One of the major limitations of VDZ is its delayed effect; while in some patients VDZ can work quickly, in the majority of patients, it can take up to 14 weeks to have full efficacy. Therefore, VDZ is often used in combination with a faster-acting agent, such as calcineurin inhibitor, in order to induce remission in those with severe, refractory disease [48, 49]. Pellet et al. [49] published a study looking at patients with ASUC refractory to steroids who were treated with tacrolimus or CyA as induction therapy and concomitant VDZ as maintenance therapy. In this study, after 1 year, 68% of patients avoided colectomy [49]. These studies are quite limited, and further research is needed to better understand the role of VDZ for patients with ASUC. Given its slow onset of action in many patients, it is possible that VDZ will be better suited in combination therapy with a faster-acting agent to induce remission.

Ustekinumab, a monoclonal antibody targeting IL12/IL23, was approved for use in patients with UC in October 2019. Ustekinumab can be considered in patients who have previously failed a TNF inhibitor such as IFX, as well as in those with concomitant skin disease, as it has shown excellent efficacy in treating psoriasis [50]. While there are no studies to date specifically looking at its use as rescue therapy in patients with severe, steroid-refractory disease, a case study was recently published, suggesting that ustekinumab may in fact be effective in this patient population. In this publication, one patient refractory to steroids and TNF inhibitors was treated with IV ustekinumab and had a dramatic improvement in symptoms within 1 week of the infusion and remained in clinical and endoscopic remission for over 1 year [51]. Although this is single-case report, further studies are necessary to evaluate the efficacy of ustekinumab to induce remission in patients with ASUC.

Small-Molecule Therapy: Tofacitinib

Tofacitinib is a rapidly acting oral small molecule that inhibits Janus kinase and is approved to treat patients with UC. As it is a cytokine-mediated therapy, tofacitinib offers a unique combination of being a fast-acting agent in an oral form. In one of the initial studies evaluating the efficacy of tofacitinib in patients with ASUC, four patients hospitalized with steroid-refractory disease were given tofacitinib (10 milligrams (mg) three times daily), and all demonstrated clinical response and improvement in CRP and avoided colectomy prior to discharge [52]. In this study, one patient had recurrent symptoms when the dose was reduced to maintenance therapy (5 mg twice daily) and ultimately required urgent colectomy [52]. In the largest study to date evaluating the efficacy of tofacitinib in patients with ASUC, 77% avoided colectomy at week 24 and 70% at week 48 with few adverse events, suggesting that tofacitinib could be used successfully as salvage therapy [53]. In a very recent study, four patients were started on tofacitinib (10 mg twice daily) as salvage therapy for steroid-refractory ASUC. In this trial, all patients had clinical improvement and maintained remission at 90 days, avoiding colectomy [54].

Of note, in July of 2019, the Federal Drug Administration issued an additional black box safety warning for tofacitinib, stating that patients over 50 years of age with a cardiac history taking the induction dosing (10 mg twice daily) are at increased risk for blood clots and death. Larger studies are necessary to further define the efficacy of tofacitinib in patients with steroid-refractory ASUC as well as the potential risks associated with this therapy. These studies suggest that tofacitinib offers significant promise for patients with severe, refractory UC. However, future studies are necessary to further clarify tofacitinib's efficacy and optimal dosing strategy in this patient population, as well as the potential risks associated with this therapy.

Immunomodulators: Tacrolimus, Azathioprine, and Methotrexate

Tacrolimus, a selective calcineurin inhibitor that impairs transcription of various cytokines including IL2 and TNFa, has been studied extensively for use as salvage therapy in patients with steroid-refractory ASUC. Both tacrolimus and cyclosporine have similar mechanisms of action, and use of one or the other is often dictated by geography. In a small retrospective study from Germany, 22 patients hospitalized with refractory severe disease were given IV tacrolimus and subsequently converted to oral therapy. In this study, colectomy-free survival rates at 1, 6, and 12 months after initiation of tacrolimus were 90.9%, 77.3%, and 68.2% with minimal side effects [4]. Similarly, in a placebo-controlled double-blind study, patients with steroid-refractory disease were randomized to either tacrolimus or placebo; after 2 weeks, clinical response from tacrolimus was 50.0% compared to 13.3% in the placebo group, and mucosal healing was seen in 43.8% of those on tacrolimus compared to 13.3% in the placebo group [55]. In a larger study including patients with moderate to severe steroid-refractory UC treated with tacrolimus, clinical remission was achieved in 72% of patients, and 14% required colectomy in the first 3 months. Interestingly, in this study, concomitant use of thiopurines was associated with a lower colectomy rate and increased remission ($p = 0.002$) [56].

While these studies specifically looked at the short-term ability of tacrolimus to induce response in patients with acute severe disease, Schmidt et al. studied the long-term outcomes of tacrolimus alone and in combination with thiopurines, demonstrating that those treated with combination therapy (tacrolimus plus thiopurine) had significantly lower rates of colectomy and longer time to relapse [57]. Finally, in terms of dosing, one study comparing tacrolimus to TNF inhibitors (IFX or adalimumab) simultaneously compared traditional tacrolimus dosing (0.5 mg/kg/day) to a rapid induction protocol (1 mg/kg/day), titrating to a goal serum tacrolimus level of 10–15 ng/mL until week 2 and 5–10 ng/mL thereafter [58]. After 12 weeks, patients receiving the rapid induction had improved clinical remission rates compared to those who received traditional dosing tacrolimus and compared to those who received the TNF inhibitor, although this difference was not statistically significant [58]. Although less commonly used, tacrolimus can potentially offer patients with ASUC another option for salvage therapy and perhaps is most effective as well as durable when combined with a thiopurine. However, given potential safety concerns with combining tacrolimus with a thiopurine, combination therapy should be restricted to short-term use.

While azathioprine is not used as acute salvage monotherapy for steroid-refractory severe UC, many studies have shown its efficacy as combination therapy with CyA or IFX for maintenance of remission. As was mentioned above, in patients treated with intravenous CyA, combination therapy with azathioprine is associated with improved long-term efficacy ($p = 0.0014$) [59]. Moreover, azathioprine has been shown to be effective as monotherapy for maintaining remission induced from intravenous CyA in patients with steroid-refractory ASUC. Domènech et al. demonstrated that in patients treated with IV CyA (4 mg/kg/day) for only 7–14 days and then started on azathioprine 2–2.5 m/g/kg/day, colectomy rates at 1, 3, and 5 years were 29%, 35%, and

42%, respectively [60]. Regardless of whether IFX or CyA is used to induce remission, azathioprine should not be introduced until the steroids have been tapered to a minimum of 20 mg, to reduce the risk of complications from exposure to three simultaneous immunosuppressive medications (the inducing agent, steroid, and the thiopurine). Given this, the azathioprine is most commonly started after discharge, often by the outpatient gastroenterologist. Although no studies have specifically evaluated the use of methotrexate in patients with steroid-refractory ASUC, Herfarth et al. performed a systematic review evaluating the use of methotrexate monotherapy in patients with UC and concluded that it overall had poor efficacy [61].

Making the Switch: Transitioning Therapies

In light of the increasing numbers of biologic and small-molecule options for the management of ulcerative colitis, prescribers must feel comfortable facilitating safe and effective shifts from one medication to another. If the decision has been made to abandon a particular biologic or small-molecule therapy in the setting of acute flare, careful consideration must be made to both the timing and selection of the new agent. It is important to ensure that sufficient time has passed in order to allow for washout to avoid overly immunosuppressing the patient. At the same time, bridge therapies, such as steroids or immunomodulators, may be indicated in order to prevent repeated flares.

The importance of a washout period was highlighted in a 2008 study by Maser et al. [62], which examined the utility of cyclosporine and infliximab as salvage therapies for one another. This study concluded that rapid crossing over from one drug to the other resulted in remission in only one third of patients and serious adverse events were seen in 16% of patients, including one death due to septic shock, likely the result of significant immunosuppression [62]. Similarly, in a multicenter study performed in Spain, IFX was studied as rescue therapy for patients with ASUC who were refractory to steroids and CyA. In this study, 60% of patients who received IFX achieved remission, 37% had partial improvement, and 30% required colectomy. However, in this group, 23% of patients reported an adverse event, including one death from infection in a postoperative patient [63]. These studies suggest that CyA should be avoided in those recently exposed to IFX and vice versa as significant immunosuppression occurs and can lead to potentially fatal infectious complications. While no minimum "washout period" has been established, future studies can help define the minimum time required between last exposure to IFX and subsequent induction with CyA (or the reverse) to prevent severe adverse events.

If drug levels are obtainable and are noted to be undetectable, it may be safe to proceed to a new drug (Table 3.1). Otherwise, studies in patients with rheumatologic and dermatologic indications for biologic therapy have demonstrated that it is advisable to

Table 3.1 Drug half-life and recommended washout period

Drug	Half-life	Recommended washout period[a]
Infliximab	7.7–9.5 days	8 weeks or negative levels
Cyclosporine	8 hours	5 days
Adalimumab	14 days (range 10–20 days)	8 weeks or negative levels
Certolizumab pegol	14 days	8 weeks or negative levels
Golimumab	14 days	8 weeks or negative levels
Vedolizumab	25 days	12 weeks or negative levels
Ustekinumab	19 days	12 weeks or negative levels
Tofacitinib	3 hours (IR form), 6–8 hours (ER form)	5 days
Tacrolimus	3.5–40.6 hours	5 days
Methotrexate	3–10 hours	7 days
Azathioprine	5 hours	7 days

[a]Pharmacologic washout is typically five half-lives. After that point, if there is drug remaining, it is likely at very low levels. The above recommendations represent consensus expert opinion

wait at least four half-lives before initiation of a new maintenance therapy [64]. Biologic medications have longer half-lives (e.g., median terminal half-life of infliximab is 7.7 to 9.5 days), whereas small molecules are cleared more quickly (e.g., tofacitinib has a half-life of 3 hours) [65].

The risks of over-immunosuppression must be weighed against the risk of inadequate disease control. In patients for whom surgery is not either an option or would pose especially high risk, it may be necessary to favor disease control without waiting the allotted washout period between drugs. In that case, particularly if the patient has been on combination therapy or steroids are being used as a bridge, it is essential to ensure patients are receiving appropriate prophylaxis against opportunistic infections, such as *Pneumocystis carinii* (PCP) [66].

Antibiotics as a bridge therapy are not advised, as their use has not been proven to be efficacious in preventing disease flares [67–69]. Studies examining the impact of antibiotics in ulcerative colitis have been limited to small, often nonrandomized trials evaluating a variety of oral antibiotics, either alone or in combination, for the treatment of non-severe ulcerative colitis [70]. The exception to avoidance of antibiotics is in the setting of active *Clostridium difficile* infection or in the case of toxic megacolon, in which case IV antibiotics are advised in order to mitigate increased risk of perforation and subsequent sepsis.

Predictors of Poor Outcomes

Both retrospective and prospective studies have clarified predictors of poor outcomes, such as prolonged hospital length of stay (longer than 7 days) and need for urgent colectomy, in patients with ASUC. These include epidemiologic findings, serologic markers, genetic predictors, and specific endoscopic features such as disease severity, location, characteristic macroscopic mucosal features, and CMV infection (Table 3.2). Furthermore, clinical efficacy declines with each subsequent biologic exposure, so patients, who previously failed multiple biologic therapies, are also at increased risk for poor outcomes and steroid refractori-

Table 3.2 Risk factors associated with poor outcomes in patients with acute severe ulcerative colitis

Risk factors associated with poor outcomes
Serum albumin <2.0
High C-reactive protein
Fecal incontinence
Frequency of stooling
Rectal bleeding
Length of prior steroid use
CMV positive
Proctitis extending to universal colitis
Severe flare in the first year of diagnosis
Failed one or more biologics

ness. Several risk-stratification models using clinical, serological, and genetic markers have been proposed, with the aim of aiding in identification of steroid nonresponse [71].

Epidemiologic factors, including race and ethnicity (black and Hispanic patients [72]), need for hospitalization [73, 74], and prior anti-TNF, thiopurine, and steroid exposure [75, 76] have all been associated with poor outcomes in patients with ASUC. Studies in the pediatric population have identified low weight percentile as an additional predictor of poor outcomes in this age group [77]. Clinical findings, such as fever, increased frequency of bowel movements, and presence of blood in stool, have been associated with risk for urgent or emergent colectomy [8–10, 78].

Heightened disease severity and extent on endoscopic examination, typified by Mayo or partial Mayo score at time of presentation, is known to be associated with increased risk for colectomy [79–82]. Furthermore, patients with rapid extension of proctitis to pancolitis are more likely to require surgical intervention [74]. Certain endoscopic features, such as bear claw denudations of mucosa (confluent superficial ulcerations), may also be suggestive of poor prognosis.

Validated histologic indices, such as the Nancy Index and the Robarts Histopathology Index, are useful in assessing disease severity, but are often only available several days following colonoscopy with biopsy; thus their utility in guiding clinical management is limited [83]. Intramucosal calprotectin, which can be identified using immunohistochemical staining, has found to be an independent predictor of disease severity [84], though it has not been found to be strongly associated as fecal calprotectin [85]. Again, delays in obtaining pathologic specimen results limit clinical usefulness of histologic findings in predicting outcomes in patients with ASUC.

Concomitant ASUC and *Clostridium difficile* infection (CDI) has been associated with increased length of stay, hospitalization frequency, risk of urgent colectomy, and colectomy within 1 year [75, 86–89] and markedly increased healthcare costs [90]. CDI infection also portends worsened prognosis for patients with UC than those with *C. diff* and Crohn's disease [91]. All ASUC patients should be tested for *Clostridium difficile* toxin at time of presentation, as steroid exposure increases risk of colectomy in infected patients with UC flare [92]. Similarly, CMV is frequently found on biopsy in patients with ASUC [93]. Though the role of CMV in propagation of inflammation in UC continues to be controversial, patients who receive antiviral therapy have decreased colectomy rates [94], suggesting that the virus should be treated if identified. Patients with concurrent CDI and CMV infection were noted to have higher endoscopic severity scores [95], and the presence of any stool infection, including parasitic infections, HHV-6, and EBV infections, in addition to CDI and CMV, have been associated with disease severity [96, 97].

Several stool and serum markers have been studied in risk-stratification research of patients with ASUC at highest risk for poor outcomes. These laboratory findings include hypoalbuminemia at time of admission, elevated CRP, ESR, and low hemoglobin (or need for blood transfusion). In particular, patients with persistently elevated CRP on day 3 of steroid exposure have been associated with poor outcomes for ASUC patients [8–10, 78, 98]. Despite this association, no single numeric cut-point has been identified [9, 99]. Furthermore, not all patients with ulcerative colitis mount an elevated CRP despite severe inflammation. Fecal calprotectin has been used to monitor response to therapy and risk of relapse in patients with UC [100], and elevated FC levels (in particular, > 1000 μg/g) have been shown to correlate with disease severity, steroid nonresponse, and increased colectomy risk [101–103], with some studies finding stronger correlation between elevated fecal calprotectin and either CRP or albumin [104]. Fecal lactoferrin levels have been found to correlate with disease severity and extent in patients with UC, but its utility in ASUC has not yet been defined [105]. In practice, utility of stool testing in patients with ASUC may be limited by prolonged turnaround times if testing requires sending out of samples, though assays themselves take only a few hours to run [106].

Serologic antibodies have been another area of investigation, with one prospective study of 187 patients with UC demonstrating association between ASCA IgA and higher risk of requirement for long-term immunosuppression [107]. Hospitalization rates were higher in patients with elevations in three or more of the following markers: antineutrophil cytoplasmic (ANCA), anti-DNA-bound lactoferrin (anti-LFS), anti-goblet cell (anti-GAB), and anti-pancreatic antibodies (PAB: anti-CUZD1 and anti-GP2) [107]. In a pediatric population with UC, elevated pANCA was associated with greater disease extent [108], but risk-stratification and colectomy rates were not delineated. Other studies have failed to show correlation with disease activity and serologic positivity [107, 109–111], and elevations of antibody levels can be seen in other pathologic processes, including intestinal tuberculosis and Behcet's disease [112]. Furthermore, use of serum antibodies for risk stratification has been limited by poor sensitivity of these tests [110, 113].

Identification of genetic predictors of disease course in IBD has proved a highly generative area of research in recent years. Several genes have been implicated in CD and UC and may prove useful in distinguishing between patients with ileal Crohn's disease, colonic Crohn's disease, and ulcerative colitis. HLA variants, in particular, may predict disease extent in patients with UC [114, 115]. However, clear associations between genetics and long-term disease behavior or colectomy risk have not yet been found in large-scale, genome-wide association studies [74, 116, 117]. Most risk models for determining steroid failure and poor outcomes involve multifactorial metrics, incorporating clinical presentation, endoscopic and imaging findings, as well as serologic and genetic markers [71]. The Pediatric Ulcerative Colitis Activity Index (PUCAI), which uses pain, bleeding, consistency, stools over a 24-hour period, and presence of nocturnal stools, is one validated index [10] and has been shown to perform better than serologic markers (including calprotectin) alone [118]. Patients identified as high-risk using both Travis and Ho scoring systems, which are calculated after 72 hours of exposure to intravenous steroids, have been found to have increased colectomy rates when compared to low-risk subjects [119]. In clinical practice, scoring systems may be cumbersome and are currently more useful for research purposes.

Surgical Consultation: Why and When?

A multidisciplinary approach to the management of ASUC, with input from gastroenterologists, radiologists, surgeons, and stoma management specialists, has been found to improve patient outcomes [120–122]. Best practices thus suggest that all patients admitted with ASUC, and, in particular, those determined to be at high risk for steroid failure, warrant early surgical consultation. Despite the development of and ready access to biologic therapies, colectomy rates (around 30% of patients with ASUC) have remained relatively stable over time [2, 8, 123].

With each sequential biologic exposure, the probability of achieving remission declines, thus increasing the potential need for surgical intervention [124]. Mortality rates and intraoperative and postoperative complications all increase in the setting of toxic megacolon or perforation [125]. Thus, all patients with ASUC should get a baseline KUB, with serial imaging and close monitoring of abdominal examination findings. If the patient has not responded to medical therapy by days 4–7 of hospitalization, colectomy should be considered a potentially lifesaving intervention [126, 127]. Mortality rates increase after day 5 of steroid-refractory clinical decline, so prolonged observation is not recommended [128, 129].

There are several surgical approaches to the patient requiring intervention [129]. Most commonly, a subtotal colectomy (STC) with end ileostomy is offered in the setting of antecedent rapid clinical deterioration [130]. Epidemiologic factors may impact the type of subtotal colectomy a patient undergoes, with one national study demonstrating decreased use of laparoscopic subtotal colectomy for lower-income patients with Medicaid payer status [131, 132].

While more recent studies have noted improved postsurgical outcomes with a less invasive, laparoscopic approach [133–136], a learning curve exists, and bowel excision in ulcerative colitis may prove more technically challenging than patients with Crohn's disease or diverticulitis undergoing STC [137]. Following colectomy, a two- or three-step staged approach, with Hartmann pouch creation and ileoanal anastomosis, can later be completed [138]. Definitive mucosal resection with total proctocolectomy with ileal pouch-anal anastomosis can be offered later in the elective setting or in patients with ASUC found to have rectal dysplasia or neoplasia at the time of acute flare [130, 139]. As has been demonstrated in patients prior to surgery, post-colectomy outcomes are improved with access to a multidisciplinary medical team [128].

Initiation of biologic therapy (specifically, with IFX) does not appear to increase postoperative complication rates in patients requiring colectomy or total proctocolectomy, so initiation of IFX need not be avoided, even in cases of severe or fulminant ulcerative colitis [140]. There is data to suggest that patients with preoperative IFX exposure, who underwent ileoanal pouch-anal anastomosis (IPAA), did exhibit increased rates of postoperative, pouch-specific complications and may therefore benefit from avoidance of primary IPAA creation [141, 142]. Furthermore, there may be a dose-dependent effect, with higher rates of pouch-specific complications seen in patients with more than three IFX infusions in the 90 days prior to surgery [143].

Looking Toward the Future

As we look toward the future of care for patients with steroid-refractory ASUC, several additional areas of study may be of interest. Several investigators are studying the sustainability and cost associated with hospitalized patients with ASUC [90, 144].

Vasudevan et al. published a study evaluating the healthcare-associated costs for patients with ASUC and concluded that IFX was associated with fewer healthcare costs at 6 months compared with early colectomy [145]. Further work, which combines clinical effectiveness with an eye toward optimization of healthcare expenditures, will be especially relevant for those patients with lower socioeconomic status (a risk factor for poor outcomes). Additionally, new modalities for assessing disease activity and severity are being developed, in order to better differentiate high- and low-risk patients. By using artificial intelligence and deep learning modeling for assessing endoscopic disease severity [146], we may be able to more accurately follow patients' clinical course and responses to new and current therapies.

Case-Based Review

The patient is a 21-year-old woman with ulcerative pancolitis, diagnosed 3 years ago. While she initially did well on IFX for 1 year, she lost insurance and access to the drug. She was then treated with adalimumab with good initial response but within 1 month developed worsened diarrhea and hematochezia and is now admitted to the hospital and on day 10 of IV steroids (albumin 2.6, still having 8–10BM per day). What is the next best step in management?

Learning Objective Recycling of biologics may be a reasonable therapeutic option in some cases.

First Choice

Retrial of IFX 10 mg/kg infused slowly over 4 hours to reduce risk of infusion reaction, with close monitoring and drug cessation if patient develops adverse symptoms. If no clinical benefit is noted after 2–3 days, repeat dose of infliximab. Since this patient has been exposed to IFX before, our clinical practice is to re-induce at 0, 4, and 8 weeks. Check levels prior to the third dose and if it is below 10, increase dose. If patient has ATIs, it may be necessary to consider another agent.

Other Approaches to Consider.
Cyclosporine: Determine when the last dose of an anti-TNF was given. If there has been at least an 8-week washout period, it is probably safe to try IV cyclosporine. Since she has already had 10 days of steroids and will likely remain on steroids for longer than 30 days, use appropriate antibiotic prophylaxis to prevent PCP pneumonia.

Tofacitinib: Initial evidence suggests that this could be used for acute steroid-refractory UC if it is obtainable in hospital and cost is not an issue. However, this patient is still in her childbearing years, and currently there is not enough evidence to support its safety in pregnancy.

Surgery: Surgery should be considered on this admission if she fails a retrial of IFX.

The patient is a 29-year-old man, initially found to have ulcerative proctitis, but now noted to have disease extending to the cecum despite topical steroids, mesalamine, and, later, vedolizumab. Four months later, he is hospitalized for failure to thrive and malnutrition, with albumin 1.8, and on day 4 of IV steroids. What is the next best step in management?

Learning Objective Understanding risk factors for colectomy (see Table 3.1).

First Choice
Surgical consult. This patient needs to understand that his risk of colectomy is very high. He has three risk factors that put him at high risk for colectomy: rapid extension of disease, hypoalbuminemia, and he has failed a reasonable trial of IV steroids.

Other Approaches to Consider
Infliximab: Consider high-dose infliximab starting with 10 mg/kg and repeating dosing after 2–3 days if he has no clinical or biomarker response. Check levels at 2 weeks, and if less than 25, consider administering the third induction dose at week 4 instead of week 6. Consider adding a thiopurine when the steroid dose has been reduced below 20 mg. Plan to keep him on the thiopurine for

less than 2 years as the risk of hepatosplenic T cell lymphoma is highest in his demographic (males <age 35).

Cyclosporine: This is a reasonable choice; however, we would need to consider an alternative maintenance drug once he is in remission. Examples include tofacitinib or oral tacrolimus.

Tofacitinib: Initial evidence suggests that this medication may be used for acute steroid-refractory UC if it is obtainable in the inpatient setting and cost to the patient post-discharge is not an issue. Its onset of action is not as rapid as infliximab or cyclosporine.

The patient is a 22-year-old woman with ulcerative colitis that was diagnosed 3 months ago. She was initially treated with mesalamine and steroids as an outpatient, but after 2 weeks of prednisone 60 mg, she presented to the hospital for continued rectal bleeding and severe cramping. She also mentions that she had new-onset right knee swelling that has improved with steroids. What is the next best step in management?

Learning Objective Choose a biologic that can treat both luminal and extraintestinal manifestations of IBD.

First Choice

This patient has severe colitis, coupled with IBD-associated arthritis. She also has aggressive disease in the first year of treatment, so combination therapy would be appropriate.

Drugs to consider include anti-TNF (IFX or adalimumab) or IV cyclosporine with 6mp or tofacitinib as maintenance therapy. Tofacitinib could be also considered; however its safety profile in pregnancy is less well established, and this patient is in her childbearing years. Therefore, it would be further down on our list of choices.

Vedolizumab and ustekinumab would not be considered as they are not helpful for arthritis. However, they could be combined with a thiopurine which does have some efficacy for arthritis.

The patient is a 40-year-old woman with left-sided ulcerative colitis, who recently visited her primary care doctor for dysuria and was diagnosed with a urinary tract infection, for which she was prescribed ciprofloxacin. A week after completing her course of antibiotics, she developed rectal bleeding and diarrhea and visited an urgent care center, where she was noted to be positive for *Clostridium difficile* toxin (first occurrence). After 5 days of oral vancomycin, her symptoms persisted, so she presented to the hospital and is now on day 3 of IV steroids.

Learning Objective Treatment of ASUC in the setting of active *C. diff* infection.

First Choice
C. difficile colitis happens frequently in patients with UC and may even be considered a marker of severe disease. Because this is her first episode of *C. diff* colitis, she should complete a course oral vancomycin. If she does not have clinical response and meets criteria for severe infection, IV metronidazole should be added. Treatment for UC should also proceed. Therefore, she should be considered for either IFX or cyclosporine as first-line treatment for ASUC. If the *C. diff* does not respond to aggressive treatment, fecal transplant may be considered.

The patient is a 72-year-old man with long-standing ulcerative colitis, pyoderma gangrenosum, and heart failure with reduced ejection fraction (EF 35%, medically optimized, stable for the last 10 years). He began having flare symptoms and was begun on azathioprine and oral steroids, without effect, so he was admitted to the hospital and is now on day 5 of IV steroids. What is the next best step in management?

Learning Objective Treatment of ASUC with pyoderma gangrenosum (PG). Treatment of ASUC in patients with heart failure.

First Choice
An anti-TNF (i.e., IFX) is typically the first choice for patients with pyoderma gangrenosum. However, this patient has heart failure. Worsening heart failure is a contraindication for anti-TNF. However, because his heart failure is stable and he is on optimal medical therapy and the other biologics and small mol-

ecules are not effective for pyoderma, anti-TNF therapy should be considered. An echocardiogram should be performed 3 months after beginning therapy. If there is any worsening of heart failure, the anti-TNF should be immediately discontinued. Dermatology should also be involved in co-management. Of note, pyoderma gangrenosum will only correlate with UC disease activity 50% of the time. Therefore, colectomy may not offer a cure for recurrent PG.

References

1. Truelove SC, Witts LJ. Cortisone in ulcerative colitis; preliminary report on a therapeutic trial. Br Med J. 1954;2:375–8.
2. Bernstein CN, Ng SC, Lakatos PL, Moum B, Loftus EV Jr. A review of mortality and surgery in ulcerative colitis: milestones of the seriousness of the disease. Inflamm Bowel Dis. 2013;19:2001–10.
3. Truelove SC, Willoughby CP, Lee EG, Kettlewell MG. Further experience in the treatment of severe attacks of ulcerative colitis. Lancet. 1978;2:1086–8.
4. Dignass A, Lindsay JO, Sturm A, Windsor A, Colombel JF, Allez M, D'Haens G, D'Hoore A, Mantzaris G, Novacek G, Oresland T, Reinisch W, Sans M, Stange E, Vermeire S, Travis S, Van Assche G. Second European evidence-based consensus on the diagnosis and management of ulcerative colitis part 2: current management. J Crohns Colitis. 2012;6:991–1030.
5. Esteve M, Gisbert JP. Severe ulcerative colitis: at what point should we define resistance to steroids? World J Gastroenterol. 2008;14:5504–7.
6. Kornbluth A, Present DH, Lichtiger S, Hanauer S. Cyclosporin for severe ulcerative colitis: a user's guide. Am J Gastroenterol. 1997;92:1424–8.
7. Travis S, Satsangi J, Lemann M. Predicting the need for colectomy in severe ulcerative colitis: a critical appraisal of clinical parameters and currently available biomarkers. Gut. 2011;60:3–9.
8. Turner D, Walsh CM, Steinhart AH, Griffiths AM. Response to corticosteroids in severe ulcerative colitis: a systematic review of the literature and a meta-regression. Clin Gastroenterol Hepatol. 2007;5:103–10.
9. Travis SP, Farrant JM, Ricketts C, Nolan DJ, Mortensen NM, Kettlewell MG, Jewell DP. Predicting outcome in severe ulcerative colitis. Gut. 1996;38:905–10.
10. Lindgren SC, Flood LM, Kilander AF, Lofberg R, Persson TB, Sjodahl RI. Early predictors of glucocorticosteroid treatment failure in severe and moderately severe attacks of ulcerative colitis. Eur J Gastroenterol Hepatol. 1998;10:831–5.

11. Gold DM, Levine JJ, Weinstein TA, Kessler B, Pettei MJ. Prolonged medical therapy for severe pediatric ulcerative colitis. Am J Gastroenterol. 1995;90:732–5.
12. Daperno M, Sostegni R, Scaglione N, Ercole E, Rigazio C, Rocca R, Pera A. Outcome of a conservative approach in severe ulcerative colitis. Dig Liver Dis. 2004;36:21–8.
13. Seah D, De Cruz P. Review article: the practical management of acute severe ulcerative colitis. Aliment Pharmacol Ther. 2016;43:482–513.
14. Sood A, Midha V, Sharma S, Sood N, Bansal M, Thara A, Khanna P. Infliximab in patients with severe steroid-refractory ulcerative colitis: Indian experience. Indian J Gastroenterol. 2014;33:31–4.
15. Jarnerot G, Hertervig E, Friis-Liby I, Blomquist L, Karlen P, Granno C, Vilien M, Strom M, Danielsson A, Verbaan H, Hellstrom PM, Magnuson A, Curman B. Infliximab as rescue therapy in severe to moderately severe ulcerative colitis: a randomized, placebo-controlled study. Gastroenterology. 2005;128:1805–11.
16. Lees CW, Heys D, Ho GT, Noble CL, Shand AG, Mowat C, Boulton-Jones R, Williams A, Church N, Satsangi J, Arnott ID. A retrospective analysis of the efficacy and safety of infliximab as rescue therapy in acute severe ulcerative colitis. Aliment Pharmacol Ther. 2007;26:411–9.
17. Gustavsson A, Jarnerot G, Hertervig E, Friis-Liby I, Blomquist L, Karlen P, Granno C, Vilien M, Strom M, Verbaan H, Hellstrom PM, Magnuson A, Halfvarson J, Tysk C. Clinical trial: colectomy after rescue therapy in ulcerative colitis – 3-year follow-up of the Swedish-Danish controlled infliximab study. Aliment Pharmacol Ther. 2010;32:984–9.
18. Nasuno M, Miyakawa M, Tanaka H, Motoya S. Short- and long-term outcomes of infliximab treatment for steroid-refractory ulcerative colitis and related prognostic factors: a single-center retrospective study. Digestion. 2017;95:67–71.
19. Hindryckx P, Novak G, Vande Casteele N, Laukens D, Parker C, Shackelton LM, Narula N, Khanna R, Dulai P, Levesque BG, Sandborn WJ, D'Haens G, Feagan BG, Jairath V. Review article: dose optimisation of infliximab for acute severe ulcerative colitis. Aliment Pharmacol Ther. 2017;45:617–30.
20. Ungar B, Mazor Y, Weisshof R, Yanai H, Ron Y, Goren I, Waizbard A, Yavzori M, Fudim E, Picard O, Loebstein R, Kopylov U, Dotan I, Chowers Y, Eliakim R, Ben-Horin S. Induction infliximab levels among patients with acute severe ulcerative colitis compared with patients with moderately severe ulcerative colitis. Aliment Pharmacol Ther. 2016;43:1293–9.
21. Seow CH, Newman A, Irwin SP, Steinhart AH, Silverberg MS, Greenberg GR. Trough serum infliximab: a predictive factor of clinical outcome for infliximab treatment in acute ulcerative colitis. Gut. 2010;59:49–54.

22. Papamichael K, Rivals-Lerebours O, Billiet T, Vande Casteele N, Gils A, Ferrante M, Van Assche G, Rutgeerts PJ, Mantzaris GJ, Peyrin-Biroulet L, Vermeire S. Long-term outcome of patients with ulcerative colitis and primary non-response to infliximab. J Crohns Colitis. 2016;10:1015–23.
23. Gibson DJ, Heetun ZS, Redmond CE, Nanda KS, Keegan D, Byrne K, Mulcahy HE, Cullen G, Doherty GA. An accelerated infliximab induction regimen reduces the need for early colectomy in patients with acute severe ulcerative colitis. Clin Gastroenterol Hepatol. 2015;13:330–5.e1
24. Choy MC, Seah D, Faleck DM, Shah SC, Chao CY, An YK, Radford-Smith G, Bessissow T, Dubinsky MC, Ford AC, Churilov L, Yeomans ND, De Cruz PP. Systematic review and meta-analysis: optimal salvage therapy in acute severe ulcerative colitis. Inflamm Bowel Dis. 2019;25:1169–86.
25. Shah SC, Naymagon S, Cohen BL, Sands BE, Dubinsky MC. There is significant practice pattern variability in the management of the hospitalized ulcerative colitis patient at a tertiary care and IBD referral center. J Clin Gastroenterol. 2018;52:333–8.
26. Lichtiger S, Present DH, Kornbluth A, Gelernt I, Bauer J, Galler G, Michelassi F, Hanauer S. Cyclosporine in severe ulcerative colitis refractory to steroid therapy. N Engl J Med. 1994;330:1841–5.
27. Hart AL, Ng SC. Review article: the optimal medical management of acute severe ulcerative colitis. Aliment Pharmacol Ther. 2010;32: 615–27.
28. Cohen RD, Stein R, Hanauer SB. Intravenous cyclosporin in ulcerative colitis: a five-year experience. Am J Gastroenterol. 1999;94:1587–92.
29. Ng SC, Shi HY, Hamidi N, Underwood FE, Tang W, Benchimol EI, Panaccione R, Ghosh S, Wu JCY, Chan FKL, Sung JJY, Kaplan GG. Worldwide incidence and prevalence of inflammatory bowel disease in the 21st century: a systematic review of population-based studies. Lancet. 2018;390:2769–78.
30. Van Assche G, D'Haens G, Noman M, Vermeire S, Hiele M, Asnong K, Arts J, D'Hoore A, Penninckx F, Rutgeerts P. Randomized, double-blind comparison of 4 mg/kg versus 2 mg/kg intravenous cyclosporine in severe ulcerative colitis. Gastroenterology. 2003;125:1025–31.
31. Sternthal MB, Murphy SJ, George J, Kornbluth A, Lichtiger S, Present DH. Adverse events associated with the use of cyclosporine in patients with inflammatory bowel disease. Am J Gastroenterol. 2008;103: 937–43.
32. Rayner CK, McCormack G, Emmanuel AV, Kamm MA. Long-term results of low-dose intravenous ciclosporin for acute severe ulcerative colitis. Aliment Pharmacol Ther. 2003;18:303–8.
33. Actis GC, Ottobrelli A, Pera A, Barletti C, Ponti V, Pinna-Pintor M, Verme G. Continuously infused cyclosporine at low dose is sufficient to

avoid emergency colectomy in acute attacks of ulcerative colitis without the need for high-dose steroids. J Clin Gastroenterol. 1993;17:10–3.
34. Toruner M, Loftus EV Jr, Harmsen WS, Zinsmeister AR, Orenstein R, Sandborn WJ, Colombel JF, Egan LJ. Risk factors for opportunistic infections in patients with inflammatory bowel disease. Gastroenterology. 2008;134:929–36.
35. Bernstein CN, Kornbluth A. Yes, we are still talking about cyclosporin vs. infliximab in steroid resistant acute severe ulcerative colitis. Am J Gastroenterol. 2017;112:1719–21.
36. Campbell S, Travis S, Jewell D. Ciclosporin use in acute ulcerative colitis: a long-term experience. Eur J Gastroenterol Hepatol. 2005;17:79–84.
37. Bojic D, Radojicic Z, Nedeljkovic-Protic M, Al-Ali M, Jewell DP, Travis SP. Long-term outcome after admission for acute severe ulcerative colitis in Oxford: the 1992–1993 cohort. Inflamm Bowel Dis. 2009;15:823–8.
38. Moskovitz DN, Van Assche G, Maenhout B, Arts J, Ferrante M, Vermeire S, Rutgeerts P. Incidence of colectomy during long-term follow-up after cyclosporine-induced remission of severe ulcerative colitis. Clin Gastroenterol Hepatol. 2006;4:760–5.
39. Laharie D, Bourreille A, Branche J, Allez M, Bouhnik Y, Filippi J, Zerbib F, Savoye G, Nachury M, Moreau J, Delchier JC, Cosnes J, Ricart E, Dewit O, Lopez-Sanroman A, Dupas JL, Carbonnel F, Bommelaer G, Coffin B, Roblin X, Van Assche G, Esteve M, Farkkila M, Gisbert JP, Marteau P, Nahon S, de Vos M, Franchimont D, Mary JY, Colombel JF, Lemann M. Ciclosporin versus infliximab in patients with severe ulcerative colitis refractory to intravenous steroids: a parallel, open-label randomised controlled trial. Lancet. 2012;380:1909–15.
40. Szemes K, Soos A, Hegyi P, Farkas N, Eros A, Eross B, Mezosi E, Szakacs Z, Marta K, Sarlos P. Comparable long-term outcomes of cyclosporine and infliximab in patients with steroid-refractory acute severe ulcerative colitis: a meta-analysis. Front Med. 2019;6:338.
41. Narula N, Marshall JK, Colombel JF, Leontiadis GI, Williams JG, Muqtadir Z, Reinisch W. Systematic review and meta-analysis: infliximab or cyclosporine as rescue therapy in patients with severe ulcerative colitis refractory to steroids. Am J Gastroenterol. 2016;111:477–91.
42. Williams JG, Alam MF, Alrubaiy L, Clement C, Cohen D, Grey M, Hilton M, Hutchings HA, Longo M, Morgan JM, Rapport FL, Seagrove AC, Watkins A. Comparison of iNfliximab and ciclosporin in STeroid resistant ulcerative colitis: pragmatic randomised trial and economic evaluation (CONSTRUCT). Health Technol Assess. 2016;20:1–320.
43. Sandborn WJ, van Assche G, Reinisch W, Colombel JF, D'Haens G, Wolf DC, Kron M, Tighe MB, Lazar A, Thakkar RB. Adalimumab induces and maintains clinical remission in patients with moderate-to-severe ulcerative colitis. Gastroenterology. 2012;142:257–65.e1–3

44. Chandra A, Kanth R, Thareja S. Efficacy and safety of adalimumab biosimilar (Exemptia) in moderate-to-severe steroid-refractory ulcerative colitis patients: real-life outcomes in resource-constrained setting at 24-weeks follow-up. Biologics Targets Therapy. 2019;13: 191–200.
45. Midha V, Mahajan R, Mehta V, Narang V, Singh A, Kaur K, Sood A. Efficacy and safety of the adalimumab biosimilar Exemptia as induction therapy in moderate-to-severe ulcerative colitis. Intest Res. 2018;16:83–9.
46. Sandborn WJ, Feagan BG, Marano C, Zhang H, Strauss R, Johanns J, Adedokun OJ, Guzzo C, Colombel JF, Reinisch W, Gibson PR, Collins J, Jarnerot G, Hibi T, Rutgeerts P. Subcutaneous golimumab induces clinical response and remission in patients with moderate-to-severe ulcerative colitis. Gastroenterology. 2014;146:85–95; quiz e14–5
47. Wiskin AE, Paul SP, Spray CH. Response to vedolizumab for children with steroid-refractory ulcerative colitis unresponsive to anti-TNF. Acta Paediatr. 2019;108:1359–60.
48. Shen CH, Chiou HY, Tung MC, Wu CC, Kao WT, Wang YH, Juang GD. Clinical and demographic characteristics among patients with urothelial carcinomas of the upper urinary tract and bladder in Taiwan. J Chin Med Assoc: JCMA. 2017;80:563–8.
49. Pellet G, Stefanescu C, Carbonnel F, Peyrin-Biroulet L, Roblin X, Allimant C, Nachury M, Nancey S, Filippi J, Altwegg R, Brixi H, Fotsing G, de Rosamel L, Shili S, Laharie D. Efficacy and safety of induction therapy with calcineurin inhibitors in combination with vedolizumab in patients with refractory ulcerative colitis. Clin Gastroenterol Hepatol. 2019;17:494–501.
50. Drugs for psoriatic arthritis. Med Lett Drugs Ther. 2019;61:203–10.
51. Chen AY, Oz HS. Rapid induction and maintenance of remission in refractory ulcerative colitis with ustekinumab. Diseases. 2019;7:55.
52. Berinstein JA, Steiner CA, Regal RE, Allen JI, Kinnucan JAR, Stidham RW, Waljee AK, Bishu S, Aldrich LB, Higgins PDR. Efficacy of induction therapy with high-intensity tofacitinib in 4 patients with acute severe ulcerative colitis. Clin Gastroenterol Hepatol. 2019;17:988–90.e1
53. Lair-Mehiri L, Stefanescu C, Vaysse T, Laharie D, Roblin X, Rosa I, Treton X, Abitbol V, Amiot A, Bouguen G, Dib N, Fumery M, Pariente B, Carbonnel F, Peyrin-Biroulet L, Simon M, Viennot S, Bouhnik Y. Real-world evidence of tofacitinib effectiveness and safety in patients with refractory ulcerative colitis. Dig Liver Dis. 2020;52:268–73.
54. Kotwani P, Terdiman J, Lewin S. Tofacitinib for rescue therapy in acute severe ulcerative colitis: a real-world experience. J Crohns Colitis. 2020;14(7):1026–8.
55. Ogata H, Kato J, Hirai F, Hida N, Matsui T, Matsumoto T, Koyanagi K, Hibi T. Double-blind, placebo-controlled trial of oral tacrolimus

(FK506) in the management of hospitalized patients with steroid-refractory ulcerative colitis. Inflamm Bowel Dis. 2012;18:803–8.
56. Schmidt KJ, Herrlinger KR, Emmrich J, Barthel D, Koc H, Lehnert H, Stange EF, Fellermann K, Buning J. Short-term efficacy of tacrolimus in steroid-refractory ulcerative colitis – experience in 130 patients. Aliment Pharmacol Ther. 2013;37:129–36.
57. Schmidt KJ, Muller N, Dignass A, Baumgart DC, Lehnert H, Stange EF, Herrlinger KR, Fellermann K, Buning J. Long-term outcomes in steroid-refractory ulcerative colitis treated with tacrolimus alone or in combination with purine analogues. J Crohns Colitis. 2016;10:31–7.
58. Matsumoto S, Kawamura H, Nishikawa T, Sagihara N, Miyatani H, Mashima H. Tacrolimus versus anti-tumor necrosis factor agents for steroid-refractory active ulcerative colitis based on the severity of endoscopic findings: a single-center, open-label cohort study. Clin Exp Gastroenterol. 2017;10:249–58.
59. Miyake N, Ando T, Ishiguro K, Maeda O, Watanabe O, Hirayama Y, Maeda K, Morise K, Matsushita M, Furukawa K, Funasaka K, Nakamura M, Miyahara R, Ohmiya N, Goto H. Azathioprine is essential following cyclosporine for patients with steroid-refractory ulcerative colitis. World J Gastroenterol. 2015;21:254–61.
60. Domenech E, Garcia-Planella E, Bernal I, Rosinach M, Cabre E, Fluvia L, Boix J, Gassull MA. Azathioprine without oral ciclosporin in the long-term maintenance of remission induced by intravenous ciclosporin in severe, steroid-refractory ulcerative colitis. Aliment Pharmacol Ther. 2002;16:2061–5.
61. Herfarth HH, Osterman MT, Isaacs KL, Lewis JD, Sands BE. Efficacy of methotrexate in ulcerative colitis: failure or promise. Inflamm Bowel Dis. 2010;16:1421–30.
62. Maser EA, Deconda D, Lichtiger S, Ullman T, Present DH, Kornbluth A. Cyclosporine and infliximab as rescue therapy for each other in patients with steroid-refractory ulcerative colitis. Clin Gastroenterol Hepatol. 2008;6:1112–6.
63. Chaparro M, Burgueno P, Iglesias E, Panes J, Munoz F, Bastida G, Castro L, Jimenez C, Mendoza JL, Barreiro-de Acosta M, Senent SG, Gomollon F, Calvet X, Garcia-Planella E, Gomez M, Hernandez V, Hinojosa J, Manosa M, Nyssen OP, Gisbert JP. Infliximab salvage therapy after failure of ciclosporin in corticosteroid-refractory ulcerative colitis: a multicentre study. Aliment Pharmacol Ther. 2012;35:275–83.
64. Hu Y, Chen Z, Gong Y, Shi Y. A review of switching biologic agents in the treatment of moderate-to-severe plaque psoriasis. Clin Drug Investig. 2018;38:191–9.
65. Cada DJ, Demaris K, Levien TL, Baker DE. Tofacitinib. Hosp Pharm. 2013;48:413–24.

66. Winthrop KL, Baddley JW. Pneumocystis and glucocorticoid use: to prophylax or not to prophylax (and when?); that is the question. Ann Rheum Dis. 2018;77:631–3.
67. Chapman RW, Selby WS, Jewell DP. Controlled trial of intravenous metronidazole as an adjunct to corticosteroids in severe ulcerative colitis. Gut. 1986;27:1210–2.
68. Mantzaris GJ, Petraki K, Archavlis E, Amberiadis P, Kourtessas D, Christidou A, Triantafyllou G. A prospective randomized controlled trial of intravenous ciprofloxacin as an adjunct to corticosteroids in acute, severe ulcerative colitis. Scand J Gastroenterol. 2001;36:971–4.
69. Mantzaris GJ, Hatzis A, Kontogiannis P, Triadaphyllou G. Intravenous tobramycin and metronidazole as an adjunct to corticosteroids in acute, severe ulcerative colitis. Am J Gastroenterol. 1994;89:43–6.
70. Nitzan O, Elias M, Peretz A, Saliba W. Role of antibiotics for treatment of inflammatory bowel disease. World J Gastroenterol. 2016;22:1078–87.
71. Silverberg MS, Satsangi J, Ahmad T, Arnott ID, Bernstein CN, Brant SR, Caprilli R, Colombel JF, Gasche C, Geboes K, Jewell DP, Karban A, Loftus EV Jr, Pena AS, Riddell RH, Sachar DB, Schreiber S, Steinhart AH, Targan SR, Vermeire S, Warren BF. Toward an integrated clinical, molecular and serological classification of inflammatory bowel disease: report of a working party of the 2005 Montreal world congress of gastroenterology. Can J Gastroenterol = Journal canadien de gastroenterologie. 2005;19(Suppl A):5A–36A.
72. Nguyen GC, Laveist TA, Gearhart S, Bayless TM, Brant SR. Racial and geographic variations in colectomy rates among hospitalized ulcerative colitis patients. Clin Gastroenterol Hepatol. 2006;4:1507–13.
73. Ananthakrishnan AN, Issa M, Beaulieu DB, Skaros S, Knox JF, Lemke K, Emmons J, Lundeen SH, Otterson MF, Binion DG. History of medical hospitalization predicts future need for colectomy in patients with ulcerative colitis. Inflamm Bowel Dis. 2009;15:176–81.
74. Waterman M, Knight J, Dinani A, Xu W, Stempak JM, Croitoru K, Nguyen GC, Cohen Z, McLeod RS, Greenberg GR, Steinhart AH, Silverberg MS. Predictors of outcome in ulcerative colitis. Inflamm Bowel Dis. 2015;21:2097–105.
75. Le Baut G, Kirchgesner J, Amiot A, Lefevre JH, Chafai N, Landman C, Nion I, Bourrier A, Delattre C, Martineau C, Sokol H, Seksik P, Nguyen Y, Marion Y, Lebreton G, Carbonnel F, Viennot S, Beaugerie L. A scoring system to determine patients' risk of colectomy within 1 year after hospital admission for acute severe ulcerative colitis. Clin Gastroenterol Hepatol. 2021;19(8):1602–10.e1
76. Dias CC, Rodrigues PP, da Costa-Pereira A, Magro F. Clinical predictors of colectomy in patients with ulcerative colitis: systematic review and meta-analysis of cohort studies. J Crohns Colitis. 2015;9:156–63.

77. Yerushalmy-Feler A, Singer D, Berkovitch G, Lubetzky R, Dotan I, Ziv-Baran T, Cohen S. Predictors for poor outcome of hospitalized children with inflammatory bowel disease. Eur J Pediatr. 2020;179:157–64.
78. Han W, Xu JM, Hu NZ, Mei Q, Liu MW. Early predictors of responses and clinical outcomes of corticosteroid treatment for severe ulcerative colitis. Scand J Gastroenterol. 2014;49:424–33.
79. Solberg IC, Lygren I, Jahnsen J, Aadland E, Hoie O, Cvancarova M, Bernklev T, Henriksen M, Sauar J, Vatn MH, Moum B. Clinical course during the first 10 years of ulcerative colitis: results from a population-based inception cohort (IBSEN study). Scand J Gastroenterol. 2009;44:431–40.
80. Barreiro-de Acosta M, Vallejo N, de la Iglesia D, Uribarri L, Baston I, Ferreiro-Iglesias R, Lorenzo A, Dominguez-Munoz JE. Evaluation of the risk of relapse in ulcerative colitis according to the degree of mucosal healing (Mayo 0 vs 1): a longitudinal cohort study. J Crohns Colitis. 2016;10:13–9.
81. Manginot C, Baumann C, Peyrin-Biroulet L. An endoscopic Mayo score of 0 is associated with a lower risk of colectomy than a score of 1 in ulcerative colitis. Gut. 2015;64:1181–2.
82. Rowan CR, Cullen G, Mulcahy HE, Sheridan J, Moss AC, Ryan EJ, Doherty GA. DUBLIN [degree of ulcerative colitis burden of luminal inflammation] score, a simple method to quantify inflammatory burden in ulcerative colitis. J Crohns Colitis. 2019;13:1365–71.
83. Mosli MH, Parker CE, Nelson SA, Baker KA, MacDonald JK, Zou GY, Feagan BG, Khanna R, Levesque BG, Jairath V. Histologic scoring indices for evaluation of disease activity in ulcerative colitis. Cochrane Database Syst Rev. 2017;5:CD011256.
84. Guirgis M, Wendt E, Wang LM, Walsh A, Burger D, Bryant RV, Kent A, Adamson R, Brain O, Travis SPL, Keshav S. Beyond histological remission: intramucosal calprotectin as a potential predictor of outcomes in ulcerative colitis. J Crohns Colitis. 2017;11:460–7.
85. Fabian O, Hradsky O, Lerchova T, Mikus F, Zamecnik J, Bronsky J. Limited clinical significance of tissue calprotectin levels in bowel mucosa for the prediction of complicated course of the disease in children with ulcerative colitis. Pathol Res Pract. 2019;215:152689.
86. Jodorkovsky D, Young Y, Abreu MT. Clinical outcomes of patients with ulcerative colitis and co-existing Clostridium difficile infection. Dig Dis Sci. 2010;55:415–20.
87. Zhang T, Lin QY, Fei JX, Zhang Y, Lin MY, Jiang SH, Wang P, Chen Y. Clostridium difficile infection worsen outcome of hospitalized patients with inflammatory bowel disease. Sci Rep. 2016;6:29791.
88. Navaneethan U, Mukewar S, Venkatesh PG, Lopez R, Shen B. Clostridium difficile infection is associated with worse long term outcome in patients with ulcerative colitis. J Crohns Colitis. 2012;6:330–6.

89. Aletaha N, Dadvar Z, Salehi B, Ketabi Moghadam P, Niksirat A, Jowkar A, Taslimi R, Allameh SF, Ebrahimi DN. Clinical and pathological features of ulcerative colitis in patients with and without Clostridium difficile infection; an observational study. Middle East J Dig Dis. 2019;11:17–23.
90. Schmidt C, Kohler F, Kraplin T, Hartmann M, Lerch MM, Stallmach A. Does the hospital cost of care differ for inflammatory bowel disease patients with or without gastrointestinal infections? A case-control study. Z Gastroenterol. 2014;52:643–8.
91. Trifan A, Stanciu C, Stoica O, Girleanu I, Cojocariu C. Impact of Clostridium difficile infection on inflammatory bowel disease outcome: a review. World J Gastroenterol. 2014;20:11736–42.
92. Solanky D, Pardi DS, Loftus EV, Khanna S. Colon surgery risk with corticosteroids versus immunomodulators or biologics in inflammatory bowel disease patients with Clostridium difficile infection. Inflamm Bowel Dis. 2019;25:610–9.
93. Lee HS, Park SH, Kim SH, Kim J, Choi J, Lee HJ, Kim WS, Lee JM, Kwak MS, Hwang SW, Yang DH, Kim KJ, Ye BD, Byeon JS, Myung SJ, Yoon YS, Yu CS, Kim JH, Yang SK. Risk factors and clinical outcomes associated with cytomegalovirus colitis in patients with acute severe ulcerative colitis. Inflamm Bowel Dis. 2016;22:912–8.
94. Park SC, Jeen YM, Jeen YT. Approach to cytomegalovirus infections in patients with ulcerative colitis. Korean J Intern Med. 2017;32:383–92.
95. Xu H, Tang H, Xu T, Xiao M, Li J, Tan B, Yang H, Lv H, Li Y, Qian J. Retrospective analysis of Clostridium difficile infection in patients with ulcerative colitis in a tertiary hospital in China. BMC Gastroenterol. 2019;19:3.
96. Iyer VH, Augustine J, Pulimood AB, Ajjampur SS, Ramakrishna BS. Correlation between coinfection with parasites, cytomegalovirus, and Clostridium difficile and disease severity in patients with ulcerative colitis. Indian J Gastroenterol. 2013;32:115–8.
97. Nahar S, Hokama A, Fujita J. Clinical significance of cytomegalovirus and other herpes virus infections in ulcerative colitis. Pol Arch Intern Medicine. 2019;129:620–6.
98. Mokhele NN, Thomson SR, Watermeyer GA. Predictors of emergency colectomy in patients admitted with acute severe ulcerative colitis. S Afr J Surg. Suid-Afrikaanse tydskrif vir chirurgie. 2017;55:20–6.
99. Vermeire S, Van Assche G, Rutgeerts P. C-reactive protein as a marker for inflammatory bowel disease. Inflamm Bowel Dis. 2004;10:661–5.
100. Theede K, Holck S, Ibsen P, Kallemose T, Nordgaard-Lassen I, Nielsen AM. Fecal calprotectin predicts relapse and histological mucosal healing in ulcerative colitis. Inflamm Bowel Dis. 2016;22:1042–8.
101. Jain S, Kedia S, Bopanna S, Sachdev V, Sahni P, Dash NR, Pal S, Vishnubhatla S, Makharia G, Travis SPL, Ahuja V. Faecal calprotectin

and UCEIS predict short-term outcomes in acute severe colitis: prospective cohort study. J Crohns Colitis. 2017;11:1309–16.
102. Wu HM, Wei J, Li J, Wang K, Ye L, Qi Y, Yuan BS, Yang YL, Zhao L, Yang Z, Yang MF, Gong JF, Wang FY. Serum procalcitonin as a potential early predictor of short-term outcomes in acute severe ulcerative colitis. Dig Dis Sci. 2019;64:3263–73.
103. Ho GT, Lee HM, Brydon G, Ting T, Hare N, Drummond H, Shand AG, Bartolo DC, Wilson RG, Dunlop MG, Arnott ID, Satsangi J. Fecal calprotectin predicts the clinical course of acute severe ulcerative colitis. Am J Gastroenterol. 2009;104:673–8.
104. Xie T, Zhao C, Ding C, Zhang T, Dai X, Lv T, Li Y, Guo Z, Gong J, Zhu W. Fecal calprotectin as an alternative to ulcerative colitis endoscopic index of severity to predict the response to corticosteroids of acute severe ulcerative colitis: a prospective observational study. Dig Liver Dis. 2017;49:984–90.
105. Rubio MG, Amo-Mensah K, Gray JM, Nguyen VQ, Nakat S, Grider D, Love K, Boone JH, Sorrentino D. Fecal lactoferrin accurately reflects mucosal inflammation in inflammatory bowel disease. World J Gastrointest Pathophysiol. 2019;10:54–63.
106. Calprotectin.co.uk. Volume 2020, 2012.
107. Kovacs G, Sipeki N, Suga B, Tornai T, Fechner K, Norman GL, Shums Z, Antal-Szalmas P, Papp M. Significance of serological markers in the disease course of ulcerative colitis in a prospective clinical cohort of patients. PLoS One. 2018;13:e0194166.
108. Spencer EA, Davis SM, Mack DR, Boyle BM, Griffiths AM, LeLeiko NS, Sauer CG, Keljo DJ, Markowitz JF, Baker SS, Rosh JR, Baldassano RN, Oliva-Hemker M, Pfefferkorn MD, Otley AR, Heyman MB, Noe JD, Patel AS, Rufo PA, Alison Marquis M, Walters TD, Collins MH, Kugathasan S, Denson LA, Hyams JS, Dubinsky MC. Serologic reactivity reflects clinical expression of ulcerative colitis in children. Inflamm Bowel Dis. 2018;24:1335–43.
109. Smids C, Horjus Talabur Horje CS, Groenen MJM, van Koolwijk EHM, Wahab PJ, van Lochem EG. The value of serum antibodies in differentiating inflammatory bowel disease, predicting disease activity and disease course in the newly diagnosed patient. Scand J Gastroenterol. 2017;52:1104–12.
110. Papp M, Altorjay I, Dotan N, Palatka K, Foldi I, Tumpek J, Sipka S, Udvardy M, Dinya T, Lakatos L, Kovacs A, Molnar T, Tulassay Z, Miheller P, Norman GL, Szamosi T, Papp J, Lakatos PL. New serological markers for inflammatory bowel disease are associated with earlier age at onset, complicated disease behavior, risk for surgery, and NOD2/CARD15 genotype in a Hungarian IBD cohort. Am J Gastroenterol. 2008;103:665–81.
111. Yao F, Fan Y, Lv B, Ji C, Xu L. Diagnostic utility of serological biomarkers in patients with Crohn's disease: a case-control study. Medicine. 2018;97:e11772.

112. Zhang S, Luo J, Wu Z, Roggenbuck D, Schierack P, Reinhold D, Li J, Zeng X, Zhang F, Qian J, Li Y. Antibodies against glycoprotein 2 display diagnostic advantages over ASCA in distinguishing CD from intestinal tuberculosis and intestinal Behcet's disease. Clin Transl Gastroenterol. 2018;9:e133.
113. Wang ZZ, Shi K, Peng J. Serologic testing of a panel of five antibodies in inflammatory bowel diseases: diagnostic value and correlation with disease phenotype. Biomed Rep. 2017;6:401–10.
114. Satsangi J, Welsh KI, Bunce M, Julier C, Farrant JM, Bell JI, Jewell DP. Contribution of genes of the major histocompatibility complex to susceptibility and disease phenotype in inflammatory bowel disease. Lancet. 1996;347:1212–7.
115. Haritunians T, Taylor KD, Targan SR, Dubinsky M, Ippoliti A, Kwon S, Guo X, Melmed GY, Berel D, Mengesha E, Psaty BM, Glazer NL, Vasiliauskas EA, Rotter JI, Fleshner PR, McGovern DP. Genetic predictors of medically refractory ulcerative colitis. Inflamm Bowel Dis. 2010;16:1830–40.
116. Cleynen I, Boucher G, Jostins L, Schumm LP, Zeissig S, Ahmad T, Andersen V, Andrews JM, Annese V, Brand S, Brant SR, Cho JH, Daly MJ, Dubinsky M, Duerr RH, Ferguson LR, Franke A, Gearry RB, Goyette P, Hakonarson H, Halfvarson J, Hov JR, Huang H, Kennedy NA, Kupcinskas L, Lawrance IC, Lee JC, Satsangi J, Schreiber S, Theatre E, van der Meulen-de Jong AE, Weersma RK, Wilson DC, Parkes M, Vermeire S, Rioux JD, Mansfield J, Silverberg MS, Radford-Smith G, DP MG, Barrett JC, Lees CW. Inherited determinants of Crohn's disease and ulcerative colitis phenotypes: a genetic association study. Lancet. 2016;387:156–67.
117. Kopylov U, Boucher G, Waterman M, Rivers CR, Patel M, Cho JH, Colombel JF, Duerr RH, Binion D, McGovern DP, Schumm PP, Brant SR, Silverberg MS, Rioux JD, Bitton A. Genetic predictors of benign course of ulcerative colitis-a north American inflammatory bowel disease genetics consortium study. Inflamm Bowel Dis. 2016;22:2311–6.
118. Turner D, Leach ST, Mack D, Uusoue K, McLernon R, Hyams J, Leleiko N, Walters TD, Crandall W, Markowitz J, Otley AR, Griffiths AM, Day AS. Faecal calprotectin, lactoferrin, M2-pyruvate kinase and S100A12 in severe ulcerative colitis: a prospective multicentre comparison of predicting outcomes and monitoring response. Gut. 2010;59:1207–12.
119. Lynch RW, Churchhouse AM, Protheroe A, Arnott ID. Predicting outcome in acute severe ulcerative colitis: comparison of the Travis and Ho scores using UK IBD audit data. Aliment Pharmacol Ther. 2016;43:1132–41.
120. Calvet X, Panes J, Alfaro N, Hinojosa J, Sicilia B, Gallego M, Perez I, Lazaro y de Mercado P, Gomollon F, Aldeguera X, Alos R, Andreu M, Barreiro M, Bermejo F, Casis B, Domenech E, Espin E, Esteve M,

Garcia-Sanchez V, Lopez-Sanroman A, Martinez-Montiel P, Luis Mendoza J, Gisbert JP, Vera M, Dosal A, Sanchez E, Marin L, Sanroman L, Pinilla P, Murciano F, Torrejon A, Ramon Garcia J, Ortega M, Roldan J. Delphi consensus statement: quality indicators for inflammatory bowel disease comprehensive care units. J Crohns Colitis. 2014;8:240–51.

121. Morar PS, Sevdalis N, Warusavitarne J, Hart A, Green J, Edwards C, Faiz O. Establishing the aims, format and function for multidisciplinary team-driven care within an inflammatory bowel disease service: a multicentre qualitative specialist-based consensus study. Frontline Gastroenterol. 2018;9:29–36.
122. Carvello M, Watfah J, Wlodarczyk M, Spinelli A. The management of the hospitalized ulcerative colitis patient: the medical-surgical conundrum. Curr Gastroenterol Rep. 2020;22:11.
123. Leijonmarck CE, Persson PG, Hellers G. Factors affecting colectomy rate in ulcerative colitis: an epidemiologic study. Gut. 1990;31:329–33.
124. Yanai H, Hanauer SB. Assessing response and loss of response to biological therapies in IBD. Am J Gastroenterol. 2011;106:685–98.
125. Kimura H, Kunisaki R, Tatsumi K, Koganei K, Sugita A, Endo I. Prolonged medical therapy increases the risk of surgical complications in patients with severe ulcerative colitis. Dig Surg. 2016;33:182–9.
126. Fornaro R, Caratto M, Barbruni G, Fornaro F, Salerno A, Giovinazzo D, Sticchi C, Caratto E. Surgical and medical treatment in patients with acute severe ulcerative colitis. J Dig Dis. 2015;16:558–67.
127. Ginanneschi U, Fabiani P, Rizzi M, Fanti G. Emergency surgical treatment of ulcerative rectocolitis and Crohn's disease of the colon. Ann Ital Chir. 1996;67:193–6.
128. Pal S, Sahni P, Pande GK, Acharya SK, Chattopadhyay TK. Outcome following emergency surgery for refractory severe ulcerative colitis in a tertiary care Centre in India. BMC Gastroenterol. 2005;5:39.
129. Seelig MH, Uhlig H, Braun J, Schumpelick V. Surgical therapy of severe colitis. Der Chirurg; Zeitschrift fur alle Gebiete der operativen Medizen. 1996;67:150–4.
130. Binderow SR, Wexner SD. Current surgical therapy for mucosal ulcerative colitis. Dis Colon Rectum. 1994;37:610–24.
131. Greenstein AJ, Romanoff AM, Moskowitz AJ, Sosunov EA, Khaitov S, Egorova NN. Payer status and access to laparoscopic subtotal colectomy for ulcerative colitis. Dis Colon Rectum. 2013;56:1062–7.
132. Bardakcioglu O, Khan A, Aldridge C, Chen J. Growth of laparoscopic colectomy in the United States: analysis of regional and socioeconomic factors over time. Ann Surg. 2013;258:270–4.
133. Gu J, Stocchi L, Remzi FH, Kiran RP. Total abdominal colectomy for severe ulcerative colitis: does the laparoscopic approach really have benefit? Surg Endosc. 2014;28:617–25.

134. Fichera A, Zoccali M. Single-incision laparoscopic total abdominal colectomy for refractory ulcerative colitis. Surg Endosc. 2012;26:862–8.
135. Fichera A, Zoccali M, Gullo R. Single incision ("scarless") laparoscopic total abdominal colectomy with end ileostomy for ulcerative colitis. J Gastrointest Surg. 2011;15:1247–51.
136. Sonoda T. The use of laparoscopic techniques in surgery for mucosal ulcerative colitis. Semin Laparosc Surg. 2003;10:169–75.
137. Wexner SD, Cera SM. Laparoscopic surgery for ulcerative colitis. Surg Clin North Am. 2005;85:35–47, viii
138. Ionescu M, Dumitrascu T, Stroescu C, Barbuta S, Tomulescu V, Popescu I. Surgical treatment in ulcerative rectocolitis. Analysis of a 24 years experience of 50 patients. Chirurgia. 2004;99:125–35.
139. Frizelle FA, Burt MJ. Review: the surgical management of ulcerative colitis. J Gastroenterol Hepatol. 1997;12:670–7.
140. Alsaleh A, Gaidos JK, Kang L, Kuemmerle JF. Timing of last preoperative dose of infliximab does not increase postoperative complications in inflammatory bowel disease patients. Dig Dis Sci. 2016;61:2602–7.
141. Kulaylat AS, Kulaylat AN, Schaefer EW, Tinsley A, Williams E, Koltun W, Hollenbeak CS, Messaris E. Association of preoperative anti-tumor necrosis factor therapy with adverse postoperative outcomes in patients undergoing abdominal surgery for ulcerative colitis. JAMA Surg. 2017;152:e171538.
142. Kuehn F, Hodin RA. Impact of modern drug therapy on surgery: ulcerative colitis. Visc Med. 2018;34:426–31.
143. Selvaggi F, Pellino G, Canonico S, Sciaudone G. Effect of preoperative biologic drugs on complications and function after restorative proctocolectomy with primary ileal pouch formation: systematic review and meta analysis. Inflamm Bowel Dis. 2015;21:79–92.
144. Kuenzig ME, Benchimol EI, Lee L, Targownik LE, Singh H, Kaplan GG, Bernstein CN, Bitton A, Nguyen GC, Lee K, Cooke-Lauder J, Murthy SK. The impact of inflammatory bowel disease in Canada 2018: direct costs and health services utilization. J Can Assoc Gastroenterol. 2019;2:S17–33.
145. Vasudevan A, Arachchi A, Scanlon C, Greenhalgh J, Van Langenberg DR. A comparison of long-term healthcare utilization and costs in patients with acute severe ulcerative colitis receiving infliximab versus early colectomy. Ther Adv Chronic Dis. 2019;10:2040622319825595.
146. Stidham RW, Liu W, Bishu S, Rice MD, Higgins PDR, Zhu J, Nallamothu BK, Waljee AK. Performance of a deep learning model vs human reviewers in grading endoscopic disease severity of patients with ulcerative colitis. JAMA Netw Open. 2019;2:e193963.

Surgical Management of Hospitalized Patients with Ulcerative Colitis

4

Evan Messaris and Daniel Wong

Introduction

Although recent advances in medical therapy for ulcerative colitis (UC) improve the ability to induce disease remission, surgical resection in UC is curative and should not be viewed as medical failure. Performing the right operation, for the right patient, at the right time is a central tenant of surgical planning and critical to success in the surgical management of the hospitalized patient with UC. The emergence of biologic therapies combined with advancements in surgical care challenges our previous understanding of outcomes and best practices in this challenging patient population. Nevertheless, several essential principles of surgery in the hospitalized patient with UC remain consistent. First is that rapid recognition and immediate operation is essential in the

E. Messaris · D. Wong (✉)
Division of Colon and Rectal Surgery, Beth Israel Deaconess Medical Center, Boston, MA, USA
e-mail: emessari@bidmc.harvard.edu; dwong3@bidmc.harvard.edu

J. D. Feuerstein, A. S. Cheifetz (eds.), *Management of Inpatient Inflammatory Bowel Disease*,
https://doi.org/10.1007/978-1-0716-1987-2_4

patient with toxic colitis. Second is that best patient care comes from collaboration within a multidisciplinary team including gastroenterologists, colorectal surgeons, and wound ostomy continence nurses among others. Finally is the acknowledgment by both the surgeon and patient that operations in the acute setting are at higher risk of complications. Frank preoperative discussions, intraoperative flexibility, and early recognition of complications are essential to optimal short- and long-term outcomes.

Overview of Surgery for UC

Surgical cure for UC requires the removal of the entire colon and rectum. Historically, total colectomy with ileorectal anastomosis and rectal surveillance was offered to patients with UC; however, most regard this operation as an inferior procedure due to the risk for ongoing proctitis and malignancy [1]. Thus total proctocolectomy (TPC) is preferred either with end ileostomy (EI) or ileal pouch anal anastomosis (IPAA) reconstruction for continent reconstruction [2]. TPC with IPAA can be performed in one, two, or three stages (Table 4.1). However, resection of the colon and rectum is the treatment for UC, and thus it is important to remember that IPAA is an elective procedure that is not appropriate for all patients, particularly those with potential issues of continence [3]. Moreover, the improvement in quality of life is mainly related to disease control, and patient satisfaction is similar regardless of the choice for IPAA or EI [4]. While less common, continent ileostomies (often called ileal Kock pouches) are an additional option following TPC when IPAA is not feasible and permanent end ileostomy is undesirable [5].

Systems-Based Approaches for Optimal Surgical Outcomes in UC

In the rapidly changing clinical landscape of IBD management, we strongly endorse a multidisciplinary approach to these determinations. Patients with UC present distinct perioperative chal-

Table 4.1 Approaches to surgical cure and ileoanal pouch reconstruction for ulcerative colitis

	Operation	Advantages	Disadvantages
Three-stage	Stage 1: Total abdominal colectomy with end ileostomy	Lower morbidity of the first operation in urgent setting	Greater number of operations
	Stage 2: Completion proctectomy with IPAA formation and diverting ileostomy	Allows time to recover and wean steroids prior to IPAA creation	Risk for rectal stump complications after stage 1
	Stage 3: Ileostomy takedown		Higher risk for readmission
Two-stage	Stage 1: Total proctocolectomy and IPAA with diverting ileostomy	Fewer operations, more efficient for patient	IPAA formation in suboptimal patient
	Stage 2: Ileostomy takedown		Higher rate of complication in urgent setting
One-stage	Total proctocolectomy with IPAA and no ileostomy	Single operation, no ileostomy	Only appropriate in select populations and not widely adopted

lenges due to their degree of immunosuppression, often prolonged steroid exposure, relative malnutrition, and increased risk for venous thromboembolism. Given this array of challenges, collaborative team management is critical to mitigate negative outcomes. Where feasible, operations for inflammatory bowel disease should be concentrated at IBD centers. Similar to other complex surgeries, operating for UC within tertiary care, high-volume centers appear to be associated with lower mortality [6–10]. Patients undergoing operations for UC should also follow enhanced recovery after surgery (ERAS) protocols [11]. While not all elements of an ERAS protocol may be possible in a hospitalized UC patient, limited data supports ERAS use in IBD patients with no evidence of harm [12, 13].

Surgical Consultation for the Hospitalized Patient with UC

Opinions about optimal timing to consult a surgeon on a hospitalized UC patient vary from immediately upon admission to after evidence of a lack of response to medical therapies [14, 15]. While rates of colectomy have decreased over time, most recent series of acute severe UC (ASUC) in the "biologic" age have a 12-month colectomy rate of around 30% [16–21]. Inpatient and 30-day colectomy rates are approximately 10–15%. Given the high risk of urgent or semi-urgent surgery, we suggest a low threshold for early surgeon consultation on patients with ASUC [22]. Framing surgery not as "failure" but an alternative therapy is essential in these settings. Ideally, these conversations occur in the outpatient setting prior to an acute hospitalization. When this is not possible, early inpatient surgical consultation allows patients adequate time to contemplate, ask questions, and adjust expectations prior to surgery. Proactive involvement of wound ostomy continence nurses (WOCN) helps to address patient concerns about the postoperative care and daily activities with a stoma.

Contemporary Colectomy Rates

Overall rates of colectomy in UC are decreasing over time [23–27]. Examining the hospitalized UC patient, two recent studies from the Nationwide Inpatient Sample highlight that emergent colectomy rates are decreasing, while elective colectomy and IPAA rates increase or remain stable [28, 29]. A recent meta-analysis of infliximab use in ASUC estimates colectomy-free survival rates at 1, 3, and 12 months of 86%, 80%, and 70%, respectively. There was no clear benefit in dose-intensified infliximab regimens for ASUC although data is limited and confounded in these populations [21]. Thus while improvements in medical therapy have reduced emergent colectomies, around one-third of patients with ASUC will require a colectomy within 12 months.

Preoperative Evaluation of the Patient

In general, patients admitted with ASUC undergo a standard workup including a complete blood count, standard chemistries, inflammatory markers, abdominal x-ray or CT scan, stool studies, and sigmoidoscopy [30, 31]. Particularly relevant results for the surgeon include hemoglobin, albumin, c-reactive protein, radiographic and endoscopic appearance of the colon and rectum, and potential treatable etiologies of the current flare such as cytomegalovirus (CMV) or *Clostridioides difficile* (*C. diff*) infection. Additionally, any uncertainty in the diagnosis between UC, indeterminate, or Crohn's colitis requires discussion within the multidisciplinary team as this may alter the surgical plan.

Aside from a standard preoperative history, special attention should be paid to dose, timing, and duration of prior steroid, biologic, or immunomodulatory therapy. The history should elucidate degree of weight loss, exercise tolerance, functional status, prior abdominal surgery, obstetrical history, family planning goals, and instances of pelvic radiation. A total abdominal colectomy with end ileostomy does not require pelvic dissection and thus does not alter the rate of fertility or fecundity. If an IPAA is being considered, one should elucidate whether there is any history of stool incontinence prior to the current flare. Fecal urgency related to the flare does not preclude patients from an IPAA. A thorough and well-documented abdominal exam is necessary to allow serial monitoring of clinical status. Description of the degree of distension, the presence of peritonitis (localized or general) in addition to tenderness, as well as documenting voluntary or involuntary guarding is necessary. Finally, a digital rectal exam should be performed with qualitative evaluation of resting and maximal sphincter pressures.

The Decision to Operate

Unfortunately robust predictive models to identify patients requiring emergent, urgent, or elective colectomies do not exist. Thus the decision to operate, except in clear and immediate indications, is individualized for each patient. A number of risk factors for requiring colectomy in patient with ASUC have been identified [17, 19, 21, 32–37]. In general, these factors correspond with markers of severe disease such as low albumin levels; elevated CRP; anemia; inflammation on histology, endoscopy, or cross-sectional imaging; duration and extent of disease; and previous treatment failures. Genetic predisposition may also influence therapeutic response; however, this is not used clinically [38]. Due to the difficulty in predicting patients who will require colectomy, clear and daily communication between the medical team, surgical team, and patient is required to determine when surgery is the right option. Importantly, prior to colectomy patients should be evaluated by a WOCN and a site marked for ostomy placement.

Indications for Immediate Surgery

The recognition of a patient requiring emergent colectomy is the surgeon's first obligation when evaluating a hospitalized patient with ASUC. Perforation, generalized peritonitis, abdominal sepsis, shock, and intractable bleeding are indications for immediate surgery. In these cases, resuscitation and emergent subtotal colectomy with end ileostomy is the safest choice. Of note, immunosuppression may lead to a masking of peritoneal findings on physical exam, and therefore one should have a low threshold for obtaining cross-sectional imaging when initially evaluating patients with ASUC. While a patient may not have a clear indication for surgery on initial evaluation, serial reevaluation for signs of systemic illness and deterioration is essential to identify patients who require surgery.

Distension with Fulminant Colitis

Several scoring systems are used to classify disease severity in UC on a combination of clinical, laboratory, and endoscopic criteria including the Truelove and Witts and Mayo score which are most commonly used now [39–41]. Patients with severe colitis have >6 bowel movements per day and evidence of systemic toxicity with fulminant classification reserved for patients with >10 bowel movements/day and some degree of colonic dilation. "Toxic megacolon" commonly refers to fulminant or severe colitis with distension of the transverse colon greater than 6 cm and signs of systemic toxicity [22]. Some identify a cecal diameter of greater than 10 cm with localized peritonitis as an indication for immediate surgery [42]. In our experience, it is difficult to anchor to any single measurement when evaluating ASUC with distension. Perforation is possible without dilation. Repeated measurements from abdominal x-rays can be misleading. Serial exams and close monitoring of the patient with severe colitis and distension are critical. Worsening clinical presentation in the setting of colonic distension or progressive distension likely prompts operative intervention as perforation in patients with fulminant colitis has a higher mortality rate.

Steroid-Refractory Patients

There is no clear answer on when to operate on patients with ASUC that do not respond to initial medical therapy. If a patient with ASUC fails to improve following 3 days of IV steroids, she or he will likely undergo salvage therapy consisting of infliximab or cyclosporine [40]. Unless the patient is systemically worsening, has contraindications to salvage medications, or has failed previous therapies, most providers will likely attempt a trial of salvage therapy before recommending surgery. Thus in our experience, there are four common trajectories for this patient:

1. Salvage therapy is successful, and the patient goes into remission.
2. Salvage therapy is initially successful, patient is discharged, steroid reduced, and semi-elective colectomy is performed if remission is not obtained.
3. Salvage therapy is unsuccessful and the patient undergoes urgent colectomy.
4. Salvage therapy is minimally effective and does not allow full recovery or steroid reduction, and the patient undergoes semi-urgent surgery in a debilitated state.

The outcomes in the first two trajectories are optimal; however given the difficulty in predicting which path a patient will follow, we must also attempt to mitigate the risks encountered in the other two trajectories.

Approximately 10–15% of patients will require colectomy within 30 days of admission for ASUC. Limited evidence suggests that rescue therapy with infliximab or cyclosporine does not increase the risk of perioperative complications in this population [43]. However, several observational studies have shown that prolonged preoperative length of stay is associated with higher postoperative morbidity in patients requiring colectomy [10, 44–47]. Whether preoperative length of stay is truly a modifiable risk factor for operative complications is unknown; nevertheless, almost all series identify preoperative steroid use, malnutrition, and anemia as risk factors for perioperative complications [45, 48–50]. Thus once it is clear that a patient is not responding to salvage medical therapy, colectomy should be performed as soon as safely possible to avoid worsening of anemia, malnutrition, and accumulation of further steroid doses.

Operations for the Hospitalized Patient with UC

Subtotal Colectomy

The optimal operation for the hospitalized patient with UC removes the colon and minimizes perioperative complications.

For most patients, the safest choice is a subtotal colectomy with an end ileostomy. This operation controls the disease while avoiding dissection within the pelvis or forming a pouch or anastomosis in an acutely inflamed and often debilitated patient. In general we do not prescribe a bowel preparation. A minimally invasive approach is preferable for the colectomy [51]. Rectal stump leakage occurs in approximately 5–10% of cases and can have significant morbidity especially if the stump is stapled and left intraperitoneal [52–54]. Options to decrease morbidity related to rectal stump leakage include creating a mucus fistula with the proximal end of the divided sigmoid colon. The stapled off distal sigmoid colon can be secured to the fascia at the incision or brought through the fascia lying in the subcutaneous tissue. In the event of a rectal stump leak, the skin can be opened superficially to avoid intra-abdominal sepsis.

Total Proctocolectomy

Although less common, total proctocolectomy with end ileostomy (TPC-EI) is sometimes performed in hospitalized patients with UC [9, 55]. This operation has the advantage of removing all of the colon and rectum in a single operation as a cure for UC. Impaired perineal wound healing is a common complication with this operation [55]. High-dose steroids increase the risk of both wound complications and reoperation; thus one must be cognizant of this when choosing this operation for a patient receiving high-dose steroid therapy. TPC-EI may be a good option for patients not eligible for IPAA or in whom surveillance of the rectal stump may be challenging.

Ileoanal Pouch Formation

Whether or not IPAA formation can occur in the hospitalized patient with UC is a subject of much debate [56]. Perioperative complications especially pelvic sepsis following IPAA can adversely affect long-term pouch function [57, 58]. National data indicates an increase in reoperation, sepsis, and organ space infections when comparing semi-urgent to elective TPC with IPAA [59]. While the data is not conclusive, many suspect that recent biologic exposure increases complications in IPAA formation [60, 61]. However, some single institutional data shows no difference in short- or long-term complications with IPAA in the elective vs hospitalized setting [7]. In general, we recommend against IPAA formation in the hospitalized UC patient although in select cases of patients with lower steroid exposure and good nutritional status, IPAA formation may be feasible. Our recommended surgical pathway is a three-stage IPAA such that the IPAA is performed while patients are off steroids and nutritionally sound.

More Rare Operations

Rescue diverting loop ileostomy (RDLI) has been proposed as an alternative to subtotal colectomy in the acute setting for severe colitis. Experience with this surgery is extremely limited although an initial series showed promising results [62]. Further investigation is warranted especially given the prospect of colon salvage. Another potential colon preserving operative therapy is appendectomy although its utility in hospitalized UC patients has yet to be seen [63]. The formation of a continent ileostomy, most commonly a Kock pouch, can be performed as an alternative to or in the setting of a failed IPAA [64]. The formation of a continent ileostomy involves the creation of an intra-abdominal reservoir with an ileal S-pouch and an intubatable valve from the intussuscepted efferent limb which is connected to the abdominal wall [5]. While the continent ileostomy offers some quality of life advantages over permanent end ileostomy, complication rates are high, and operative expertise in their creation is limited to a few centers [65]. In general, we recommend against the creation of any ileal reservoir in a non-optimized, hospitalized patient with UC.

Postoperative Management

Most hospitalized patients with UC undergoing surgery will follow a standard enhanced recovery pathway. This includes opiate sparing pain multimodal medication, conservative intravenous fluids, and early ambulation. Venous thromboembolism prophylaxis is essential in these patients as their risk for deep vein thrombosis or pulmonary embolus is high [66]. We generally treat patients with low molecular weight heparin prophylaxis during the postoperative admission and for an additional month after discharge. We emphasize early stoma nurse involvement to assist patients in learning how to manage an ileostomy and monitor stoma output. These are essential to preventing readmission for dehydration [67]. Most, if not all, patients will have undergone some degree of steroid treatment prior to their operation. Preoperative dosage and duration helps dictate the postoperative wean [68]. Most postoperative tapers will continue for a number of weeks following discharge, and thus ensuring adequate outpatient follow-up is important.

Recognizing Complications

Complications are common in surgery for hospitalized patients with UC [7, 9, 10, 43, 45, 46, 50, 69, 70] (Table 4.2). Similar to risk factors for colectomy, many of these factors such as immunosuppression, anemia, and malnutrition are reflective of worse disease at the time of operation. Other common factors such as age, American Society of Anesthesiologist (ASA) classification, and preexisting conditions are not modifiable. Therefore, the focus should be on early recognition and intervention of postoperative complications to minimize effect. Infectious complications in the immunosuppressed are common. Early urinary catheter removal and prophylactic negative pressure therapy on closed incisions may help to reduce complications [71]. In the setting of rising leukocytosis, persistent ileus, or instability, there should be a low

Table 4.2 Operative morbidity in hospitalized patients with UC

Author	Operation	Complications	Notes
Hicks et al. [7]	Colectomy with ileostomy (30%) TPC w/ IPAA (70%)	Abdominal sepsis: 18% Ileus: 30%	Pouch failure: 7%
Nelson et al. [43]	Colectomy	Noninfectious: 34% Infectious: 24% Pelvic abscess: 5%	No difference between IV steroids and cyclosporine or infliximab
Schineis et al. [50]	Colectomy with ileostomy	Overall: 28% Rectal stump leak: 6% Abscess: 2%	Mortality: 0.5%
Feuerstein et al. [9]	Colectomy with ileostomy (62%) TPC with IPAA (20%) TPC with EI (19%)	Minor complication: 38% Major complication: 16% Abscess/collection: 4%	Mortality: 1.2%
Coakley et al. [45]	Colectomy with ileostomy	Any complication: 27% Deep infection: 9% Sepsis: 2%	Prolonged preoperative hospitalization associated with complication
Leeds et al. [46]	Total abdominal colectomy	Any complication: 68% Sepsis: 34% 10% mortality	Early colectomy associated with decreased mortality
Andrew et al. [70]	Total colectomy	Any complication: 10% for steroids only 21% for infliximab Abscess: 5%	Low rate of infliximab use (16%)

threshold to obtaining a CT of the abdomen and pelvis to rule rectal stump leakage or intra-abdominal abscess. Due to the high risk for venous thromboembolic disease, we recommend the usage of IV contrast to evaluate for portal or mesenteric thrombus as well as having a low threshold to also obtaining a CT of the chest. Readmission is common in this patient population occurring in as many as 20–30% of cases [7, 9]. We see patients in follow-up within 1–2 weeks of discharge in conjunction with a WOCN appointment in an attempt to address issues early on and prevent readmission.

Summary

Despite a number of advances in the treatment of UC, once a patient is hospitalized, surgery is required in ~30% of patients within 1 year and associated with a higher complication rate than elective procedures. Patients are almost universally immunosuppressed and often malnourished and debilitated. In these settings, the goal is to remove the majority of the disease in a safe and effective surgery, which for the majority of patients consists of a laparoscopic subtotal colectomy with end ileostomy. In rare cases, a total proctocolectomy with ileoanal pouch formation can be pursued, but it is the authors' preference to perform an IPAA as a three-stage procedure. Complications are common and early recognition and intervention is key to limiting associated morbidity. Finally, due to the complexity of these patients and high rate of eventual colectomy, early collaboration within a multidisciplinary team is absolutely critical to providing the best care to patients.

Clinical Vignette

A 60-year-old woman with a 10-year history of ulcerative colitis is hospitalized for hematochezia and diarrhea. She was recently switched from infliximab to vedolizumab (most recent dose 3 weeks ago) and takes oral prednisone 30 mg/day. She presented

3 days ago with 10 bloody bowel movements per day and was started on IV methylprednisolone. A flexible sigmoidoscopy performed during the hospitalization revealed ulcerated and friable mucosa with contact bleeding. She is afebrile, with mild tenderness on deep palpation of the abdomen and no distension. She reports a 15-pound weight loss over the last 6 months, her albumin is 3.4, and hemoglobin is 10. She is Cdiff negative and CMV status from colonic biopsies are pending. She denies any incontinence to stool or gas and does not want an ostomy. What surgical therapy should be recommended to this patient?

Learning Objective Understand the safest and most effective surgical therapy in hospitalized patients with ulcerative colitis.

First Choice Laparoscopic total abdominal colectomy with end ileostomy. The patient should undergo colectomy, wean from steroids, and be considered for pouch reconstruction or completion proctectomy in 3 months if doing well.

Alternative Choices Total proctocolectomy with end ileostomy is another option; however, the addition of proctectomy and inherent pelvic dissection increases operative time and potential complications. If the patient has a concomitant rectal cancer, a proctocolectomy at the initial operation is required. Limited experience supports that diverting loop ileostomy is feasible as a bridge to definitive therapy in ASUC although this would not be considered the standard of care.

Would Avoid Ileoanal pouch construction. Given her recent biologic dosing and steroid exposure as well as malnourishment, attempting ileoanal pouch reconstruction even with diversion would be an unnecessary risk. Colectomy with ileorectal anastomosis would be also be a poor choice since any anastomosis under these circumstances would be high risk for leak.

Other Considerations Perioperative patients with ulcerative colitis are at high risk for venous thrombosis including deep vein thrombosis, pulmonary embolus, and mesenteric venous thrombosis. Appropriate prophylaxis pre- and postoperatively is essential. Avoiding a stoma in patients with severe ulcerative colitis is not possible. Preoperative consultation of enterostomal nurses for education and preoperative stoma marking is critical.

References

1. Uzzan M, Cosnes J, Amiot A, et al. Long-term follow-up after ileorectal anastomosis for ulcerative colitis. Ann Surg. 2017;266(6):1029–34. https://doi.org/10.1097/SLA.0000000000002022.
2. Parks A, Nicholls R. Proctocolectomy without ileostomy. Br Med J. 1978;2(July):85–8.
3. Chang S, Shen B, Remzi F. When not to pouch: important considerations for patient selection for ileal pouch-anal anastomosis. Gastroenterol Hepatol. 2017;13(8):466–75.
4. Murphy PB, Khot Z, Vogt KN, Ott M, Dubois L. Quality of life after total proctocolectomy with ileostomy or IPAA: a systematic review. Dis Colon Rectum. 2015;58(9):899–908. https://doi.org/10.1097/DCR.0000000000000418.
5. Aytac E, Ashburn J, Dietz DW. Is there still a role for continent ileostomy in the surgical treatment of inflammatory bowel disease? Inflamm Bowel Dis. 2014;20(12):2519–25. https://doi.org/10.1097/MIB.0000000000000160.
6. Ananthakrishnan AN, McGinley EL. Weekend hospitalisations and post-operative complications following urgent surgery for ulcerative colitis and Crohn's disease. Aliment Pharmacol Ther. 2013;37(9):895–904. https://doi.org/10.1111/apt.12272.
7. Hicks CW, Hodin RA, Bordeianou L. Semi-urgent surgery in hospitalized patients with severe ulcerative colitis does not increase overall J-pouch complications. Am J Surg. 2014;207(2):281–7. https://doi.org/10.1016/j.amjsurg.2013.06.006.
8. Ordás I, Domènech E, Mañosa M, et al. Post-operative morbidity and mortality of a cohort of steroid refractory acute severe ulcerative colitis: nationwide multicenter study of the GETECCU ENEIDA registry. Am J Gastroenterol. 2018;113(7):1009–16. https://doi.org/10.1038/s41395-018-0057-0.
9. Feuerstein JD, Curran T, Alosilla M, Cataldo T, Falchuk KR, Poylin V. Mortality is rare following elective and non-elective surgery for ulcerative colitis, but mild postoperative complications are common. Dig Dis Sci. 2018;63(3):713–22. https://doi.org/10.1007/s10620-018-4922-x.
10. Leeds IL, Truta B, Parian AM, et al. Early surgical intervention for acute ulcerative colitis is associated with improved postoperative outcomes. J

Gastrointest Surg. 2017;21(10):1675–82. https://doi.org/10.1007/s11605-017-3538-3.
11. Carmichael JC, Keller DS, Baldini G, et al. Clinical practice guidelines for enhanced recovery after colon and rectal surgery from the American Society of Colon and Rectal Surgeons and Society of American Gastrointestinal and Endoscopic Surgeons. Dis Colon Rectum. 2017;60(8):761–84. https://doi.org/10.1097/DCR.0000000000000883.
12. Liska D, Bora Cengiz T, Novello M, et al. Do patients with inflammatory bowel disease benefit from an enhanced recovery pathway? Inflamm Bowel Dis. 2020;26(3):476–83. https://doi.org/10.1093/ibd/izz172.
13. D'Andrea AP, Khetan P, Miller R, Sylla P, Divino CM. Outcomes after bowel resection for inflammatory bowel disease in the era of surgical care bundles and enhanced recovery. J Gastrointest Surg. 2020;24(1):123–31. https://doi.org/10.1007/s11605-019-04362-2.
14. Shah SC, Naymagon S, Cohen BL, Sands BE, Dubinsky MC. There is significant practice pattern variability in the management of the hospitalized ulcerative colitis patient at a tertiary care and IBD referral center. J Clin Gastroenterol. 2018;52(4):333–8. https://doi.org/10.1097/MCG.0000000000000779.
15. Carvello M, Watfah J, Włodarczyk M, Spinelli A. The management of the hospitalized ulcerative colitis patient: the medical–surgical conundrum. Curr Gastroenterol Rep. 2020;22(3):4–11. https://doi.org/10.1007/s11894-020-0750-1.
16. Choy MC, Seah D, Faleck DM, et al. Systematic review and meta-analysis: optimal salvage therapy in acute severe ulcerative colitis. Inflamm Bowel Dis. 2019;25(7):1169–86. https://doi.org/10.1093/ibd/izy383.
17. Choy MC, Seah D, Gorelik A, et al. Predicting response after infliximab salvage in acute severe ulcerative colitis. J Gastroenterol Hepatol. 2018;33(7):1347–52. https://doi.org/10.1111/jgh.14072.
18. Vedamurthy A, Xu L, Luther J, et al. Long-term outcomes of immunosuppression-naïve steroid responders following hospitalization for ulcerative colitis. Dig Dis Sci. 2018;63(10):2740–6. https://doi.org/10.1007/s10620-018-5176-3.
19. Kopylov U, Papamichael K, Katsanos K, et al. Impact of infliximab and cyclosporine on the risk of colectomy in hospitalized patients with ulcerative colitis complicated by cytomegalovirus – a multicenter retrospective study. Inflamm Bowel Dis. 2017;23(9):1605–13. https://doi.org/10.1097/MIB.0000000000001160.
20. Powar MP, Martin P, Croft AR, et al. Surgical outcomes in steroid refractory acute severe ulcerative colitis: the impact of rescue therapy. Color Dis. 2013;15(3):374–9. https://doi.org/10.1111/j.1463-1318.2012.03188.x.
21. Nalagatla N, Falloon K, Tran G, et al. Effect of accelerated infliximab induction on short- and long-term outcomes of acute severe ulcerative

colitis: a retrospective multicenter study and meta-analysis. Clin Gastroenterol Hepatol. 2019;17(3):502–9.e1. https://doi.org/10.1016/j.cgh.2018.06.031.
22. Ross H, Steele SR, Varma M, et al. Practice parameters for the surgical treatment of ulcerative colitis. Dis Colon Rectum. 2014;57(1):5–22. https://doi.org/10.1097/DCR.0000000000000030.
23. Jeuring SFG, Bours PHA, Maurice P, et al. Disease outcome of ulcerative colitis in an era of changing treatment strategies: results from the Dutch population-based IBDSL cohort. J Crohns Colitis. 2015:837–45. https://doi.org/10.1093/ecco-jcc/jjv129.
24. Rungoe C, Langholz E, Andersson M, et al. Changes in medical treatment and surgery rates in inflammatory bowel disease: a nationwide cohort study 1979–2011. Gut. 2014;63:1607–16. https://doi.org/10.1136/gutjnl-2013-305607.
25. Reich KM, Chang H, Rezaie A, et al. Alimentary pharmacology and therapeutics the incidence rate of colectomy for medically refractory ulcerative colitis has declined in parallel with increasing anti-TNF use: a time-trend study. Aliment Pharmacol Ther. 2014;40:629–38. https://doi.org/10.1111/apt.12873.
26. Frolkis AD, Dykeman J, Negrón ME, et al. Risk of surgery for inflammatory bowel diseases has decreased over time: a systematic review and meta-analysis of population-based studies. Gastroenterology. 2013;145(5):996–1006. https://doi.org/10.1053/j.gastro.2013.07.041.
27. Kaplan GG, Seow CH, Ghosh S, et al. Decreasing colectomy rates for ulcerative colitis: a population-based time trend study. Am J Gastroenterol. 2012;107:1879–87. https://doi.org/10.1038/ajg.2012.333.
28. Ghoz H, Kesler A, Hoogenboom SA, et al. Decreasing colectomy rates in ulcerative colitis in the past decade: improved disease control? J Gastrointest Surg. 2020;24(2):270–7. https://doi.org/10.1007/s11605-019-04474-9.
29. Kayal M, Saha A, Poojary P, et al. Emergent colectomy rates decreased while elective ileal pouch rates were stable over time: a nationwide inpatient sample study. Int J Color Dis. 2019;34(10):1771–9. https://doi.org/10.1007/s00384-019-03375-2.
30. Andrew RE, Messaris E. Update on medical and surgical options for patients with acute severe ulcerative colitis: what is new? World J Gastrointest Surg. 2016;8(9):598. https://doi.org/10.4240/wjgs.v8.i9.598.
31. Fudman DI, Sattler L, Feuerstein JD. Inpatient management of acute severe ulcerative colitis. J Hosp Med. 2019;14(12):766–73. https://doi.org/10.12788/jhm.3207.
32. Cushing KC, Kordbacheh H, Gee MS, Kambadakone A, Ananthakrishnan AN. CT-visualized colonic mural stratification independently predicts the need for medical or surgical rescue therapy in hospitalized ulcerative

colitis patients. Dig Dis Sci. 2019;64(8):2265–72. https://doi.org/10.1007/s10620-019-05520-x.

33. Lynch RW, Churchhouse AMD, Protheroe A, Arnott IDR. Predicting outcome in acute severe ulcerative colitis: comparison of the Travis and Ho scores using UK IBD audit data. Aliment Pharmacol Ther. 2016;43(11):1132–41. https://doi.org/10.1111/apt.13614.
34. Le Baut G, Kirchgesner J, Amiot A, et al. A scoring system to determine patients' risk of colectomy within 1 year after hospital admission for acute severe ulcerative colitis. Clin Gastroenterol Hepatol. 2021;19(8):1602–10.e1. https://doi.org/10.1016/j.cgh.2019.12.036.
35. Borren NZ, Khalili H, Luther J, Colizzo FP, Garber JJ, Ananthakrishnan AN. Second-look endoscopy in hospitalized severe ulcerative colitis: a retrospective cohort study. Inflamm Bowel Dis. 2019;25(4):751–5. https://doi.org/10.1093/ibd/izy282.
36. Chao CY, Al Khoury A, Aruljothy A, et al. High-dose infliximab rescue therapy for hospitalized acute severe ulcerative colitis does not improve colectomy-free survival. Dig Dis Sci. 2019;64(2):518–23. https://doi.org/10.1007/s10620-018-5358-z.
37. Al-Darmaki A, Hubbard J, Seow CH, et al. Clinical predictors of the risk of early colectomy in ulcerative colitis: a population-based study. Inflamm Bowel Dis. 2017;23(8):1272–7. https://doi.org/10.1097/MIB.0000000000001211.
38. Burke KE, Khalili H, Garber JJ, et al. Genetic markers predict primary nonresponse and durable response to anti-tumor necrosis factor therapy in ulcerative colitis. Inflamm Bowel Dis. 2018;24(9):1840–8. https://doi.org/10.1093/ibd/izy083.
39. Strong SA. Management of acute colitis and toxic megacolon. Clin Colon Rectal Surg. 2010;23(4):274–84. https://doi.org/10.1055/s-0030-1268254.
40. Feuerstein JD, Isaacs KL, Schneider Y, Siddique SM, Falck-Ytter Y, Singh S. AGA clinical practice guidelines on the management of moderate to severe ulcerative colitis. Gastroenterology. 2020:1–12. https://doi.org/10.1053/j.gastro.2020.01.006.
41. Truelove S, Witts L. Cortisone in ulcerative colitis. Br Med J. 1955;2(4947):1041–8. https://doi.org/10.1136/bmj.2.4952.1386-b.
42. Rothenberger DA, Dunn KB. Surgery for toxic megacolon. In: Fisher JA, Jones DB, Pomposelli FB, Upchurch GB, editors. Fischer's mastery of surgery. 6th ed. Philadelphia: Lippincott Williams & Wilkins: A Wolters Kulwer; 2012. p. 1621–31.
43. Nelson R, Liao C, Fichera A, Rubin DT, Pekow J. Rescue therapy with cyclosporine or infliximab is not associated with an increased risk for postoperative complications in patients hospitalized for severe steroid-refractory ulcerative colitis. Inflamm Bowel Dis. 2014;20(1):14–20. https://doi.org/10.1097/01.MIB.0000437497.07181.05.
44. Bartels SAL, Gardenbroek TJ, Bos L, et al. Prolonged preoperative hospital stay is a risk factor for complications after emergency colectomy for

severe colitis. Color Dis. 2013;15(11):1392–8. https://doi.org/10.1111/codi.12328.
45. Coakley BA, Telem D, Nguyen S, Dallas K, Divino CM. Prolonged preoperative hospitalization correlates with worse outcomes after colectomy for acute fulminant ulcerative colitis. Surg (United States). 2013;153(2):242–8. https://doi.org/10.1016/j.surg.2012.08.002.
46. Leeds IL, Sundel MH, Gabre-Kidan A, et al. Outcomes for ulcerative colitis with delayed emergency colectomy are worse when controlling for preoperative risk factors. Dis Colon Rectum. 2019;62(5):600–7. https://doi.org/10.1097/DCR.0000000000001276.
47. Randall J, Singh B, Warren BF, Travis SPL, Mortensen NJ, George BD. Delayed surgery for acute severe colitis is associated with increased risk of postoperative complications. Br J Surg. 2010;97(3):404–9. https://doi.org/10.1002/bjs.6874.
48. Gu J, Stocchi L, Remzi F, Kiran RP. Factors associated with postoperative morbidity, reoperation and readmission rates after laparoscopic total abdominal colectomy for ulcerative colitis. Color Dis. 2013;15(9):1123–9. https://doi.org/10.1111/codi.12267.
49. Nguyen GC, Du L, Chong RY, Jackson TD. Hypoalbuminaemia and postoperative outcomes in inflammatory bowel disease: the NSQIP surgical cohort. J Crohns Colitis. 2019;13(11):1433–8. https://doi.org/10.1093/ecco-jcc/jjz083.
50. Schineis C, Lehmann KS, Lauscher JC, et al. Colectomy with ileostomy for severe ulcerative colitis-postoperative complications and risk factors. Int J Color Dis. 2020;35(3):387–94. https://doi.org/10.1007/s00384-019-03494-w.
51. Messenger DE, Mihailovic D, Macrae HM, O'Connor BI, Victor JC, McLeod RS. Subtotal colectomy in severe ulcerative and Crohn's colitis: what benefit does the laparoscopic approach confer? Dis Colon Rectum. 2014;57(12):1349–57. https://doi.org/10.1097/DCR.0000000000000238.
52. Bedrikovetski S, Dudi-Venkata N, Kroon HM, et al. Systematic review of rectal stump management during and after emergency total colectomy for acute severe ulcerative colitis. ANZ J Surg. 2019;89(12):1556–60. https://doi.org/10.1111/ans.15075.
53. Gu J, Stocchi L, Remzi F, Kiran RP. Intraperitoneal or subcutaneous: does location of the (colo)rectal stump influence outcomes after laparoscopic total abdominal colectomy for ulcerative colitis? Dis Colon Rectum. 2013;56(5):615–21. https://doi.org/10.1097/DCR.0b013e3182707682.
54. Gu J, Stocchi L, Ashburn J, Remzi FH. Total abdominal colectomy vs. restorative total proctocolectomy as the initial approach to medically refractory ulcerative colitis. Int J Color Dis. 2017;32(8):1215–22. https://doi.org/10.1007/s00384-017-2836-2.
55. Balachandran R, Tøttrup A. Safety of proctocolectomy for ulcerative colitis under elective and non-elective circumstances: preoperative cortico-

steroid treatment worsens outcome. Dig Surg. 2015;32(4):251–7. https://doi.org/10.1159/000381033.
56. Hicks CW, Hodin RA, Bordeianou L. Possible overuse of 3-stage procedures for active ulcerative colitis. JAMA Surg. 2013;148(7):658. https://doi.org/10.1001/2013.jamasurg.325.
57. Kiely JM, Fazio VW, Remzi FH, Shen B, Kiran RP. Pelvic sepsis after IPAA adversely affects function of the pouch and quality of life. Dis Colon Rectum. 2012;55(4):387–92. https://doi.org/10.1097/DCR.0b013e318246418e.
58. Farouk R, Dozois RR, Pemberton JH, Larson D. Incidence and subsequent impact of pelvic abscess after ileal pouch-anal anastomosis for chronic ulcerative colitis. Dis Colon Rectum. 1998;41(10):1239–43. https://doi.org/10.1007/bf02258220.
59. McKenna NP, Bews KA, Mathis KL, Lightner AL, Habermann EB. Surgery during admission for an ulcerative colitis flare: should pouch formation be considered? J Surg Res. 2019;239:216–23. https://doi.org/10.1016/j.jss.2019.02.014.
60. Selvaggi F, Pellino G, Canonico S, Sciaudone G. Effect of preoperative biologic drugs on complications and function after restorative proctocolectomy with primary ileal pouch formation: systematic review and meta-analysis. Inflamm Bowel Dis. 2015;21(1):79–92. https://doi.org/10.1097/MIB.0000000000000232.
61. Yang Z, Wu Q, Wu K, Fan D. Meta-analysis: pre-operative infliximab treatment and short-term post-operative complications in patients with ulcerative colitis. Aliment Pharmacol Ther. 2010;31(4):486–92. https://doi.org/10.1111/j.1365-2036.2009.04204.x.
62. Russell TA, Dawes AJ, Graham DS, Angarita SAK, Ha C, Sack J. Rescue diverting loop ileostomy: an alternative to emergent colectomy in the setting of severe acute refractory IBD-colitis. Dis Colon Rectum. 2018;61(2):214–20. https://doi.org/10.1097/DCR.0000000000000985.
63. Sahami S, Wildenberg ME, Koens L, et al. Appendectomy for therapy-refractory ulcerative colitis results in pathological improvement of colonic inflammation: short-term results of the PASSION study. J Crohns Colitis. 2019;13(2):165–71. https://doi.org/10.1093/ecco-jcc/jjy127.
64. Kock NG. Intra-abdominal "reservoir" in patients with permanent ileostomy. Arch Surg. 1969;99:223–31.
65. Nessar G, Fazio VW, Tekkis P, et al. Long-term outcome and quality of life after continent ileostomy. Dis Colon Rectum. 2006;49(3):336–44. https://doi.org/10.1007/s10350-005-0285-4.
66. Wilson MZ, Connelly TM, Tinsley A, Hollenbeak CS, Koltun WA, Messaris E. Ulcerative colitis is associated with an increased risk of venous thromboembolism in the postoperative period: the results of a matched cohort analysis. Ann Surg. 2015;261(6):1160–6. https://doi.org/10.1097/SLA.0000000000000788.

67. Nagle D, Pare T, Keenan E, Marcet K, Tizio S, Poylin V. Ileostomy pathway virtually eliminates readmissions for dehydration in new Ostomates. Dis Colon Rectum. 2012;55(12):1266–72. https://doi.org/10.1097/DCR.0b013e31827080c1.
68. Lightner AL, Shen B. Perioperative use of immunosuppressive medications in patients with Crohn's disease in the new "biological era". Gastroenterol Rep. 2017;5(3):165–77. https://doi.org/10.1093/gastro/gow046.
69. Wong DJ, Roth EM, Feuerstein JD, Poylin VY. Surgery in the age of biologics. Gastroenterol Rep. 2019;7(2):77–90. https://doi.org/10.1093/gastro/goz004.
70. Andrew RE, Lauria A, Puleo FJ, Berg A, Stewart DB. Inpatient infliximab is ineffective at preventing colectomy for steroid refractory extensive colitis. J Surg Res. 2017;219:18–24. https://doi.org/10.1016/j.jss.2017.05.077.
71. Curran T, Alvarez D, Pastrana Del Valle J, Cataldo TE, Poylin V, Nagle D. Prophylactic closed-incision negative-pressure wound therapy is associated with decreased surgical site infection in high-risk colorectal surgery laparotomy wounds. Color Dis. 2019;21(1):110–8. https://doi.org/10.1111/codi.14350.

Management of the Hospitalized Patient with Inflammatory and Stricturing Crohn's Disease

5

Parul Tandon and Adam V. Weizman

Introduction

Crohn's disease (CD) is a transmural inflammatory condition of the gastrointestinal tract that can result in significant morbidity and mortality [1]. The early stages of the disease consist of intestinal inflammation which can lead to symptoms such as fatigue, abdominal pain, and diarrhea. Over time, over half of all patients progress from this inflammatory phenotype to a stricturing and/or fistulizing phenotype that can then lead to complications such as abscesses, fistulas, and intestinal strictures [2, 3]. In fact, a significant number of patients require hospitalization for the management of these complications [4].

Stricturing complications in particular are associated with significant morbidity and remain a common cause of hospitalization

P. Tandon · A. V. Weizman (✉)
Division of Gastroenterology and Hepatology, Mount Sinai Hospital, Department of Medicine, University of Toronto, Toronto, ON, Canada
e-mail: Parul.tandon@mail.utoronto.ca; adam.weizman@sinaihealth.ca

J. D. Feuerstein, A. S. Cheifetz (eds.), *Management of Inpatient Inflammatory Bowel Disease*,
https://doi.org/10.1007/978-1-0716-1987-2_5

for patients with CD [2, 4]. A stricture, as per the Montreal classification, is defined as a chronic luminal narrowing with associated obstructive symptoms and/or prestenotic dilatation [5]. These can occur anywhere in the gastrointestinal tract, but most commonly develop in the terminal ileum among patients with Crohn's disease [6, 7].

Approximately 5–10% of patients with CD have evidence of stricturing disease at time of diagnosis [3, 8], and almost half develop obstructive symptoms by 20 years after IBD diagnosis [9]. Though recent data suggests that emergency-room visits and inpatient surgeries for stricturing CD have decreased from 2003 to 2014, outpatient stricture dilatations have increased over the same time period [10]. As such, a thorough understanding of stricture management, particularly inpatient care, is required to prevent associated morbidity.

This chapter will review the clinical presentation, diagnosis, and management of hospitalized patients with inflammatory and stricturing Crohn's disease. The management of hospitalized patients with fistulizing CD, and associated abscesses, will be discussed in Chap. 6.

Natural History

Crohn's disease typically affects the small bowel in up to 80% of patients. In particular, it can result in ileocolitis in 40% of patients, ileitis only in 30% of patients, colitis only in 20% of patients, and foregut disease in 10% of patients [2]. Furthermore, a quarter of patients may also have perianal CD [2]. Regardless of the disease location however, less than 15% of patients develop progression to another anatomical location over time [2].

Small bowel and perianal diseases often reflect a more aggressive phenotype with an increased risk of stricturing and penetrating complications compared to those with colonic disease only [3]. Though early in the disease CD reflects a predominantly inflammatory process, over half of all patients eventually develop stricturing and penetrating complications, with a majority requiring intestinal resective surgery at 10-year follow-up [2–4, 11].

Intestinal strictures can be divided into inflammatory, fibrotic, or mixed subtypes. Though the exact mechanisms for their development remain unknown, the combination of mesenchymal cell (i.e., fibroblast, myofibroblast, smooth muscle cell) proliferation and collagen-rich extracellular matrix accumulation contributes to bowel wall thickening and eventual fibrosis [12, 13]. Several risk factors predispose patients to the development of stricturing CD. These include clinical factors (age < 40, concurrent perianal disease, active small bowel disease, active smoking) and endoscopic factors such as deep mucosal ulcerations [7, 12, 14]. Furthermore, serologic markers such as antimicrobial and anti-*Saccharomyces cerevisiae* antibodies may predict future development of fibrostenotic stricturing disease, particularly in the Asian population [7].

Almost half of patients who develop stricturing CD require surgical intervention for obstructive symptoms [11]. Several factors may predict a more aggressive course and an accelerated time to surgery. Anastomotic strictures, compared to de novo intestinal strictures, may be associated with overall poor short-term outcomes and quality of life, although they are more likely to be amenable to endoscopic balloon dilatation [15, 16]. Furthermore, stricture length (>3 cm) and greater prestenotic dilatation (>2.9 cm) is associated with increased risk of need for surgical intervention [17]. In fact, every 1 cm increase in stricture length may increase the risk of future surgery by almost 8% [15]. Finally, strictures in the upper gastrointestinal tract (i.e., duodenum, proximal jejunum) have poor short-term outcomes and progress toward surgery more quickly compared to strictures elsewhere [15].

A proportion of CD patients will require urgent assessment and hospitalization for obstructive symptoms such as nausea, vomiting, and/or abdominal discomfort. Despite improvement in CD-related therapies and the introduction of biological agents as a treatment option, recent evidence suggests there has been no decline in CD-related hospitalization [18].

Clinical Presentation

The clinical presentation of severe inflammatory CD requiring hospitalization is variable and dependent on disease location. Those with ileal-predominant CD often present with abdominal pain, weight loss, diarrhea, and cramping with bowel movements, whereas those with colonic-predominant disease may also have watery/loose or bloody bowel movements and associated urgency [19]. Furthermore, signs of significant transmural inflammation can manifest as fever, or in the case of the development of a complication, peritonitis may be present requiring emergent assessment. Though less common, those with upper gastrointestinal CD may present with foregut symptoms such as nausea and vomiting and may have signs of bleeding such as coffee-ground emesis or hematemesis. Malnutrition in some patients can be significant, regardless of disease location. Finally, extraintestinal manifestations such as oral ulcers or joint pain may also reflect the degree of underlying inflammation.

Similarly, the clinical presentation of stricturing CD is dependent on anatomical location. Intestinal strictures may be found incidentally in 20% of patients who remain asymptomatic from obstructive symptoms [6]. More commonly however, strictures are accompanied by postprandial abdominal pain and discomfort, weight loss, and fatigue. Constipation, with no change in flatus, may be the predominant symptoms of colonic strictures [13]. Interestingly, some partial-obstructive symptoms may be in fact present years before the diagnosis of stricturing CD [20]. Furthermore, in cases of concurrent penetrating disease and/or abdominal abscess, systemic symptoms such as fevers, chills, or night sweats may be present. Finally, nausea and vomiting, constipation, obstipation, and hyperactive bowel sounds may indicate acute bowel obstruction, which remains the most common surgical emergency in the inpatient management of IBD [21, 22]. These patients require emergent hospitalization and surgical consultation.

Investigation of Active Inflammatory Crohn's Disease

Patients presenting to the emergency department with symptoms suggestive of active inflammatory CD require emergent assessment and investigations to facilitate appropriate management. A thorough history and physical examination should be performed to confirm hemodynamic stability and assess for emergencies such as sepsis and peritonitis. Physical examination demonstrating abdominal mass, abdominal pain, or fever is suggestive of a severe presentation. Assessment of volume status as well as nutritional status, using the subjective global assessment, is important and should be repeated throughout the course of a disease flare [23]. Laboratory investigations, such as complete blood cell count, electrolytes, and renal function, may also assist in determining the overall severity of the presentation. In addition, serum inflammatory markers such as C-reactive protein (CRP) and albumin may assist in determining the burden of inflammatory disease [23]. Stool cultures should be obtained to exclude infectious etiology particularly *Clostridium difficile* (*C. difficile*) [24]. Finally, where available, fecal calprotectin, a noninvasive marker of inflammatory activity, may be used to detect active colonic inflammation, though its utility in small intestinal CD remains less clear [25].

Early cross-sectional imaging compliments the clinical assessment and allows for identification of affected intestinal segments. Important principles for accurate radiological assessment of intestinal inflammation include the requirement of fasting prior to the examination, adequate bowel distention with large amount of intraluminal contrast agents, and prevention of peristalsis via antiperistalsis agents [26, 27]. Both computed tomography enterography (CTE) and magnetic resonance enterography (MRE) have excellent sensitivity and specificity in identifying acute inflammation in patients with CD [28]. In addition, these modalities can assist in differentiating inflammatory from non-inflammatory fibrostenotic disease. Features suggestive of active inflammation may include bowel wall thickening, lymph node enlargement, and peri-intestinal hypervascularity.

More recently, small bowel ultrasound has been used in the acute setting to detect inflammation [29]. Increased bowel wall thickness and vascularization on ultrasonography are suggestive of acute inflammation [30], with a sensitivity and specificity of 80% and 97%, respectively [29]. Though this technique is safe, easily available, and quick to perform, its diagnostic performance is often limited by body habitus and operator technique. As such, it should only be performed by those with specialized training in bowel wall ultrasonography.

For those with symptoms suggestive of inflammatory colonic CD, ileocolonoscopy remains the gold-standard method to assess for the burden of inflammatory disease. If safe to perform, ileocolonoscopy with biopsies should be performed early in the hospitalization to guide further management. The simple endoscopic score for CD (SES-CD) can be used to grade the severity of disease (Table 5.1). Each segment (terminal ileum, right colon, transverse colon, left colon, and rectum) should be scored separately on the presence of ulcers, degree of affected area, degree of ulcerated area, and presence of narrowing. A score of 16 or more is suggestive of severe CD.

Table 5.1 Simple endoscopic score for Crohn's disease. Each segment of the colon (ileum, right colon, transverse colon, left colon, and rectum) should be scored separately with a maximum possible score of 60

	Points			
	0	1	2	3
Presence and size of ulcers	None	Aphthous (0.1–0.5 cm)	Large (0.5–2 cm)	Very large (> 2 cm)
Surface area affected by disease activity	0%	<50%	50–75%	>75%
Surface area affected by ulcers	0%	<10%	10–30%	>30%
Presence of narrowing	None	Single, can be passed	Multiple, can be passed	Cannot be passed

Investigation of Stricturing Crohn's Disease

Though endoscopy is typically relied on to make a diagnosis of IBD, it remains insufficient in the setting of stricturing CD, as not all strictures may be easily accessible by routine endoscopic techniques. Furthermore, in acute bowel obstructions, endoscopic assessment is often avoided due to intolerability and significant risk of complications such as perforation. As such, cross-sectional imaging modalities are relied upon in various clinical scenarios such as acute bowel obstruction, stricture identification, and characterization. Plain abdominal radiography should be the initial assessment tool of choice in the emergency department when bowel obstruction is suspected [31].

Cross-Sectional Imaging in Suspected Bowel Obstruction

In suspected bowel obstruction, plain abdominal radiography is the first-line modality to confirm the diagnosis [31]. Typical features of bowel obstruction on radiography include small bowel distention and the presence of air-fluid levels (particularly wider than 2.5 cm) [31]. Furthermore, upright films can accurately identify free air suggestive of perforation. However, radiography has poor diagnostic accuracy in identifying partial or high-grade intestinal obstructions, with a sensitivity and specificity of only 69% and 57%, respectively [31, 32]. Furthermore, this modality cannot typically identify the transition site of the bowel obstruction which may be required prior to surgical intervention.

In this setting, computed tomography (CT), particularly with multidetector technique, improves the overall accuracy of identifying partial obstructions and the transition point. Typical features of obstruction on CT include dilatation of small bowel loops >2.5 cm [33] and the presence of the "small bowel feces" sign (i.e., gas bubbles mixed with particulate matter proximal to obstruction) [34]. Overall, multidetector CT techniques have a sensitivity and specificity as high as 95%, respectively, for diagnosing small bowel obstructions and are often essential prior to surgical intervention [35].

Finally, ultrasonography, though not commonly applied in patients with suspected obstructions, has in fact excellent sensitivity in this setting. Features of acute bowel obstruction on ultrasonography include luminal dilatation more than 3 cm, segment length more than 10 cm, and increase in upstream peristalsis [31, 36].

Cross-Sectional Imaging in Stricture Diagnosis

In patients whom stricturing CD is suspected based on subacute symptoms, cross-sectional imaging is used for identification and prognostication. Key radiographic principles in stricture identification include bowel lumen narrowing with prestenotic dilatation and/or bowel wall thickening.

Transabdominal ultrasound has a sensitivity of 79–100% and a specificity of 63–92% in stricture identification [37, 38]. Contrast enhancement using gas-filled microbubbles improves organ visualization and bowel vasculature. This can improve the overall sensitivity and specificity of stricture detection to 98% and 100%, respectively [39].

Advanced modalities such as CT enterography (CTE) and MR enterography (MRE) are useful tests for identification of stricturing CD. Compared to conventional CT or MR abdominal imaging, enterography techniques involve adequate bowel distention with oral contrast agents and small bowel distention using antiperistalsis agents [26, 27]. The sensitivity and specificity of CTE for stricture identification are as high as 100%, respectively [37, 40]. Similarly, the sensitivity and specificity of MRE for stricture identification are 100% and 96%, respectively [37, 41]. Though either of these techniques may be used to diagnose intestinal strictures, MRE may be the preferred approach due to lack of exposure to ionizing radiation.

Inflammatory vs. Fibrostenotic Strictures

An important principle of inpatient management of stricturing CD is the differentiation of inflammatory and fibrostenotic strictures. This differentiation is important as it can have a significant impact on overall management. Whereas inflammatory strictures may in part be reversible and managed with medical therapy, fibrostenotic strictures may be more likely to require surgical intervention. Unfortunately, despite advancements in cross-sectional imaging techniques, this stratification remains challenging [42]. Furthermore, most imaging modalities, other than perhaps MRI, have demonstrated poor diagnostic performance in predicting the burden of fibrosis in stricturing CD [43].

Transabdominal ultrasound, with contrast enhancement, may be able to identify features of acute inflammation in stricturing CD. Though the sensitivity is as high as 100%, the specificity of fibrosis detection however remains poor at 63% [38]. The use of contrast enhancement may improve the accuracy of ultrasonography in identifying inflammatory strictures [44]. Again, body habitus and sonographer skill limit the use of this modality, particularly for the evaluation of deep small bowel segments.

CTE is often ordered in the emergency setting due to availability to differentiate inflammatory from fibrostenotic stricturing CD. Features of inflammatory strictures on CT imaging include mural enhancement, mesenteric vascularization, and associated fat stranding. The sensitivity and specificity of CTE for fibrosis detection are 77% and 79%, respectively [45]. However, ionizing radiation cxposurc, particularly in young patients, often limits the repeated use of this modality for stricture characterization in patients with frequent hospitalizations due to underlying stricturing CD.

As such, MRI offers an alternative and relatively safer approach to distinguish inflammatory from fibrostenotic strictures. In particular, contrast-enhanced MRI techniques have demonstrated excellent diagnostic ability in determining the type of stricture in patients with CD [46, 47]. On T2-weighted images, layered enhancement may indicate predominant fibrosis, whereas homogenous mural enhancement may indicate predominantly inflammatory strictures [46]. Furthermore, the presence of abscess may predict predominantly inflammatory strictures [46, 47].

Management of Hospitalized Inflammatory Crohn's Disease

The management of severe inflammatory CD often requires hospitalization due to severity of symptoms, inability to maintain oral intake or hydration, malnutrition, or the urgent need to rule out complications such as obstruction, perforation, or sepsis due to intra-abdominal abscesses. Initial management involves volume resuscitation, physical examination, and consideration of imaging to assess disease activity and location as well as the presence of complications. These patients should be managed concurrently by gastroenterologists and general surgeons with early surgical intervention if required. Antibiotic therapy should be reserved for patients with documented infections such as intra-abdominal abscesses or *C. difficile*. In patients with *C. difficile* infection in particular, oral vancomycin is considered first-line therapy for 10–14 days, though prolonged duration of therapy may prevent recurrence rates within 8 weeks of antibiotic discontinuation [24, 48].

Once infection has been ruled out, induction medical therapy can be considered to reduce morbidity associated with severe inflammation. The inpatient management of inflammatory CD requires early treatment ideally with agents that have strong evidence in the hospitalized setting, have a rapid onset of action, are reasonably tolerable, and are readily accessible. Several therapies may offer these benefits.

Corticosteroids, such as prednisone, have been demonstrative as effective agents to induce clinical remission in active CD [49, 50] and may be considered first-line for many hospitalized scenarios. For those with more severe disease or inability to tolerate oral therapy, intravenous methylprednisolone is recommended, at doses of 40–60 mg of prednisone equivalent per day [49, 51].

Though these agents are effective in inducing remission in those with severe inflammatory CD, their ongoing use is associated with numerous side effects which include insomnia, delirium, hyperglycemia, hypertension, ache, bony fractures, and relative adrenal insufficiency [48]. Furthermore, about 20% of patients experience steroid-refractory disease. In these cases, steroid-sparing agents should be considered during the hospitalization.

Antitumor necrosis factor (anti-TNF) agents, particularly infliximab in the inpatient setting, remain the cornerstone therapy to induce clinical remission in patients with steroid-refractory severe inflammatory CD [52–54]. Infliximab therapy may improve clinical symptoms as early as 2 weeks after initiation and is associated with minimal adverse events. Doses of 5 mg/kg intravenously are typically administered. Furthermore, concurrent therapy with immunomodulators may prevent immunogenicity and improve rates of clinical remission [53–55]. Prior to the use of anti-TNF therapy, assessments for opportunistic infections should be performed including work-up for latent/active tuberculosis and hepatitis B [49].

Although infliximab remains the most well-studied biologic agent for the treatment of hospitalized Crohn's disease, in patients with prior nonresponse or loss of response to this agent or a relative contraindication to anti-TNF therapy, novel classes of biologics could be considered. Anti-integrin therapy, such as vedolizumab, can be considered in patients who have achieved some degree of clinical response to corticosteroid therapy during the hospitalization and require ongoing maintenance therapy. By preventing leukocyte trafficking from blood vessels into the gut, vedolizumab therapy has been shown to induce clinical remission, particularly corticosteroid-free remission [56]. Vedolizumab therapy has not been associated with significant immunogenicity and has a favorable safety profile. Anti-interleukin 12/23 agents, such as ustekinumab, may also be considered for use in patients with moderate-severe inflammatory CD who have responded to inpatient corticosteroid therapy. Ustekinumab use has been associated with improved rates of clinical response and remission as induction therapy for the outpatient management of patients with moderate-severe CD who have failed previous anti-TNF therapy

[49, 57]. While these novel agents remain treatment options, the use of ustekinumab and vedolizumab in patients hospitalized with steroid-refractory inflammatory CD has not been well-studied, and its role in this setting remains to be determined.

Finally, immunomodulators, such as azathioprine and 6-mercaptopurine, are effective steroid-sparing agents that may induce long-term clinical remission in patients with severe CD. However, their use is limited to the maintenance setting due to the relatively slow onset of action (8–12 weeks) and lack of evidence to support their use as induction agents. As such, immunomodulators should primarily be used as steroid-sparing maintenance agents in those who have achieved response to corticosteroid therapy or in combination with anti-TNF therapies to reduce immunogenicity.

Management of Hospitalized Stricturing Crohn's Disease

The inpatient management of stricturing CD requires early diagnosis and differentiation of inflammatory and fibrostenotic subtypes. Furthermore, a multidisciplinary approach, including gastroenterologists, colorectal surgeons, radiologists, and allied healthcare teams, is necessary for high-quality care delivery.

Hospital admission is required for those presenting with acute bowel obstruction secondary to presumed stricturing CD. Correction of electrolyte abnormalities, intravenous hydration, and complete bowel rest improve overall outcomes and, in some instances, may result in resolution of the obstruction [37, 58]. In patients at risk of aspiration due to large-volume emesis, nasogastric tube decompression may be required. Furthermore, those presenting with fever and leukocytosis, suggesting of possible sepsis, may require broad-spectrum antibiotic coverage.

Patients should be closely monitored in hospital with frequent serial abdominal examinations. If there is no improvement in 48–72 hours and cross-sectional imaging suggests predominantly inflammatory stricturing disease, intravenous corticosteroids and/

or optimization of biologic therapy may reduce intestinal edema and inflammation [37]. The duration and dose of corticosteroid therapy in this setting has not been well-studied and depends on patient factors such as age and presence of comorbidities. In those patients with a lack of improvement despite these measures, predominantly fibrotic strictures resulting in complete bowel obstruction, or those with acute peritonitis, an early surgical consultation is warranted for possible intervention [37].

Finally, a dietary assessment for possible malnutrition is critical in all patients admitted with complications of CD, particularly those with bowel obstructions [59]. Malnutrition is common in patients with CD due to increasing metabolic demands and reduced oral intake. Consequently, malnutrition in the inpatient setting is associated with an increase in hospital length of stay, postsurgical complications, and overall mortality [60]. In patients with asymptomatic intestinal stricturing disease, a modified diet low in insoluble fiber is usually recommended [59, 61]. Those with symptomatic strictures often require softer consistency diets with nutritional and fluid supplementation [59]. Finally, in those with acute bowel obstruction requiring nil per os, parenteral nutrition may improve the nutritional status and reduce the risk of postoperative complications, though emergent surgery should not be delayed if warranted [62].

Conclusion

Patients with presenting inflammatory or stricturing Crohn's disease often require hospitalization for resuscitation, nutritional support, and medical or surgical management of disease. Emergent indications for surgery including perforation or nonresolving obstruction need to always be considered. A multidisciplinary approach is needed to determine when surgical management and/or medical management is most appropriate. Imaging studies can be helpful in guiding management, and familiarity with modalities available at a particular center may determine the best available test.

References

1. Lewis JD, Gelfand JM, Troxel AB, Forde KA, Newcomb C, Kim H, et al. Immunosuppressant medications and mortality in inflammatory bowel disease. Am J Gastroenterol. 2008;103:1428–36.
2. Peyrin-Biroulet L, Loftus EV Jr, Colombel J-F, Sandborn WJ. The natural history of adult Crohn's disease in population-based cohorts. Am J Gastroenterol. 2010;105:289–97.
3. Cosnes J, Cattan S, Blain A, Beaugerie L, Carbonnel F, Parc R, et al. Long-term evolution of disease behavior of Crohn's disease. Inflamm Bowel Dis. 2002;8:244–50.
4. Bernstein CN, Loftus EV Jr, Ng SC, Lakatos PL, Moum B. Epidemiology, hospitalizations and surgery in Crohn's disease. Gut. 2012;61:622–9.
5. Satsangi J, Silverberg MS, Vermeire S, Colombel JF. The Montreal classification of inflammatory bowel disease: controversies, consensus, and implications. Gut. 2006;55:749–53.
6. Hansel SL, McCurdy JD, Barlow JM, Fidler J, Fletcher JG, Becker B, et al. Clinical benefit of capsule endoscopy in Crohn's disease: impact on patient management and prevalence of proximal small bowel involvement. Inflamm Bowel Dis. 2018;24:1582–8.
7. Rieder F, Lawrance IC, Leite A, Sans M. Predictors of fibrostenotic Crohn's disease. Inflamm Bowel Dis. 2011;17:2000–7.
8. Louis E, Collard A, Oger AF, Degroote E, Aboul Nasr El Yafi FA, et al. Behaviour of Crohn's disease according to the Vienna classification: changing pattern over the course of the disease. Gut. 2001;49:777–82.
9. Rieder F, Zimmermann EM, Remzi FH, Sandborn WJ. Crohn's disease complicated by strictures: a systematic review. Gut. 2013;62:1072–84.
10. Rahman A, Jairath V, Feagan BG, Khanna R, Shariff SZ, Allen BN, et al. Declining hospitalization and surgical intervention rates in patients with Crohn's disease: a population-based cohort. Aliment Pharmacol Ther. 2019;50:1086–93.
11. Frolkis AD, Dykeman J, Negrón ME, Debruyn J, Jette N, Fiest KM, et al. Risk of surgery for inflammatory bowel diseases has decreased over time: a systematic review and meta-analysis of population-based studies. Gastroenterology. 2013;145:996–1006.
12. Rieder F, Fiocchi C. Mechanisms of tissue remodeling in inflammatory bowel disease. Dig Dis. 2013;31:186–93.
13. Rieder F, Fiocchi C, Rogler G. Mechanisms, management, and treatment of fibrosis in patients with inflammatory bowel diseases. Gastroenterology. 2017;152:340–50.
14. Loly C, Belaiche J, Louis E. Predictors of severe Crohn's disease. Scand J Gastroenterol. 2008;43:948–54.
15. Bettenworth D, Rieder F. Medical therapy of stricturing Crohn's disease: what the gut can learn from other organs – a systematic review. Fibrogenesis Tissue Repair. 2014;7:5.

16. Lian L, Stocchi L, Remzi FH, Shen B. Comparison of endoscopic dilation vs surgery for anastomotic stricture in patients with Crohn's disease following ileocolonic resection. Clin Gastroenterol Hepatol. 2017;15:1226–31.
17. Bouhnik Y, Carbonnel F, Laharie D, Stefanescu C, Hebuteme X, Abitbol V, et al. Efficacy of adalimumab in patients with Crohn's disease and symptomatic small bowel stricture: a multicentre, prospective, observational cohort (CREOLE) study. Gut. 2018;67:53–60.
18. Murthy SK, Begum J, Benchimol EI, Bernstein CN, Kaplan GG, McCurdy JD, et al. Introduction of anti-TNF therapy has not yielded expected declines in hospitalisation and intestinal resection rates in inflammatory bowel diseases: a population-based interrupted time series study. Gut. 2020;69:274–82.
19. Perler B, Ungaro R, Baird G, Maliette M, Bright R, Shah S, et al. Presenting symptoms in inflammatory bowel disease: descriptive analysis of a community-based inception cohort. BMC Gastroenterol. 2019;19:47.
20. Burgmann T, Clara I, Graff L, Walker J, Lix L, Rawsthorne P, et al. The Manitoba inflammatory bowel disease cohort study: prolonged symptoms before diagnosis – how much is irritable bowel syndrome. Clin Gastroenterol Hepatol. 2006;4:614–20.
21. Pellino G, Nicolai E, Catalano OA, Campione S, D'Amineto FP, Salvatore M, et al. PET/MR versus PET/CT imaging: impact on the clinical Management of small-bowel Crohn's disease. J Crohns Colitis. 2016;10:277–85.
22. Berg DF, Bahadursingh AM, Kaminski DL, Longo WE. Acute surgical emergencies in inflammatory bowel disease. Am J Surg. 2002;184:45–51.
23. Chang S, Malter L, Hudesman D. Disease monitoring in inflammatory bowel disease. World J Gastroenterol. 2015;21:11246–59.
24. Khanna S, Shin A, Kelly CP. Management of Clostridium difficile infection in inflammatory bowel disease: expert review from the clinical practice updates committee of the AGA Institute. Clin Gastroenterol Hepatol. 2017;15:166–74.
25. Zittan E, Kelly OB, Gralnek IM, Silverberg MS, Hillary SA. Fecal calprotectin correlates with active colonic inflammatory bowel disease but not with small intestinal Crohn's disease activity. JGH Open. 2018;2:201–6.
26. Low RN, Francis IR, Politoske D, Bennett M. Crohn's disease evaluation: comparison of contrast-enhanced MR imaging and single-phase helical CT scanning. J Magn Reson Imaging. 2000;11:127–35.
27. Balthazar EJ. CT of the gastrointestinal tract: principles and interpretation. AJR Am J Roentgenol. 1991;156:23–32.
28. Lee SS, Ha HK, Yang SK, Kim AY, Kim TK, Kim PN, et al. CT of prominent pericolic or perienteric vasculature in patients with Crohn's disease: correlation with clinical disease activity and findings on barium studies. AJR Am J Roentgenol. 2002;179:1029–36.

29. Calabrese E, Maaser C, Zorzi F, Kannengiesser K, Hanauer SB, Bruining DH, et al. Bowel ultrasonography in the management of Crohn's disease. A review with recommendations of an international panel of experts. Inflamm Bowel Dis. 2016;22:1168–83.
30. Rigazio C, Ercole E, Laudi C, Daperno M, Lavagna A, Crocella L, et al. Abdominal bowel ultrasound can predict the risk of surgery in Crohn's disease: proposal of an ultrasonographic score. Scand J Gastroenterol. 2009;44:585–93.
31. Silva AC, Pimenta M, Guimaraes LS. Small bowel obstruction: what to look for. Radiographics. 2009;29:423–39.
32. Maglinte DD, Gage SN, Harmon BH, Kelvin FM, Hage FP, Chua GT, et al. Obstruction of the small intestine: accuracy and role of CT in diagnosis. Radiology. 1993;188:61–4.
33. Fukuya T, Hawes DR, Lu CC, Chang PJ, Barloon TJ. CT diagnosis of small-bowel obstruction: efficacy in 60 patients. AJR Am J Roentgenol. 1992;158:765–72.
34. Mayo-Smith WW, Wittenberg J, Bennett GL, Gervais DA, Gazelle GS, Mueller PR. The CT small bowel faeces sign: description and clinical significance. Clin Radiol. 1995;50:765–7.
35. Maglinte DDT, Heitkamp DE, Howard TJ, Kelvin FM, Lappas JC. Current concepts in imaging of small bowel obstruction. Radiol Clin N Am. 2003;41:263–vi.
36. Baker SR. ACR appropriateness criteria on small-bowel obstruction: a critique of the term and its terms. J Am Coll Radiol. 2007;4:443–5.
37. Lu C, Holubar SD, Rieder F. How I approach the management of stricturing Crohn's disease. Am J Gastroenterol. 2019;114:1181–4.
38. Maconi G, Carsana L, Fociani P, Sampietro GM, Ardizzone S, et al. Small bowel stenosis in Crohn's disease: clinical, biochemical and ultrasonographic evaluation of histological features. Aliment Pharmacol Ther. 2003;18:749–56.
39. Kumar S, Hakim A, Alexakis C, Chhaya V, Tzias D, Pilcher J, et al. Small intestinal contrast ultrasonography for the detection of small bowel complications in Crohn's disease: correlation with intraoperative findings and magnetic resonance enterography. J Gastroenterol Hepatol. 2015;30:86–91.
40. Vogel J, da Luz MA, Baker M, Hammel J, Einstein D, Stocci L, et al. CT enterography for Crohn's disease: accurate preoperative diagnostic imaging. Dis Colon Rectum. 2007;50:1761–9.
41. Pous-Serrano S, Frasson M, Palasi Gimenez R, Sanchez-Jorda G, Pamies-Guilabert J, et al. Accuracy of magnetic resonance enterography in the preoperative assessment of patients with Crohn's disease of the small bowel. Color Dis. 2017;19:126–33.
42. Adler J, Punglia DR, Dillman JR, Polydorides AD, Dave M, Al-HAwary MM, et al. Computed tomography enterography findings correlate with tissue inflammation, not fibrosis in resected small bowel Crohn's disease. Inflamm Bowel Dis. 2012;18:849–56.

43. Bettenworth D, Bokemeyer A, Baker M, Mao R, Parker CE, Nguyen T, et al. Assessment of Crohn's disease-associated small bowel strictures and fibrosis on cross-sectional imaging: a systematic review. Gut. 2019;68:1115–26.
44. Ripolles T, Rausell N, Paredes JM, Grau E, Martinez MJ, Vizuete J. Effectiveness of contrast-enhanced ultrasound for characterization of intestinal inflammation in Crohn's disease: a comparison with surgical histopathology analysis. J Crohns Colitis. 2013;7:120–8.
45. Chiorean MV, Sandrasegaran K, Saxena R, Maglinte DD, Nakeeb A, Johnson CS. Correlation of CT enteroclysis with surgical pathology in Crohn's disease. Am J Gastroenterol. 2007;102:2541–50.
46. Rimola J, Plannel N, Rodriguez S, Delgado S, Ordas I, Ramirez-Morros A, et al. Characterization of inflammation and fibrosis in Crohn's disease lesions by magnetic resonance imaging. Am J Gastroenterol. 2015;110:432–40.
47. Li XH, Mao R, Huang SY, Sun CH, Cao QH, Fang ZN, et al. Characterization of degree of intestinal fibrosis in patients with Crohn disease by using magnetization transfer MR imaging. Radiology. 2018;287:494–503.
48. Lei DK, Ollech JE, Andersen M, Weisshof R, Zmeter N, Sossenheimer P, et al. Long-duration oral vancomycin to treat Clostridioides difficile in patients with inflammatory bowel disease is associated with a Low rate of recurrence. Am J Gastroenterol. 2019;114:1904–8.
49. Lichtenstein GR, Loftus EV, Isaacs KL, Regueiro MD, Gerson LB, Sands BE. ACG clinical guideline: management of Crohn's disease in adults. Am J Gastroenterol. 2018;113:481–517.
50. Benchimol EI, Seow CH, Steinhart AH, Griffiths AM. Traditional corticosteroids for induction of remission in Crohn's disease. Cochrane Database Syst Rev. 2008;2008:CD006792.
51. Chun A, Chadi RM, Korelitz BI, Colonna T, Felder JB, Jackson MH, et al. Intravenous corticotrophin vs. hydrocortisone in the treatment of hospitalized patients with Crohn's disease: a randomized double-blind study and follow-up. Inflamm Bowel Dis. 1998;4:177–81.
52. Hanauer SB, Feagan BG, Lichtenstein GR, Mayer LF, Schreiber S, Colombel JF, et al. Maintenance infliximab for Crohn's disease: the ACCENT I randomized trial. Lancet. 2002;359:1541–9.
53. Kawalec P, Mikrut A, Wiśniewska N, Pilc A. Tumor necrosis factor-α antibodies (infliximab, adalimumab and certolizumab) in Crohn's disease: systematic review and meta-analysis. Arch Med Sci. 2013;9:765–79.
54. Akobeng AK, Zachos M. Tumor necrosis factor-alpha antibody for induction of remission in Crohn's disease. Cochrane Database Syst Rev. 2004:CD003574.
55. Colombel JF, Sandborn WJ, Reinisch W, Mantzaris GJ, Kornbluth A, Rachmilewitz D, et al. Infliximab, azathioprine, or combination therapy for Crohn's disease. N Engl J Med. 2010;362:1383–95.

56. Sandborn WJ, Feagan BG, Rutgeerts P, Hanauer S, Colombel JF, Sands BE, et al. Vedolizumab as induction and maintenance therapy for Crohn's disease. N Engl J Med. 2013;369:711–21.
57. Feagan BG, Sandborn WJ, Gasink C, Jacobstein D, Lang Y, Friedman JR, et al. Ustekinumab as induction and maintenance therapy for Crohn's disease. N Engl J Med. 2016;375:1946–60.
58. Guo S-B, Duan Z-J. Decompression of the small bowel by endoscopic long-tube placement. World J Gastroenterol. 2012;18:1822–6.
59. Forbes A, Escher J, Hébuterne X, Klek S, Krznaric Z, Schneider S, et al. ESPEN guideline: clinical nutrition in inflammatory bowel disease. Clin Nutr. 2017;36:321–47.
60. Nguyen GC, Munsell M, Harris ML. Nationwide prevalence and prognostic significance of clinically diagnosable protein-calorie malnutrition in hospitalized inflammatory bowel disease patients. Inflamm Bowel Dis. 2008;14:1105–11.
61. Wedlake L, Slack N, Andreyev HJN, Whelan K. Fiber in the treatment and maintenance of inflammatory bowel disease: a systematic review of randomized controlled trials. Inflamm Bowel Dis. 2014;20:576–86.
62. Adamina M, Gerasimidis K, Sigall-Boneh R, Zmora O, de Buck van Overstraeten A, et al. Perioperative dietary therapy in inflammatory bowel disease. J Crohns Colitis. 2021;14(4):431–44.

Management of Hospitalized Patients with Fistulizing Crohn's and Crohn's-Related Abscess

6

R. Chibbar and S. N. Flier

Introduction

Inflammatory bowel disease (IBD) is a chronic relapsing-remitting inflammatory disorder of the gastrointestinal tract, consisting of two primary entities: Crohn's disease (CD) and ulcerative colitis (UC). Although CD and UC are distinct disease, the goal of therapy for both is to maintain a corticosteroid-free deep remission. This goal may be more challenging in CD as transmural inflammation can lead to the development of fistulas and strictures, thereby impacting the choice of induction and maintenance therapy, which is guided by severity and disease phenotype. Although significant advances have been made in the management of CD – and

R. Chibbar
Division of Gastroenterology, Department of Medicine, University of Alberta, Edmonton, AB, Canada

S. N. Flier (✉)
Division of Gastroenterology, Beth Israel Deaconess Medical Center, Boston, MA, USA
e-mail: Sflier1@bidmc.harvard.edu

J. D. Feuerstein, A. S. Cheifetz (eds.), *Management of Inpatient Inflammatory Bowel Disease*,
https://doi.org/10.1007/978-1-0716-1987-2_6

specifically fistulizing disease – complications still arise requiring hospitalization and expert multidisciplinary care.

Fistulas are connections that occur between any segment of the intestine and the skin or adjacent organ, including the bladder and vagina [1]. Fistulas also develop between loops of the bowel. The precise pathogenesis for fistula formation is unknown but is thought to be due to mucosal and transmural inflammation combined with luminal bacteria allowing the inflammation to penetrate into adjacent organs, tissue, or skin [2]. Up to 40% of patients with CD will develop a fistula (range 17–85%), and up to 15% will first present with penetrating disease, fistula, abscess, or phlegmom [3]. Those with rectal or colonic disease and young age at the time of diagnosis are at increased risk [4, 5]. Classification of fistulas is based on the location and connection with contiguous organs, which affects both the clinical presentation and treatment considerations. Internal fistulas terminate into adjacent organs (enteroenteric, enterovesical, ileocolic, gastrocolic, rectovaginal), whereas external fistulas terminate on the body surface (enterocutaneous, perianal, peristomal). Internal fistulas account for one-third of the fistulizing disease and can be further subclassified as "major" or "minor." While minor fistulas (ileocecal or ileoileal) are typically asymptomatic, major fistulas – such as gastrocolic fistulas – may lead to a functional short gut syndrome by bypassing the majority of the luminal tract [6].

Perianal fistulas are a unique entity in CD. They are defined as an abnormal communication between the rectum or anal canal and the external perianal or ischioanal skin. They occur in one-quarter of patients with CD and may be the presenting complaint in up to 10% [3, 7] of patients with approximately two-thirds developing gastrointestinal symptoms within a year [8]. Perianal fistulas most commonly develop among those with rectal disease (92%) and are least likely to occur with ileal involvement (12%) [7]. The presence of perianal CD increases the risk of poor outcomes. Risk factors for more complicated disease include younger age of onset, smoking, longer disease duration, early need for corticosteroids, anemia, hypoalbuminemia, elevated inflammatory markers (CRP, fecal calprotectin), endoscopic disease burden, and location of associated luminal disease. Anorectal strictures have been significantly associated with increased prevalence of perianal fistulas (61 vs 34%, $p > 0.001$) [8]. They carry a cumulative risk of 21% at 10 years and 26% at 20 years. A complicated perianal fistula is defined as having multiple and/or branching fistula tracts, rectovaginal fistula, and/or fistulas associated with active rectal disease or anal stenosis. Furthermore, 75% require surgical management, while >30% have recurrent disease.

Perianal fistulas have been classically characterized by the Parks classification based on the course of the fistula tract in relation to the external sphincter levator plate [8]; however, this was later revised to simple or complex perianal fistulas. Most are simple fistulas, presented as fistula-in-ano, which are superficial and low-lying (anal sphincter above the fistula tract) and have one external opening, and include low-intersphincteric and low-transsphincteric fistulas, and are typically not associated with abscess formation and lack rectal involvement [6, 9]. Complex fistulas are considered those with multiple orifices that are high with internal openings above the dentate line with horseshoe tracts or high blind extensions. They also include recurrent fistulas following fistulotomy, suprasphincteric, extrasphincteric, and fistulas that cross the sphincter at a high level. Active proctitis is independently associated with reduced rates of healing and recurrence [8]. Combined medical and surgical therapy is superior to medical therapy alone for complicated perianal CD [8, 10] and specifically among those requiring abscess drainage or seton placement.

Clinical manifestations vary based on fistula location and the amount of bowel bypassed. For example, enteroenteric fistulas involving only a short segment of the bowel may be asymptomatic, while ileosigmoid fistulas have symptoms of diarrhea, weight loss, or abdominal pain. Gastrocolic fistulas may cause diarrhea secondary to bacterial overgrowth and malabsorption [11]. Less than one percent of patients have symptoms of anorexia, weight loss, abdominal pain, and occasionally feculent belching [12]. Approximately 10 percent will develop fistulas between the bowel and the urinary system, most frequently originating from the ileum or as a complication of an anastomotic leak or abscess. These patients classically present with recurrent urinary tract infections, pneumaturia, fecaluria, and dysuria [13]. In addition to cross-sectional imaging, cystoscopy may demonstrate bullous edema around the fistula opening. Rectovaginal fistulas occur in approximately 10% of patients and are usually associated with active rectal disease and will require management as complex fistulas if side tracts to the perineum are present [11]. They typically respond well to medical management [11]. Enterovaginal fistulas usually develop following proctocolectomy with ileal pouch-to-anal anastomosis for presumed ulcerative colitis and imply a missed diagnosis of CD [14]. Patients with previous hysterectomy are at risk for fistula formation between the vagina and ileal or sigmoid CD. While symptoms may vary, they classically present with discharge of fecal or gas material from the vagina, dyspareunia, perineal pain, drainage of purulent material, and yeast infections. Enterovesical fistulas occur in ~5.6% of IBD patients and most commonly with ileal disease [6]. They can arise from inflammation in the adjacent ileum or sigmoid colon. Classically, they may present with dysuria, pneumaturia, fecaluria, and recurrent urinary tract infections. They have also been associated with recurrent cystitis and pyelonephritis. While cross-sectional imaging can delineate a fistula tract, a filling defect in the bladder may be seen on intravenous pyelograms and retrograde cystograms.

Perianal fistulas, on the other hand, typically present with anorectal pain, swelling, purulent drainage, rectal bleeding, recurrent urinary tract infections and/or fecal incontinence, as well as reduced quality of life [9]. Symptomatic remission is measured by the presence of complications, such as anal stenosis, perianal abscess, systemic sepsis, fecal incontinence, and need for fecal diversion or proctectomy. Symptoms are not a validated method to determine healing but can be used to monitor response to therapy.

Evaluation

Proper evaluation is critical to determine the fistula complexity, location, severity, and subsequent management. Imaging aids detect abscess formation and collections requiring drainage and monitoring response to therapy. The primary modes of evaluation are EUS or MRI pelvis, for which observational studies and small RCTs demonstrated good accuracy [3]. Overall, CT and MRI were found to be superior to US. US has demonstrated a sensitivity of 74% and specificity of 95% compared with 79% sensitivity and 97% specificity of CT and 76% sensitivity and 96% specificity of MRI [3]. CT is not recommended as it carries a risk of radiation exposure and it is inferior to MRI. EUS, MRI, and exam under anesthesia (EUA) demonstrate >85% accuracy in classification of fistulas, improving to 100% with any combination of two tests [15]. However, available local expertise directs choice of either EUS or MRI [15, 16]. In small RCTs, EUS was associated with reduced drainage, earlier dose escalation of medical therapy, and rapid fistula healing. The data regarding the durability of healing demonstrated on MRI and its correlation with clinical and endoscopic response is not conclusive [17, 18]. It is important to note there is no role for serial imaging [10], and endoscopy is recommended to evaluate active luminal disease [19] as it has downstream effects on choice of therapy and surgical options.

Pelvic MRI is considered the gold standard for imaging modalities to examine fistula characteristics. T2-weighted images identify fluid content in fistula tracts or abscesses, while gadolinium-enhanced images distinguish granulation tissue from purulent buildup [8, 20, 21], which is relevant to assess fistula healing following therapy. The Van Assche score is the most commonly used tool, using both the anatomical fistula features and MRI findings to determine the response to therapy in a standardized manner. It determines the number of fistula tracts, location, extension, hyperintensity on T2-weighted images, presence of collections or abscesses, and rectal wall involvement. Though this correlates well with clinical improvement [8, 18, 22, 23], the association between T2 signal and fistula healing has not been validated. Van Assche scores may improve as fluid collections resolve despite the fistula tract remaining active. While a decrease of gadolinium in the fistula tract is significantly associated with fistula healing [8, 24], there is limited data to support the use of imaging in follow-up as well as appropriate timing of repeat imaging. Overall monitoring of clinical symptoms is recommended, while repeat MRI is encouraged in those that fail to demonstrate healing clinically.

Exam under anesthesia is recommended to evaluate abscess formation and indication for drainage. Surgeons are also able to unroof fistula tracts and curette-infected granulation tissue, which is then sent for culture and histologic assessment for carcinoma, a concern among those with recurrent fistulizing disease. In those at high risk for fistulotomy, long-term seton placement is an effective alternative. To facilitate communication with CRS, fistula descriptions should include the type of fistula, location of external and internal openings, and the presence of secondary branches and abscesses [8].

Management

The overall management of fistulas must consider the type and severity of fistula, disease activity, nutritional status, and comorbidities. The general goal of therapy is healing, defined as no drainage with gentle compression on the external fistula orifice for a duration of 1 month [6]. In the acute phase, the primary focus is first to gain source control of sepsis followed by inducing remission of active luminal disease and achieving mucosal healing [25, 26]. Abscesses requiring drainage occur in approximately 60% of CD patients with perianal involvement [27, 28]. Two-thirds of perirectal abscesses heal following drainage, while the other one-third will develop into a fistula [27]. Multidisciplinary care between gastroenterology and surgery is important for perianal fistulas, specifically exam under anesthesia, abscess drainage, and seton placement.

Assessment of fistula severity and response to therapy lacks a validated endpoint, and thus it is measured through a combination of clinical scores, physical examination, biomarkers of inflammation, pelvic MRI, and endoscopy. The most commonly referenced score is the Perianal Disease Activity Index, which has been validated per physician and patient global assessments. It is based on quality of life and fistula severity (discharge, pain, type of perianal disease, and degree of induration). However, it is limited by the lack of an established cutoff equivalent to clinical response. The Anal Disease Activity Index identified spontaneous pain, pain-limiting movement, and pain at defecation as symptoms to monitor clinical improvement [29]. The Fistula Drainage Assessment is a tool to assess fistula activity and clinical response. Though it simplifies fistulas as open (drainage) or closed (no drainage with gentle finger compression), they may be classified as clinically closed, while an active tract remains in more proximal areas. Given the limitations of clinical scores, additional MR imaging may be used as an objective measure to assess for fistula healing with the limitations as previously discussed. EUA is critical to evaluate the extent of proctitis, preventing postoperative nonhealing wounds, and surgical planning [30].

Medical Management

Although corticosteroids are effective to induce Crohn's disease remission, their use is associated with worsening of fistula discharge and increased need for surgical management (prednisone >60 g/d or equivalent) [6, 8, 31]. Furthermore, a study of combination therapy with corticosteroids and cyclosporin A (CyA) demonstrated that 56% of patients relapsed following clinical response once CyA was discontinued and corticosteroids continued at a low dose [8, 32]. There is a paucity of data to support the use of aminosalicylates in the management of CD, especially in fistulizing disease [8].

The use of antibiotics for fistulizing CD is derived from case series and uncontrolled trials. They are associated with improved symptoms; specifically early studies of ciprofloxacin demonstrated improvement in both symptoms and physician and patient global assessments [33, 34]. Retrospective studies demonstrated clinical efficacy with complete healing in 10/18 patients and significant healing in another 5; however, the effect was lost once the dose was reduced [9]. A follow-up study demonstrated that only 28% of patients successfully discontinued metronidazole [35]. Combination therapy with ciprofloxacin and metronidazole provides coverage against anaerobic bacteria and gram-negative organisms, respectively [25]. However, following cessation of 12 weeks of metronidazole 500–1500 mg daily and ciprofloxacin 1000–1500 mg daily, symptoms recurred requiring repeat courses of antibiotics. To date, the sole prospective, double-blind, placebo-controlled trial in perianal CD was underpowered and noted no significant difference between patients randomized to metronidazole (7), ciprofloxacin (10), and placebo (5). A randomized, placebo-controlled trial of topical metronidazole in 74 patients demonstrated no significant difference in PDAI scores [25, 36]. There is also concern for adverse events, including paresthesias, which are reversible and dose-related [6, 9, 33, 37–42]. Ciprofloxacin has also been associated with risk for spontaneous Achilles tendon rupture. In addition, the long-term use of antibiotics raises concern for developing antibiotic resistance.

Though antibiotics are considered first-line for control of sepsis, their effectiveness as combination therapy has also been evaluated. When used in conjunction with AZA, 48% achieved clinical response compared to 15% of those using either ciprofloxacin or metronidazole alone [43, 44]. Two studies evaluated the use of combination antibiotics and anti-TNF therapies. Combination therapy with ciprofloxacin and infliximab was more effective than infliximab monotherapy to achieve fistula response; however, this difference was not statistically significant (p 0.12) [8, 45], while combination ciprofloxacin and adalimumab significantly demonstrated better efficacy than adalimumab monotherapy (P 0.047) [3, 46]. However, it is unclear if ciprofloxacin carries immunosuppressive properties as perianal fistulas are colonized with gram-positive organism, and thus ciprofloxacin does not alter the bacterial flora [47]. Given the lack of data and durability, their use is considered as an adjunct to reduce fistula drainage and as a bridge to more definitive therapy [8, 48].

Evidence for the use of immunomodulators in fistulizing perianal CD is limited. AZA is a prodrug and nonenzymatically converted to 6-MP; both proved effective to improve clinical response, fistula healing, and need for corticosteroid use; however, there was no significant difference compared to placebo [6]. In an uncontrolled follow-up study, 100% of patients responded; however, following healing >70% of those that discontinued medication developed fistula recurrence. Initial uncontrolled studies demonstrated effect for both internal and external fistulas. Subgroup analysis of those with baseline perianal fistulizing disease from a meta-analysis of the use of AZA or 6-MP noted healing in 54% of patients compared to placebo (OR 4.44, 95% CI 1.5–13.2) [49]. When used in combination with antibiotics compared to antibiotics alone, at least a 50% reduction in draining fistulas was noted in 48% of patients (*p* 0.03) [50].

Though methotrexate has demonstrated efficacy in the management of CD, there is limited data regarding its use in treating fistulizing disease [6]. Two uncontrolled case series both suggested efficacy in fistulizing CD [8, 51, 52]. However, methotrexate should be considered when other therapies have failed to work.

Cyclosporin A (CyA) inhibits IL-2 T-helper lymphocytes. It has demonstrated clinical efficacy at higher doses (7.6 mg/kg) to induce remission of CD, while at a lower dose of 5 mg/kg, the effect was similar to placebo. However, there is a lack of evidence to support its use in fistula closure. A series of 16 patients found that 7 had completed closure and 14 (88%) had a clinical response. The mean response time was 7.4 days and 9/10 patients without response to immunomodulators responded to CyA. Three placebo-controlled trials of IV CyA failed to demonstrate efficacy in fistulizing CD [3]. Overall, it is used as a bridge to maintenance therapy with an immunomodulator, and there is a concern for disease relapse once it has been discontinued [8]. Cochrane meta-analysis of four controlled trials failed to demonstrate support for its use in fistulizing CD [53]. Moreover, patients relapsed once it was discontinued, likely due to inadequate bridging with maintenance therapy [54, 55].

Tacrolimus is a *Streptomyces*-derived macrolide antibiotic and also inhibits IL-2 T-helper lymphocytes. Initial case reports showed efficacy, and one randomized clinical trial found that standard dose (0.2 mg/kg) significantly resulted in closure of >50% of external openings compared to placebo (*p* 0.004) over the 10-week study period. However, only 10% of patients had complete fistula closure compared to 8% of those given placebo [8, 56], and it is unclear if the study duration was too short to appreciate a significant difference. The study was also limited by nephrotoxicity in the tacrolimus group, with subsequent dose reduction. Topical tacrolimus did not demonstrate efficacy in perianal CD [57]. Overall, it may improve symptoms, but does not aid in healing fistulizing perianal CD.

Mycophenolate mofetil inhibits lymphocyte proliferation by selectively blocking guanosine nucleotide synthesis in T cells. In addition to its use in steroid-refractory CD, uncontrolled studies have shown benefit in fistulizing disease.

Biologics have considerably changed the management of IBD, specifically antitumor necrosis factor antibodies (TNFa). Infliximab was purposely studied for fistulizing Crohn's disease with 68% of patients receiving 5 mg/kg (*p* 0.002) and 56% of patients receiving 10 mg/kg (*p* 0.002) both significantly achieving the primary endpoint of no drainage and closure of >50% of fistula tracts present at baseline in two consecutive visits within 18 weeks. It is highly efficacious for both internal and external fistulas and the first treatment to significantly achieve fistula closure in a randomized, multicenter, double-blind, placebo-controlled trial [6, 58]. Patients that received doses of both 5 mg/kg and 10 mg/kg were able to statistically significantly reach the primary endpoint of a decrease in 50% or greater of the number of open draining fistulas, as well as closure of all fistulas compared to placebo. In addition, those in the infliximab arms (5 and 10 mg/kg) were significantly more likely to achieve complete remission, or no drainage from the fistula tracts. The median duration of fistula closure was 3 months [8]. In a follow-up maintenance study (ACCENT II), those that responded to induction therapy at 5 mg/kg were randomized to placebo or a maintenance dose every 8 weeks. Infliximab maintenance was significantly associated with fistula healing compared to placebo (*p* 0.009) [59]. There is growing evidence to support the use of therapeutic drug monitoring to dose-optimized infliximab, especially in fistulizing perianal disease in which higher levels are associated with healing [7, 60]. A retrospective study of 36 patients found that 23 patients with fistula response had higher levels at week 30 and significantly higher levels at weeks 2, 6, and 14. IFX levels of 9.25 mg/mL at week 2 and 8.6ug/mL at week 6 predicted response at week 30 [61]. A retrospective cohort also demonstrated that higher IFX levels (10–20 μg/mL) were associated with fistula healing, lower CRP levels, higher rates of mucosal healing, and male gender [62].

Efficacy with adalimumab and certolizumab was inferred from studies with infliximab. Retrospective studies demonstrated fistula healing with standard induction therapy, confirmed by MRI [63]. However, the data were less supportive with complex fistulas, with only 41% achieving clinical remission. CHARM included 117 patients with draining fistulas at screening and baseline randomly assigned to either adalimumab (n = 70) or placebo (n = 47), with significantly higher fistula closure in the anti-TNF group (*p* 0.016). CLASSIC I demonstrated that those treated with ADA were more likely to achieve fistula closure; however, this effect was not dose dependent [64].

Certolizumab is a pegylated anti-TNF agent, and PRECISE I and II studies failed to demonstrate significant difference in perianal fistulizing CD [8, 65–67]. Though 36% of patients maintained fistula closure at 26 weeks compared to 17% in the placebo arm, there was no statistically significant difference noted [9]. Further study showed benefit for initial treatment of perianal disease in biologic-naïve patients [7].

Vedolizumab is an α4β7, anti-integrin therapy. It provides a different mechanism to induce and maintain remission; however, it has a delayed onset of action and requires bridging with another therapy typically corticosteroids or calcineurin inhibitors [68]. Initial studies of anti-integrin therapy showed efficacy in induction and maintenance of CD. In fistulizing disease, there was a significant benefit with vedolizumab (p 0.03) [69]. Post hoc analysis of the GEMINI II study found that those treated with VDZ had higher rates of fistula closure at week 52 and faster time to fistula closure; however, this was not associated with VDZ levels [70]. The concern with VDZ in an inpatient setting is the time to medication onset, compared to anti-TNF agents improving symptoms within days of receiving the loading dose.

Ustekinumab (UST) is a monoclonal antibody to the p40 subunit of IL-12 and IL-23. Retrospective studies have demonstrated efficacy in perianal disease with lower off-label dosing regimens. Post hoc analysis found complete fistula closure in 14.1% of the pooled placebo group, but no statistically significant difference

[71]. Further dedicated studies are needed to evaluate UST in fistulizing CD, including the use of combination therapy.

Surgical Therapy

Surgery is an important component of inpatient management of fistulizing Crohn's disease. Up to 70% of CD patients will require surgical intervention, and approximately 31% with perianal disease will end up with a permanent stoma [72]. EUA is especially critical in perianal disease. In addition to full evaluation including endoscopy and cross-sectional imaging, the distinction between simple and complex fistulas and presence of active proctitis are important to guide the management and surgical decisions.

Proper evaluation of fistula location is critical in preparation for surgery, specifically in relation to the anal sphincter. Superficial fistulas and those below the anal sphincter may be managed with incision and drainage or excision, while a transvaginal or intra-abdominal approach is recommended for fistulas that cross the anal sphincter [73]. For example, vaginal fistulas involving the ileum or cecum may require resection of the involved bowel segment; proctocolectomy is recommended in women with severe colonic and anorectal disease refractory to medical therapy or previous failed surgeries [11]. While the majority of simple fistulas can be managed with curative fistulotomy, complex fistulas or those involving greater than 30% of the external sphincter require sphincter-sparing procedures [74].

Management of Perianal Fistulas

Active perianal fistulizing disease is frequently associated with abscess, and setons in combination with medical therapy are recommended. Setons provide a viable treatment option for complex fistulas with associated local sepsis or rectal disease complementary to medical therapy. They function by creating granulation tissue leading to fistula closure over time. They are able to maintain patency of the fistula tract, prevent premature closure of the external orifice, and reduce abscess recurrence while preserving sphincter function [8, 75, 76]. Furthermore, loose setons are recommended as they preserve the external anal sphincter function. Multiple studies of setons have demonstrated fistula healing without need for further surgical management; however, there is a lack of consensus regarding duration as there is a risk for recurrence following removal. ACCENT II found a recurrence rate of 15% when setons were removed at 2 weeks, while a prospective study demonstrated no recurrence with combination therapy with infliximab [8]. Thus, the use of a combined medical and surgical approach is recommended until induction therapy is completed, with the goal of complete closure of the fistula tract following seton removal. This dual approach is also associated with quicker time to healing and delays in time to relapse than infliximab or surgical intervention alone [77].

Fistulotomy involves a surgical longitudinal opening of a fistulous tract and is recommended for superficial and occasionally low intersphincteric fistulas that have not responded to a trial of antibiotics and are without active proctitis. Choice of surgical therapy should always consider preservation of continence especially in women with low anterior transsphincteric fistulas (known to have a high risk of incontinence) [8].

Fibrin glue is comprised of fibrinogen and thrombin, which when mixed form a fibrin clot in the lumen of the fistula tract. This subsequently leads to sealing of the tract and creates a framework for fibroblast growth and collagen deposition. Though initial observational studies of a small number of patients were promising, a prospective randomized open label study of 77 patients failed to demonstrate benefit [8, 78–83]. Overall there was a significant improvement in drainage at week 8 (38% vs 16%, p 0.04), but no statistically significant difference among those with complex fistulas, and they were more likely to recur after 8 weeks. Combination of fibrin glue with antibiotics, flap repair, or suture closure of the internal opening did not improve efficacy [84].

Bioprosthetic plugs are made with collagen or porcine intestinal submucosa that fill the fistula tract and seal the internal opening. Systematic review of 20 observational and retrospective studies did not conclusively demonstrate their clinical efficacy in

CD. An open-label randomized controlled trial of 106 patients also failed to support the use of bioprosthetic plugs. 31.5% of those in the treatment arm and 23.1% in the control group achieved fistula closure at week 12 [85, 86].

A mucosal advancement flap is a piece of rectal tissue (mucosa, submucosa, circular muscle) used to cover the internal opening without involving the sphincter. It is recommended in those without proctitis, cavitary ulceration, stenosis, local abscess, complicated anal disease, rectovaginal fistulas, or perineal fistulas. Reoperation is used to manage recurrent fistulizing disease. In a systematic review with mean follow-up of 29 months, 64% of patients demonstrated clinical efficacy, but 50% required reoperation [87].

Ligation of the intersphincteric tract involves ligation of the fistula tract at the level of the intersphincteric space close to the internal opening and removal of the intersphincteric tract, followed by curettage and removal of granulation tissue and suturing of the defect at the external sphincter muscle. A prospective study of 15 patients found that 67% were healed at 12 months and none were complicated by fecal incontinence. However, its use is limited by the high rate of treatment failure, associated with rectal inflammation [88].

Fecal diversion is a temporary measure that prevents recurrence by restoring fecal transit following resection; however, most patients develop recurrent perianal disease following stoma closure. This technique is recommended in those with severe perianal sepsis despite drainage and seton placement, those completing induction of biologic therapy, or those awaiting proctectomy [8, 89]. While >60% of patients respond to fecal diversion, >25% will need reoperation without proctectomy within 6 months of restoration [7]. The presence of rectal disease and inflammation significantly increases the risk of failed restoration [90, 91]. This approach is often required in those with complex disease, biologics failure, and failure of combination therapy.

Proctectomy with a permanent stoma is considered as a last resort for severe refractory fistulizing perianal disease and for sphincter damage with subsequent incontinence and disability. It is still required in up to 20% of patients despite use of anti-

TNF. Major complications include poor wound healing and perineal sinus tracts in 25% of patients [8, 85, 89, 92].

Management of Internal Fistulas

Ileocolonic, specifically ileocecal and ileosigmoid, fistulas are the most common type of enteroenteric fistulas. They are typically asymptomatic unless associated with active disease or septic or obstructive complications [6]. Surgery is reserved for cases refractory to medical therapy; however, the approach to treatment remains similar to external fistulas, and sepsis ideally requires combined medical and surgical management. Though anorectal fistulas are associated with a higher risk of recurrence, those with a superficial tract can be laid open, while transsphincteric and extrasphincteric fistulas have had good response [6, 73, 93] to mucosal advancement flaps. In the presence of significant rectal disease, an anocutaneous flap is recommended. One study found that a transvaginal approach yielded durable efficacy [6]. Management of enterovesical fistulas requires treating both the acute infectious process with appropriate antibiotics and the fistula with conventional medical therapy for IBD. Sepsis is unlikely to occur in these cases, but if present is suggestive of an abscess, and thus requires management as such. Surgical therapy typically involves bowel resection to remove the diseased portion of the bowel. However, if multiple fistulas are present, proximal bowel diversion is a temporizing measure, and definitive surgical intervention is required. Following dissection of the bladder from the segment of inflamed bowel and resection, overall risk of recurrence is low [6].

Bowel resection is recommended in the setting of fistulizing disease due to active Crohn's disease and the length of resection is dependent on the affected disease segment, such as ileal resection for active ileal CD [6]. A subtotal colectomy with ileorectal anastomosis is recommended if there is active colonic involvement but sparing of the rectum and ileum. Proximal diversion is considered a temporizing measure to allow healing of the bowel in addition to medical therapy, as disease recurrence is frequent following reversal. Proctocolectomy is considered when other options fail, and specifically a colectomy with rectal preservation and possible completion proctectomy in the setting of severe proctitis or perianal abscess. In general, a two-stage procedure is recommended if sepsis or inflammation is present, as they may impair wound healing.

A multidisciplinary approach is central to care for this patient population. Equally important is preoperative optimization to correct anemia, fluid depletion, electrolyte imbalance, and malnutrition. Total parental nutrition allows for bowel rest and correction of nutritional deficiencies. It can also treat fistulizing disease, while enteral nutrition reduces postoperative septic complications, based on case reports and small retrospective series [25]. It is also important to note that these studies focus on enterocutaneous fistulas and not specifically in CD. Elemental and polymeric diets have not proven effective in fistulizing CD, and a Cochrane systematic review found prednisolone more effective than enteral diets and NNT of 4 [3].

Hyperbaric oxygen therapy (HBOT) is intermittent inhalation of 100% oxygen at pressure > 1 atmosphere, which increases oxygen tension in inflamed tissue, thereby enhancing healing through fibroblast proliferation and targeting white blood cells [94, 95]. Four small prospective open-label series showed variable efficacy. More importantly, though it was associated with reduction in pro-inflammatory cytokines, this effect was not durable, and they returned to baseline levels following completion of therapy [25].

Important considerations in preoperative planning include optimizing medications and nutritional status. Corticosteroids are associated with superficial surgical site infections, deep space infections, and anastomotic leaks. It is recommended that the dose be tapered to less than 20 mg per day [96]. Immunomodulators are not associated with adverse postoperative outcomes. Biologics are not independent risk factors for increased complications [96]. Weight loss is common in CD due to a hypermetabolic state, nutrient losses, reduced oral intake, and previous surgeries. Low albumin is a risk factor for intra-abdominal septic complications. Early enteral nutrition within 24 hours of surgery is associated with improved outcomes [97]. Parental nutrition is recommended if they are unable to tolerate enteral nutrition.

As knowledge is gained about fistulizing CD, the approach to management also evolves. Inpatient treatment requires a comprehensive medical and surgical approach. The first step is to determine if fistula is present with or without abscess formation. If an abscess is present, drainage and antibiotics are recommended for source control, followed by fistula treatment. The first step in fistula management is to distinguish between simple or complex and symptomatic or asymptomatic fistulas. Observation is recommended for asymptomatic fistulas, simple or complex. If symptomatic, then pelvic imaging, possible small bowel imaging, and EUA are recommended to delineate the fistula tract. Treatment will vary depending on the findings and the individual's disease course. Further work-up may be required to determine the extent of active disease and response to current therapy with therapeutic drug monitoring. Early involvement of colorectal surgery is encouraged, especially for patients failing to respond to conservative measures. Long-term management will depend on response to medical therapy, need for surgical intervention, and disease course.

Brief Case/Vignette

A 20-year-old female presents with a 2-year history of abdominal pain, nausea, vomiting, and diarrhea. She reports eight to ten loose, non-bloody bowel movements daily with associated nocturnal symptoms and a 15-lb weight loss over the past 6 weeks. She has an uncle and two cousins with Crohn's disease. On exam, she is afebrile with normal BP and HR. Her abdominal exam is notable for right lower quadrant tenderness to deep palpation but no rebound or guarding. There is a fullness in the right lower quadrant but not hepatosplenomegaly. She also has an actively draining perianal fistula without associated fluctuance. Her bloodwork shows microcytic anemia, elevated WBC, and elevated CRP. Fecal calprotectin is elevated at 754. CTAP shows hyperemia of the distal small bowel mucosa and bowel wall thickening (4–5 mm) and query interloop fistula tract between the small bowel and right lower quadrant. Colonoscopy shows ileocolonic Crohn's disease with rectal sparing. Pelvic MRI demonstrates an intersphincteric fistula and 6 cm abscess. She is started on antibiotics and surgery is consulted for drainage of the abscess. What is the best management approach?

(A) Seton
(B) Biologics
(C) Seton + biologics
(D) Fistulotomy

Answer: C

Acutely, the primary goal of therapy is to obtain source control followed by inducing remission of the active luminal disease. Following drainage of the abscess and initiation of antibiotics, seton placement in combination with medical therapy is recommended for active perianal fistulizing disease. Response to therapy is assessed using a combination of clinical scores, physical examination, biomarkers, pelvic MRI, and endoscopy. Setons maintain patency of the fistula tract while reducing abscess recurrence. Setons in combination with infliximab prevented recurrence and were associated with quicker time to healing and delay in time to relapse compared to infliximab or surgical intervention, independently.

Corticosteroids are not recommended in this setting as their use is associated with worsening fistula discharge, need for surgical intervention, and increased risk of relapse. There is a paucity of data for aminosalicylates and immunomodulators in fistulizing Crohn's disease. Antibiotics improve symptoms, as well as physician and patient global assessments. However, their effect lacks durability and symptoms recurred once they have been discontinued. Biologics, such as infliximab, are associated with both healing of luminal disease and fistula closure.

References

1. Pellino G, Selvaggi F. Surgical treatment of perianal fistulizing Crohn's disease: from lay-open to cell-based therapy – an overview. Sci World J. 2014;2014:1–8.
2. Lee MJ, Parker CE, Taylor SR, et al. Efficacy of medical therapies for fistulizing Crohn's disease: systematic review and meta-analysis. Clin Gastroenterol Hepatol. 2016;16:1879–92. (CD BC-4)
3. Gomollon F, Dignass A, Annnese A, et al. 3rd European evidence-based consensus on the diagnosis and management of Crohn's disease 2016: part 1: diagnosis and medical management. J Crohn's Colitis. 2017;11:3–25.
4. Hellers G, Bergstrand O, Ewerth S, et al. Occurrence and outcome after primary treatment of anal fistulae in Crohn's disease. Gut. 1980;21:525–7.
5. Ingle SB, Loftus EV Jr. The natural history of perianal Crohn's disease. Dig Liver Dis. 2007;39:963–9.
6. Lichtenstein G. Treatment of fistulizing Crohn's disease. Gastroenterology. 2000;119:1132–47.
7. Rackovsky O, Hirten R, Ungaro R, Colombel JF. Clinical updates on perianal fistulas in Crohn's disease. Expert Rev Gastroenterol Hepatol. 2018;12(6):597–605.
8. Panes J, Rimola J. Perianal fistulizing Crohn's disease: pathogenesis, diagnosis and therapy. Nat Rev Gastroenterol Hepatol. 2017;14:652–64.
9. Juncadella AC, Alame AM, Sands LR, Deshpande AR. Perianal Crohn's disease: a review. Postgrad Med. 2015;127(3):266–72.
10. Steinhart AH, Panaccione R, Targownik L, et al. Clinical practice guideline for the medical management of perianal fistulizing Crohn's disease: the Toronto consensus. Inflamm Bowel Dis. 2019;25:1–13.
11. Levy C, Tremaine WJ. Management of internal fistulas in Crohn's disease. Inflamm Bowel Dis. 2002;8(2):106–11.
12. Greenstein A, Present D, Sachar D, et al. Gastric fistulas in Crohn's disease. Report of cases. Dis Colon Rectum. 1998;32:888–92.
13. Saint-Marc O, Tiret E, Vaillant J, et al. Surgical management of internal fistulas in Crohn's disease. J Am Coll Surg. 1996;183:97–100.
14. Ricart E, Panaccione R, Loftus E, et al. Successful management of Crohn's disease of the ileoanal pouch with infliximab. Gastroenterology. 1999;117:429–32.
15. Schwartz DA, Wiersma MJ, Dudiak KM, et al. A comparison of endoscopic ultrasound, magnetic resonance imaging, and exam under anesthesia for evaluation of Crohn's perianal fistulas. Gastroenterology. 2001;121:1064–72.
16. Wiese DM, Schwartz DA. Managing perianal Crohn's disease. Curr Gastroenterol Rep. 2012;14:153–61.

17. Ng SC, Plamondon S, Gupta A, et al. Prospective evaluation of anti-tumor necrosis factor therapy guided by magnetic resonance imaging for Crohn's perianal fistulas. Am J Gastroenterol. 2009;104:2973–86.
18. Kamiris K, Bielen D, Van Vanbeckevoort D, et al. Long-term monitoring of infliximab therapy for perianal fistulizing Crohn's disease by suing magnetic resonance imaging. Clin Gastroenterol Hepatol. 2011;9:130–6.
19. Ruffolo C, Citton M, Scarpa M, et al. Perianal Crohn's disease: is there something new? World J Gastroenterol. 2011;17:1939–46.
20. Sheedy SP, Bruining DH, Dozios EJ, et al. MR imaging of perianal Crohn's disease. Radiology. 2017;282:628–45.
21. Horsthuis K, et al. Evaluation of an MRI-based score of disease activity in perianal fistulizing Crohn's disease. Clin Imaging. 2011;35:360–5.
22. Van Assche G, et al. Magnetic resonance imaging of the effects of infliximab on perianal fistulizing Crohn's disease. Am J Gastroenterol. 2003;98:332–9.
23. Horsthuis K, Lavini C, Bipat S, et al. Perianal Crohn disease: evaluation of dynamic contrast-enhanced MR imaging as an indicator of disease activity. Radiology. 2009;251:38–387.
24. Savoye-Collet C, Savoye G, Koning E, et al. Fistulizing perianal Crohn's disease: contrast-enhanced imaging assessment at 1 year on maintenance anti-TNF-a therapy. Inflamm Bowel Dis. 2011;17:1751–8.
25. Schwartz DA, Ghazi LJ, Regueiro M. Guidelines for medical treatment of Crohn's perianal fistulas: critical evaluation of therapeutic trials. Inflamm Bowel Dis. 2015;21(4):737–52.
26. Spinelli A, Armuzzi A, Ciccocioppo R, et al. Management of patients with complex perianal fistulas in Crohn's disease: optimal patient flow in the Italian clinical reality. Dig Liver Dis. 2020;52:506–15.
27. Michelassi F, Melis M, Rubin M, Hurst RD. Surgical treatment of anorectal complications in Crohn's disease. Surgery. 2000;128(4):597–603.
28. Sangwan YP, Schoetz DJ Jr, Murray JJ, et al. Perianal Crohn's disease: results of local surgical treatment. Dis Colon Rectum. 1996;39(5):529–35.
29. Allan A, Linares L, Spooner HA, Alexander-Williams J. Clinical index to quantitate symptoms of perianal Crohn's disease. Dis Colon Rectum. 1992;35:656–61.
30. Wolkomir AF, Luchtefeld MA. Surgery for symptomatic hemorrhoids and anal fissures in CD. Dis Colon Rectum. 1993;36:545–7.
31. Lennard-Jones JE. Toward optimal use of corticosteroids in ulcerative colitis and Crohn's disease. Gut. 1983;24:177–81.
32. Hinterleitner TA, et al. Combination of cyclosporine, azathioprine and prednisolone for perianal fistulas in Crohn's disease. Z Gastroenterol. 1997;35:603–8.
33. Turunen U, Farkkila M, Seppala K. Long-term treatment of perianal or fistulous Crohn's disease with ciprofloxacin (suppl 148). Scand J Gastroenterol. 1989;24:144.

34. Wolf J. Ciprofloxacin may be useful in Crohn's disease (abstr). Gastroenterology. 1990;98:A212.
35. Wolf BG, Culp CE, Beart RW Jr, et al. Anorectal Crohn's disease – a long-term prospective. Dis Colon Rectum. 1985;28(10):709–11.
36. Maeda Y, et al. Randomized clinical trial of metronidazole ointment versus placebo in perianal Crohn's disease. Br J Surg. 2010;97:1340–7.
37. Brandt L, Bernstein L, Boley S, Frank M. Metronidazole therapy for perianal Crohn's disease: a follow-up study. Gastroenterology. 1982;83:383–7.
38. Jakobvits J, Schuster MM. Metronidazole therapy for Crohn's disease and associated fistulae. Am J Gastroenterol. 1984;79:533–40.
39. Stahlberg D, Barany F, Einarsson K, et al. Neurophysiologic studies of patients with Crohn's disease on long-term treatment with metronidazole. Scand J Gastroenterol. 1991;26:219–24.
40. Ursing B, Kamme C. Metronidazole for Crohn's disease. Lancet. 1975;1:775–7.
41. Korelitz BI, Present DH. Combination of ciprofloxacin and metronidazole in severe perianal Crohn's disease. Can J Gastroenterol. 1993;7:571–3.
42. Thia KT, Mahadevan U, Feagan BG, et al. Ciprofloxacin or metronidazole for the treatment of perianal fistulas in patients with Crohn's disease: a randomized double-blind, placebo-controlled pilot study. Inflamm Bowel Dis. 2009;15:17–24.
43. Pellino G, Sciaudone G, Patturelli M, et al. Relatives of Crohn's disease patients and breast cancer: an overlooked condition. Int J Surg. 2014;12(1):S156–8.
44. Nielsen OH, Rogler G, Hahnloser D, Thomsen OO. Diagnosis and management of fistulizing Crohn's disease. Nat Clin Pract Gastroenterol Hepatol. 2009;6(2):92–106.
45. West RL, et al. Clinical and endosonographic effect of ciprofloxacin on the treatment of perianal fistulae in Crohn's disease with infliximab: a double-blind placebo-controlled study. Aliment Pharmacol Ther. 2004;20:1329–36.
46. Dewint P, et al. Adalimumab combined with ciprofloxacin is superior to adalimumab monotherapy in perianal fistulae closure in Crohn's disease: a randomized double-blind, placebo-controlled trial. Gut. 2014;63:292–9.
47. West RL, Van der Woude CJ, Endtz H, et al. Perianal fistulas in Crohn's disease are predominantly colonized by skin flora: implications for antibiotic treatment? Dig Dis Sci. 2005;50:1260–3.
48. Gold SL, Cohen-Mekelburk S, Schneider Y, Steinlauf A. Perianal fistulas in patients with Crohn's disease, part 1: current medical management. Gastroenterol Hepatol. 2018;14(8):470–81.
49. Pearson DC, May GR, Fick GH, Sutherland LR. Azathioprine and 6-mercaptopurine in Crohn disease. A meta-analysis. Ann Intern Med. 1995;123:132–42.

50. Dejaco C, et al. Antibiotics and azathioprine for the treatment of perianal fistulas in Crohn's disease. Aliment Pharmacol Ther. 2003;18:1113–20.
51. Mahadevan U, Marion JF, Present DH. Fistula response to methotrexate in Crohn's disease: a case series. Aliment Pharmacol Ther. 2003;18:1003–8.
52. Schroder O, Blumenstein I, Schulte-Bockholt A, Stein J. Combining infliximab and methotrexate in fistulizing Crohn's disease resistant or intolerant to azathioprine. Aliment Pharmacol Ther. 2004;19:295–301.
53. McDonald JW, Feagan BG, Jewell D, et al. Cyclosporine for induction of remission in Crohn's disease. Cochrane Database Syst Rev. 2005;2:CD000297.
54. Sandborn WJ. A critical review of cyclosporine therapy in inflammatory bowel disease. Inflamm Bowel Dis. 1995;1:48–63.
55. Egan LJ, Sandborn WJ, Tremaine WJ. Clinical outcome following treatment of refractory inflammatory and fistulizing CD with intravenous cyclosporine. Am J Gastroenterol. 1998;3:442–8.
56. Sandborn WJ, et al. Tacrolimus for the treatment of fistulas in patients with Crohn's disease: a randomized placebo-controlled trial. Gastroenterology. 2003;125:380–8.
57. Hart AL, Plamondon S, Kamm MA. Topical tacrolimus in the treatment of perianal Crohn's disease: exploratory randomized controlled trial. Inflamm Bowel Dis. 2007;13:245–53.
58. Present DH, Rutgeers P, Targan S, et al. Infliximab for the treatment of fistulas in patients with Crohn's disease. N Engl J Med. 1999;340: 1398–405.
59. Sands BE, et al. Infliximab maintenance therapy for fistulizing Crohn's disease. N Engl J Med. 2004;350:876–85.
60. Samaan M, Campbell S, Cunningham G, et al. Biologic therapies for Crohn's disease: optimizing the old and maximizing the new. F1000Res. 2019;8:1210.
61. Davidov Y, Ungar B, Bar-Yoseph H, et al. Association of induction infliximab levels with clinical response in perianal Crohn's disease. J Crohns Colitis. 2017;11(5):549–55.
62. Yarur AJ, Kanagala V, Stein DJ, et al. Higher infliximab trough levels are associated with perianal fistula healing inn patients with Crohn's disease. Aliment Pharmacol Ther. 2017;45(7):933–40.
63. Castano-Milla C, Chaparro M, Saro C, et al. Effectiveness of adalimumab in perianal fistulas in Crohn's disease patients naïve to anti-TNF therapy. J Clin Gastroenterol. 2015;49(1):34–40.
64. Hanauer SB, Sandborn WJ, Rutgeerts P, et al. Human anti-tumor necrosis factor monoclonal antibody (adalimumab) in Crohn's disease: the CLASSIC-1 trial. Gastroenterology. 2006;130(2):323–33.
65. Schreiber S, et al. Randomised clinical trial: certolizumab pegol for fistulas in Crohn's disease- subgroup results from a placebo-controlled study. Aliment Pharmacol Ther. 2011;33:185–93.

66. Sandborn WJ, Feagan BG, Stoinov S, et al. Certolizumab pegol for the treatment of Crohn's disease. N Engl J Med. 2007;357:228–38.
67. Schreiber S, Khaliq-Kareemi M, Lawerence IC, et al. Maintenance therapy with certolizumab pegol for CD. N Engl J Med. 2007;357:239–50.
68. Christensen B, Gibson PR, Micic D, et al. Safety and efficacy of combination treatment with calcineurin inhibitors and vedolizumab in patients with refractory inflammatory bowel disease. Clin Gastroenterol Hepatol. 2019;17(3):486–93.
69. Sandborn WJ, et al. Vedolizumab as induction and maintenance therapy for Crohn's disease. N Engl J Med. 2013;369:711–21.
70. Feagan BG, Schwartz D, Danese S, et al. Efficacy of vedolizumab in fistulizing Crohn's disease: exploratory analyses of data from GEMINI 2. J Crohns Colitis. 2018;12:621–6.
71. Sands BE, Gasink C, Jacobsein D, et al. Fistula healing in pivotal studies of ustekinumab in Crohn's disease. Gastroenterology. 2017;152(5):1.
72. Mueller MH, Geis M, Glatzle J, et al. Risk of fecal diversion in complicated perianal Crohn's disease. J Gastrointest Surg. 2007;11(4):529–37.
73. Radcliffe A, Ritchie J, Hawley P, et al. Anovaginal and rectovaginal fistulas in Crohn's disease. Dis Colon Rectum. 1988;31:94–9.
74. Alexander-Williams J, Steinberg DM, Fielding JS, et al. Proceedings: perianal Crohn's disease. Gut. 1974;15:822–3.
75. Reguerio M, Mardini H. Treatment of perianal fistulizing Crohn's disease with infliximab alone or as an adjunct to exam under anesthesia with seton placement. Inflamm Bowel Dis. 2003;9:98–103.
76. Sciaudone G, et al. Treatment of complex perianal fistulas in Crohn's disease: infliximab, surgery or combined approach. Can J Surg. 2010;53:299–304.
77. Park EJ, Song K-H, Baik SH, et al. The efficacy of infliximab combined with surgical treatment of fistulizing perianal Crohn's disease: comparative analysis according to fistula subtypes. Asian J Surg. 2018;41:438–47.
78. Gaertner WB, et al. Results of combined medical and surgical treatment of recto-vaginal fistula in Crohn's disease. Color Dis. 2011;13:678–83.
79. Abel ME, Chiu YS, Russell TR, Volpe PA. Autologous fibrin glue in the treatment of rectovaginal and complex fistulas. Dis Colon Rectum. 1993;36:447–9.
80. Zmora O, et al. Fibrin glue sealing in the treatment of perianal fistulas. Dis Colon Rectum. 2003;46:584–9.
81. Loungnarath R, et al. Fibrin glue treatment of complex anal fistulas has low success rate. Dis Colon Rectum. 2004;47:432–6.
82. Lindsey I, Smilgin-Humphreys MM, Cunningham C, et al. A randomized, controlled trial of fibrin glue versus conventional treatment for anal fistulas. Dis Colon Rectum. 2002;45:1608–15.
83. Grimaud JC, et al. Fibrin glue is effective healing perianal fistulas in patients with Crohn's disease. Gastroenterology. 2010;138:2275–81.e1

84. Singer M, et al. Treatment of fistulas in-ano with fibrin sealant in combination with intra-adhesive antibiotics and/or surgical closure of the internal fistula opening. Dis Colon Rectum. 2005;48:799–808.
85. O'Riordan JM, Datta I, Johnston C, Baxter NN. A systematic review of the anal fistula plus for patients with Crohn's and non-Crohn's related fistula-in-ano. Dis Colon Rectum. 2012;55:351–8.
86. Senejoux A, et al. Fistula plug in fistulizing ano-perianal Crohn's disease: a randomized controlled trial. J Crohns Colitis. 2016;10:141–8.
87. Gionchetti P, et al. 3rd European evidence-based consensus on the diagnosis and management of Crohn's disease 2016: part 2: surgical management and special situations. J Crohns Colitis. 2016;11:135–49.
88. Kaminski JP, Zaghiyan K, Fleshner P. Increasing experience of ligation of the intersphincteric fistula tract for patients with Crohn's disease: what have we learned? Color Dis. 2017;19(8):750–5.
89. Singh S, et al. Systematic review with meta-analysis: Faecal diversion for management of perianal Crohn's disease. Aliment Pharmacol Ther. 2015;42:783–92.
90. Gu J, Valente MA, Remzi FH, et al. Factors affecting the fate of faecal diversion in patients with perianal Crohn's disease. Color Dis. 2015;17(1):66–72.
91. Regimbeau JM, Panis Y, Cazaban L, et al. Long-term results of faecal diversion for refractory perianal Crohn's disease. Color Dis. 2001;3(4):232–7.
92. Yamamoto T, Allan RN, Keighley MR. Effect of fecal diversion alone on perianal Crohn's disease. World J Surg. 2000;24:1258–62.
93. Joo JS, Weiss EG, Nogueras JJ, Wexner SD. Endorectal advancement flap in perianal Crohn's disease. Br J Surg. 1988;85:1695–8.
94. Grim PS, Gottlieb LJ, Boddie A, et al. Hyperbaric oxygen therapy. JAMA. 1990;263:2216–20.
95. Noyer CM, Brandt LJ. Hyperbaric oxygen therapy for perianal Crohn's disease. Am J Gastroenterol. 1999;94:318–21.
96. Barnes EL, Lightner AL, Regueiro M. Perioperative and postoperative management of patients with Crohn's disease and ulcerative colitis. Clin Gastroenterol Hepatol. 2020;18(6):1356–66.
97. Herbert G, Perry R, Andersen HK, et al. Early enteral nutrition within 24 hours of lower gastrointestinal surgery versus later commencement for length of hospital stay and postoperative complications. Cochrane Database Syst Rev. 2018;10:CD004080.

7 Surgical Management of Hospitalized Patients with Crohn's Disease

Michael J. Grieco and Feza H. Remzi

Introduction

Crohn's disease (CD) is a chronic relapsing-remitting inflammatory bowel disease (IBD) which has been increasingly prevalent across the globe [1]. Along with an increasing incidence of CD, the hospitalization rate for CD increased from 44.2 to 59.7 per 100,000 population from 2003 to 2013 [2]. In the last few decades, major surgery was required in 40% to 50% of CD patients within 10 years of diagnosis [3]. Surgery may be indicated to manage CD complications including obstruction, strictures, intra-abdominal abscess, gastrointestinal bleeding, malignancy, and perianal and intra-abdominal fistulas. The authors recommend specialized multidisciplinary care for CD, and within that framework surgery has a significant role. Crohn's disease patients admitted to the hospital have a higher than average risk of CD-associated complications and should be monitored for malnutrition, acute kidney injury, electrolyte derangement, cardiac complications, and venous thromboembolism. If a patient has

M. J. Grieco (✉) · F. H. Remzi
NYU Langone Health, NYU Grossman School of Medicine, New York, NY, USA
e-mail: Michael.grieco@nyulangone.org; Feza.Remzi@nyumc.org

J. D. Feuerstein, A. S. Cheifetz (eds.), *Management of Inpatient Inflammatory Bowel Disease*,
https://doi.org/10.1007/978-1-0716-1987-2_7

been treated at outside institutions, efforts should be made to obtain outside records with attention to imaging, endoscopy, surgical reports, pathology, and medication histories. Since surgery palliates but does not cure Crohn's disease, it is important to plan surgical management on a particular admission within the longer lifetime goals of long-term quality of life and bowel preservation. This chapter addresses surgical management of patients with Crohn's disease with special consideration to those who are hospitalized.

Obstruction

Approximately one third of patients with CD will form strictures in the first 10 years of the disease [4]. Crohn's patients present with obstruction due to primary stricture, anastomotic stricture, cancer, or surgical adhesions. Although an initial flat plate can be useful to rule out a rare case of perforation, cross-sectional imaging is an important initial imaging to discerning the differential diagnosis of obstruction. The natural history of CD bowel stricture is initially inflammatory, but inflammation eventually leads to fibrosis, and eventually the stricture can become entirely fibrotic scar without inflammation. Purely inflammatory stricture should be treated with medical, and purely scar should be treated with mechanical dilation, strictureplasty, or surgical resection. No one test or collection of tests is perfectly sensitive or specific to discern inflammation vs scar. Initial lab work should include CBC, complete metabolic panel, prealbumin, and C-reactive protein (CRP) to assess for infection, renal dysfunction, electrolyte abnormalities, malnutrition, and inflammation, respectively. Like any small bowel obstruction, Crohn's small bowel obstruction should be initially managed with nasogastric tube, resuscitation, clinical assessment, and cross-sectional imaging to rule out nonviable bowel, perforation, and closed-loop obstruction and locate stricture. Small bowel obstruction is managed differently than large bowel obstruction (Fig. 7.1).

Large bowel obstruction is commonly managed with emergent surgical resection or staged resection with initial diversion before

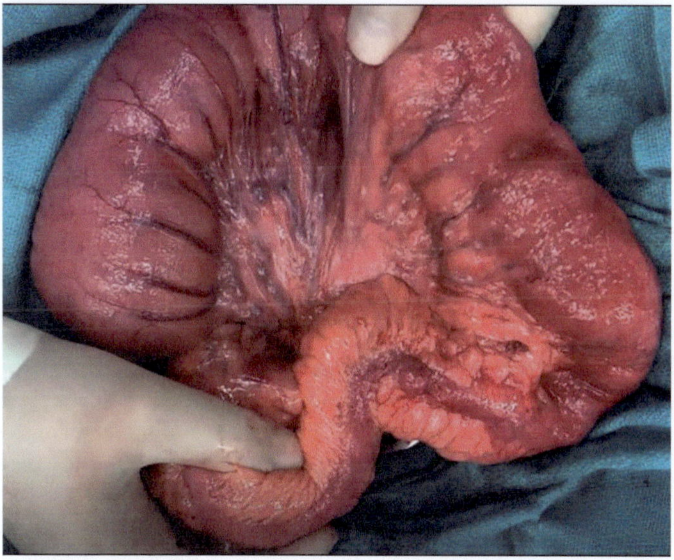

Fig. 7.1 Untimely referral, dilated small bowel proximal to ileal stricture

resection for left-sided obstruction, but endoscopic stents should be avoided. Medical therapy for the treatment of large bowel obstruction is futile since the etiology is most commonly fibrotic stricture or cancer. Although strictureplasty for colonic stricture has been described, the limited literature shows no better functional results for colonic strictureplasty compared to colonic resection [5]. The incidence of invasive adenocarcinoma incidentally found in resections for Crohn's colorectal strictures is 1.2% of cases [6]. We do not recommend colonic strictureplasty since the function of colonic strictureplasty is no better than resection, and colonic strictureplasty carries a small but significant risk of disseminating cancer.

We do recommend a multidisciplinary approach with the surgery and gastroenterology teams to coordinate the management of small bowel obstruction with the medical therapy, endoscopic dilation, or surgery. Ideal candidates for endoscopic balloon dilation (EBD) of CD strictures are those whose strictures are fibrotic (as opposed to inflammatory), symptomatic, straight (i.e., not angulated), shorter than 4 cm, and without associated abscess, fistula, or malignancy [7]. Although there is a role for endoscopic dilation, it should be appreciated that 80.6% of patients will require repeat dilation over 5 years [8]. The decision to offer endoscopic balloon dilation should be made in coordination between the GI and surgical team, since balloon dilation carries a risk of perforation that requires surgical management. A review of the safety profile of endoscopic balloon dilation showed four studies with a 0% perforation rate, but the remaining 13 studies had a perforation rate ranging from 2 to 11% [9]. Patients who could be expected to tolerate perforation particularly poorly should be considered poor candidates for endoscopic dilation. In our opinion, this can be an option in the setting of recurrent anastomotic stricture rather than a first-line modality for primary disease. Although self-expanding metal stent (SEMS) have been described in the management of Crohn's small bowel obstruction, there is not yet a robust body of literature on the topic. A review of the role of stents in CD found only only 65 patients across 19 studies [10]. Given the paucity of data, we do not recommend SEMS for Crohn's small bowel obstruction.

Surgical options for small bowel obstruction due to stricture refractory to medical management are either resection or strictureplasty. Strictureplasty avoids bowel resection by stricture lysis and widening of the bowel lumen, which is analogous to the pyloroplasty upon which the technique was based. Strictureplasty conserves the bowel and decreases risk of developing short bowel syndrome. Strictureplasty should be considered in the setting of multiple strictures, duodenal strictures, previous small bowel resection (>100 cm), recurrent ileocolic anastomotic strictures, recurrent strictures within 12 months of previous surgery, strictures at previous anastomotic sites, growth retardation, and short bowel syndrome [11]. Contraindications to strictureplasty are sepsis, diffuse peritonitis, concern for malignancy, malnutrition, hypoalbuminemia, strictureplasty under tension intestinal perforation, fistula, and phlegmonous inflammation at the intended strictureplasty site. A meta-analysis of 1112 patients who underwent 3259 strictureplasties

(Heineke-Mikulicz, 81 percent; Finney, 10 percent; side-to-side isoperistaltic, 5 percent) noted a 4% rate of septic complications, namely, leak, fistula, or abscess [12].

The type of strictureplasty should be tailored to the pathology of the stricture. A Heineke-Mikulicz strictureplasty should be performed for strictures <10 cm, Finney strictureplasty for strictures 10–20 cm, and a side-to-side isoperistaltic strictureplasty for strictures >20 cm long. In each type of the strictureplasty, the enterotomy should be on antimesenteric border extending 1–2 cm proximal and distal to the stricture, areas suspicious for cancer should be biopsied, and after completion the patency of the lumen should be confirmed [13]. In the Heineke-Mikulicz strictureplasty, after making the longitudinal enterotomy, seromuscular corner sutures of 3-0 or 2-0 polyglactin are placed on each side of the midpole of the enterotomy and are left long and then tagged with curved snaps to orient the enterotomy which is closed transversely with a single interrupted seromuscular bite of 3-0 or 2-0 polyglactin suture. Although 3-0 polyglactin suture is commonly used, for thicker or edematous tissue, 2-0 should be used since it may tear less than 3-0. The Finney is suited to 10–20 cm strictures in the bowel that is folded on itself, and the enterotomy is made along the antimesenteric border. Both the inner walls are sutured to each other in two layers with running layer followed by interrupted sutures both of either 3-0 or 2-0 polyglactin suture, and then the outer walls are sutured to each other interrupted 3-0 or 2-0 polyglactin suture. We are not advocates of a stapled Finney strictureplasty and prefer a hand-sewn technique.

The side-to-side isoperistaltic strictureplasty is created by making a full-thickness transverse division of the bowel at the midpoint of the stricture between non-crushing clamps, and the ends are spatulated and then overlapped until they each reach beyond the proximal and distal ends of the stricture (Fig. 7.2). Linear enterotomies are made on each of the two overlapping limbs from beyond the ends of the stricture by 1–2 cm and extended to the initial transverse enterotomy. Then they are closed with interrupted seromuscular bites of 3-0 or 2-0 polyglactin sutures. In the setting of multiple strictures, it is our practice to run the whole small bowel with 5 cc inflated balloon Foley

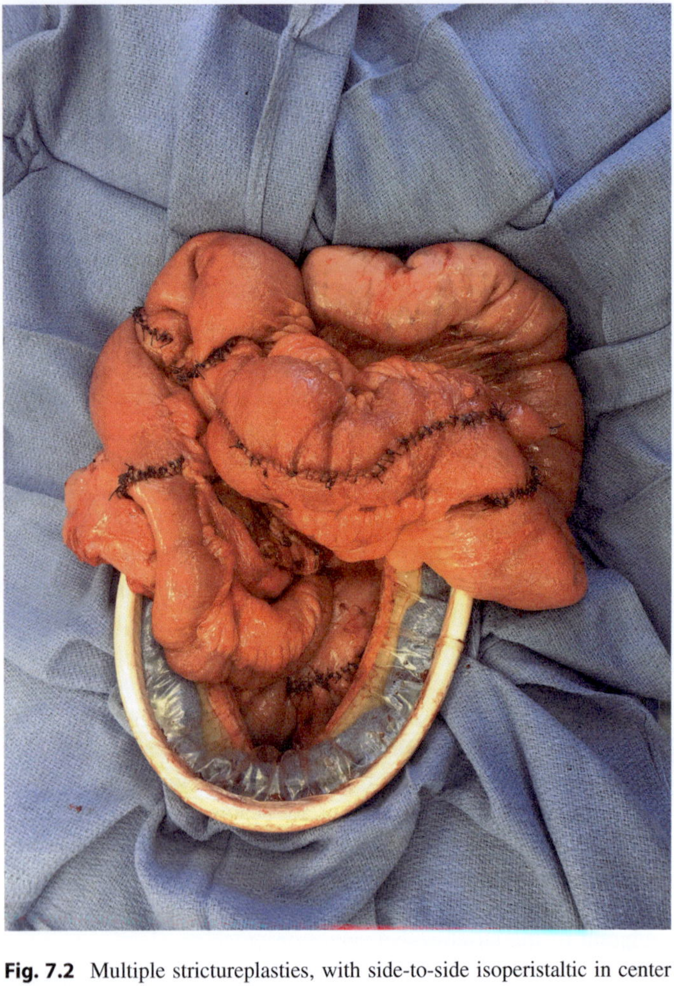

Fig. 7.2 Multiple strictureplasties, with side-to-side isoperistaltic in center of image

catheter through one or many of the enterotomies, from ligament of Treitz down the ileocecal valve.

Symptomatic strictures not amenable to medical therapy, endoscopic dilation, or strictureplasty require resection. To avoid early recurrence of disease, we recommend small bowel resection margins should be determined by a pinch test, resecting where the mesentery under the small bowel no longer feels thickened when pinching between the thumb and forefinger. In our experience this has been the best way to assess the margins rather than getting a frozen section [14].

Either stapled or sutured anastomosis can be performed, although we recommend sutured anastomosis particularly if the bowel is abnormal since surgical staplers are designed and tested on normal bowel. This is especially true in the setting of small bowel-to-small bowel anastomosis. In the setting of ileocolic resection, our preferred stapled technique has been end-to-side ileocolic anastomosis if tissues are appropriate for a stapled anastomosis. We recommend diverting loop ileostomy proximal to the anastomosis in settings of glucocorticoids, biologic therapy, anemia, malnutrition, chronic bowel obstruction, active sepsis, prior bowel resection, or surgeon judgment. It is important that the patient, surgeon, and multidisciplinary colleagues appreciated that diversion, although it does have its own morbidity and burden on the patient, is not a failure and can be the best avenue to giving the patient long-term quality of life and avoid abdominal catastrophes. Timing for the surgery in the setting of obstruction is a multidisciplinary decision; we prefer to convert an emergent admission to an elective surgical resection with medical therapy if feasible. However, in our opinion for a patient who has been hospitalized with a small bowel obstruction, long-term medical therapy is likely to be futile, and surgery will eventually be required.

Abscess

Up to a quarter of Crohn's patients will develop an intra-abdominal abscess secondary to CD in their lifetimes [15]. Although most Crohn's intra-abdominal abscess patients will ultimately require surgical management, emergent surgery is only indicated for unstable patients with generalized peritonitis or those who are clinically deteriorating despite nonoperative management. Cross-sectional imaging is important in evaluation to discern discrete abscess from phlegmon (Fig. 7.3). While phlegmon can be

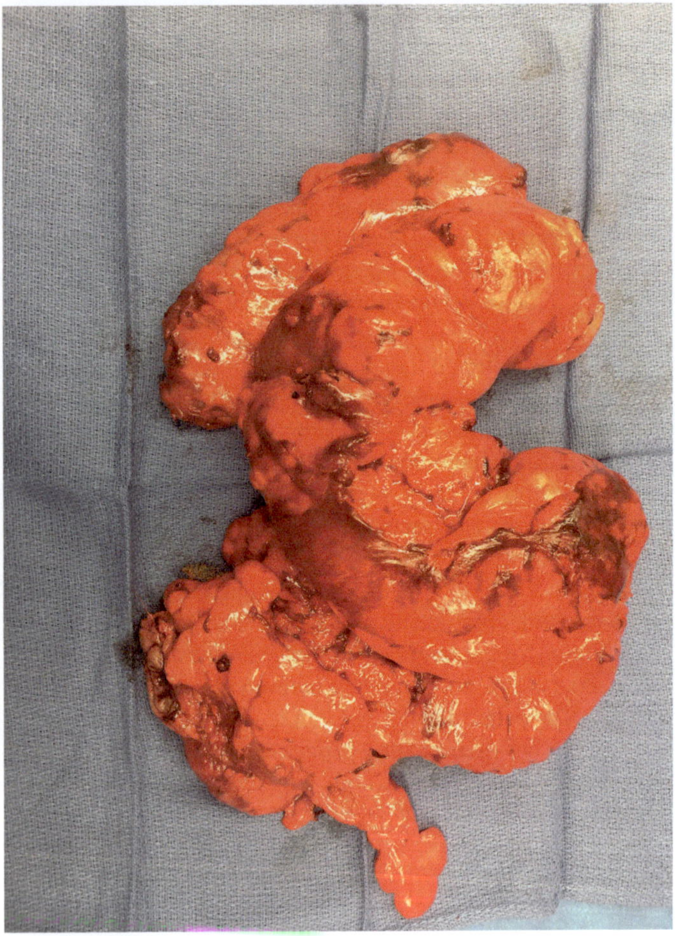

Fig. 7.3 Ileocecal phlegmon

initially treated with antibiotics alone, abscess should be initially treated with antibiotics and evaluation for percutaneous drainage by interventional radiology. The surgeon should note that the definition of "not amenable to percutaneous drainage" can be subjective and if an abscess is initially deemed "not drainable," then talking with your interventional radiologist colleague to discuss their concerns or inquiring about a second opinion might be of value. At times, a radiologist may deem an abscess "not amenable to percutaneous drainage" out of concern about causing a fistula or entering the bowel. The radiologist understanding the surgeon's eventual surgical plan of bowel resection after the patient has been optimized by percutaneous drainage and antibiotics may allay their concerns and convince them to make an attempt at drainage (Fig. 7.4). Patients with abscesses that are truly deemed "not ame-

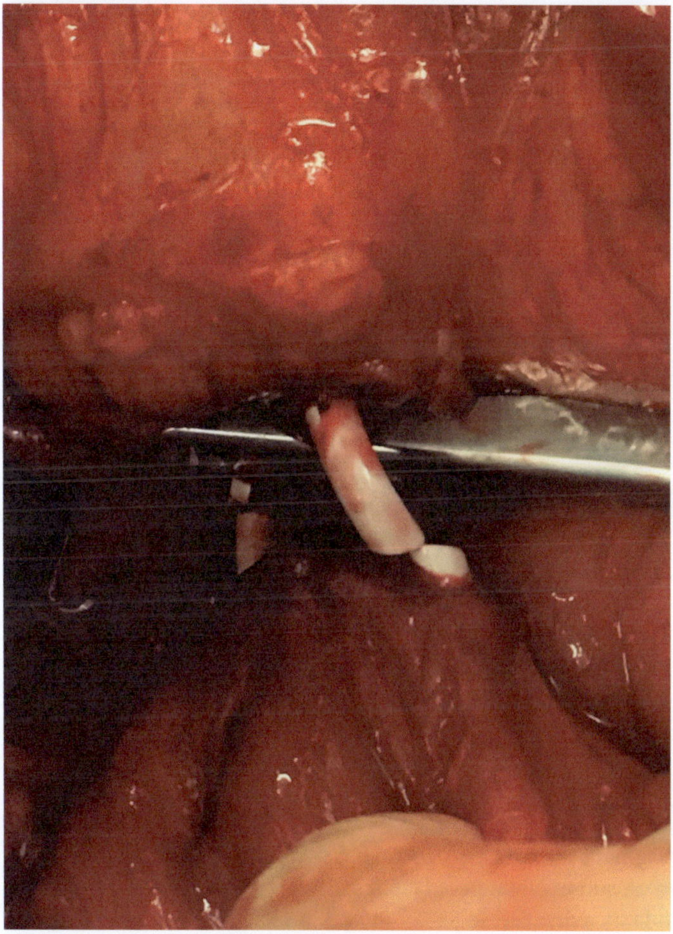

Fig. 7.4 Abscess percutaneously drained as bridge to surgery

nable to percutaneous drainage" may be managed with IV antibiotics alone but should be observed closely as an inpatient for continued improvement in clinical and laboratory criteria until they can be bridged for operative management. Once sepsis is controlled with IV antibiotics with or without percutaneous drainage, then elective resection is planned for 6–8 weeks later. In a retrospective series of CD patients with spontaneous intra-abdominal abscess managed with initial percutaneous drainage, 30% ultimately went on to not undergo surgical resection within the observation period [16, 17]. However, we recommend surgery in these settings because we consider long-term medical therapy to be futile and advocate resection to give the patient a clean start. At the time of the surgery, retreat can be a sign of excellent surgical judgment, and if a patient has substantial abscess burden that can't be adequately drained preoperatively or if the patient is not physiologically ready to tolerate a required resection, then "bailing out" with diversion and drainage can be a lifesaving next step on the road toward long-term quality of life. A definitive resection can be considered 6 months after the initial attempt.

Fistula

Fistulas, an abnormal communication between two epithelial surfaces, are a significant source of morbidity for CD patients. Asymptomatic fistulas do not require treatment. Within a year of diagnosis, 20% of CD patients will present with fistulas, and after two decades that number increases to 50% [18, 19]. Fistulas in CD are classified as anal, rectovaginal, enterocutaneous, or internal [20]. Internal fistulas can extend from bowel to bowel or from bowel to other organs such as the bladder, vagina, stomach, duodenum, or other retroperitoneal structures such as the psoas muscle or even to ureters. A retrospective series noted that relative incidence of fistulas' location is anal 55%, internal 31%, rectovaginal 9%, and enterocutaneous 6% [18] (Figs. 7.5, 7.6 and 7.7).

A subset of enterocutaneous fistula, the entero-atmospheric fistula, is a dreaded sequela of CD (Fig. 7.8). Patients are at significant risk for malnutrition, kidney injury secondary to dehydration,

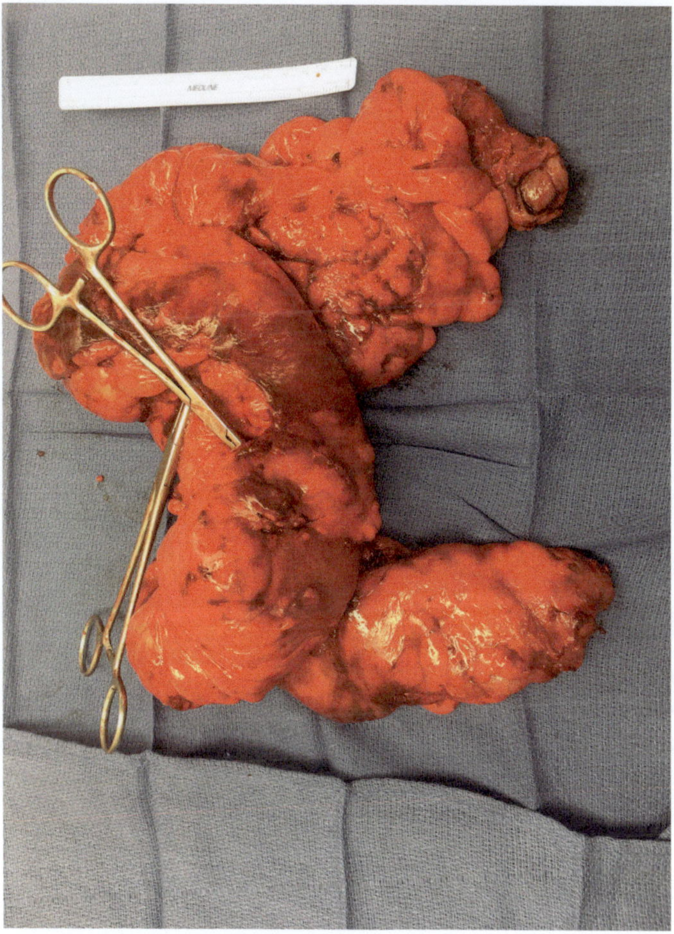

Fig. 7.5 Phlegmon with clamps marking fistulas

and electrolyte disturbances. The wound care management can be quite complex and benefits from certified wound care nursing if available. Patients require careful optimization before consideration of eventual operation, likely including peripherally inserted central catheter (PICC) for total parenteral nutrition. Efforts should be made to obtain and review imaging and opera-

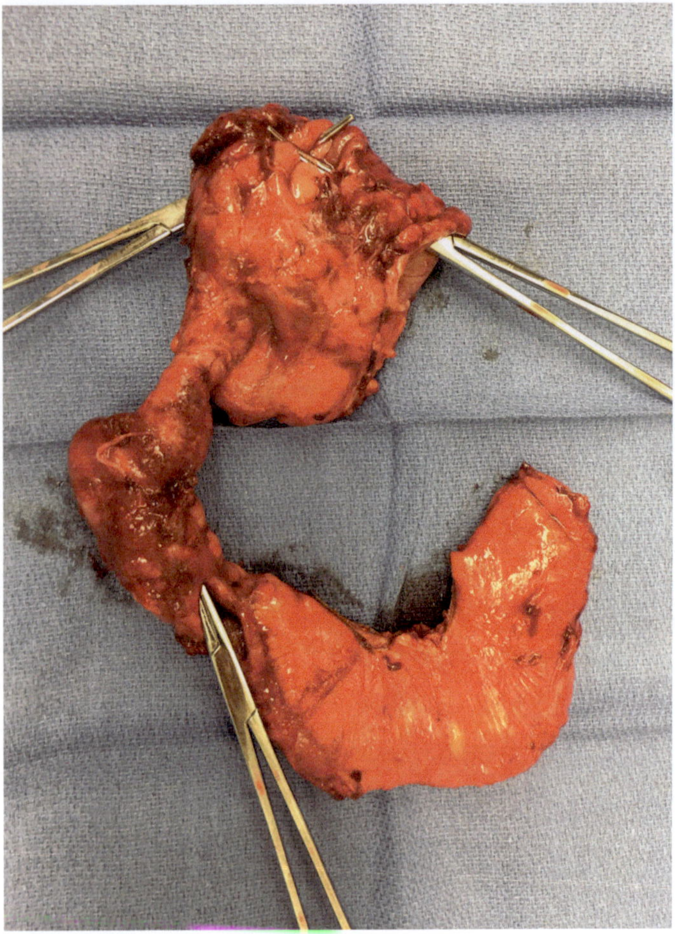

Fig. 7.6 Multiple small bowel fistulas, clamps marking each fistula

tive and pathology reports from previous hospitalizations. In addition to morbidity from fluid shifts and electrolyte abnormalities, sepsis secondary to PICC line infection is a significant source of morbidity leading up to reoperation. The duration of TPN should be decided in a multidisciplinary setting, but we recommend at least 7–10 days preoperatively. MR enterography and water-

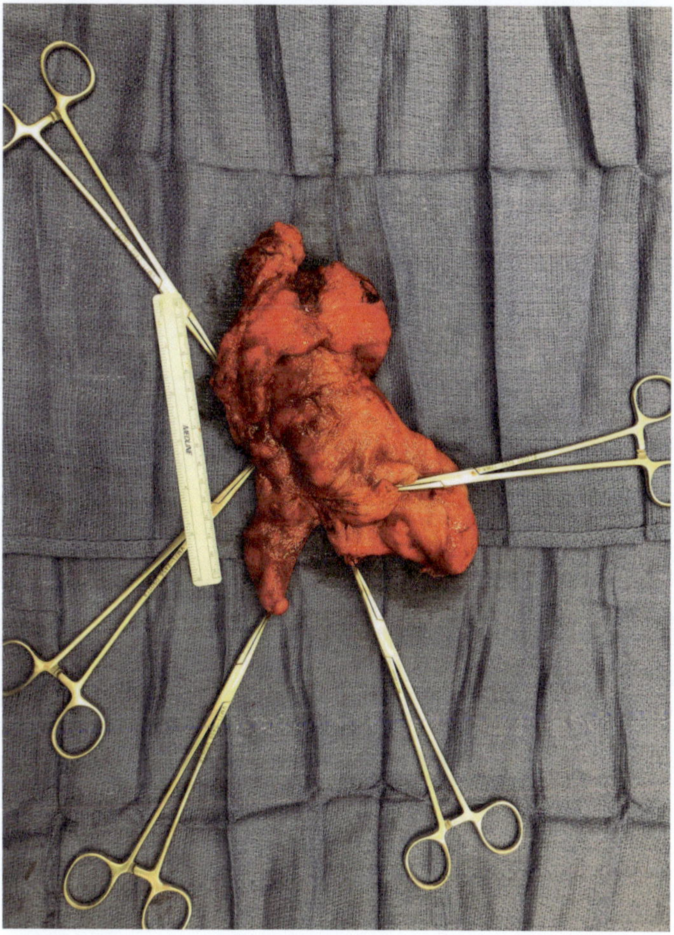

Fig. 7.7 Multiple enteroenteric fistulas with clamps marking each fistula

soluble fluoroscopy should be performed to assess extent of inflammation, stricture, fistulas, and anatomy for reconstruction. Multivisceral resection planned with non-digestive tract organs should be planned in conjunction with specialists for those organs.

The most common type of intra-abdominal fistula is entero-enteric fistula, and the most common of that subset is the ileo-

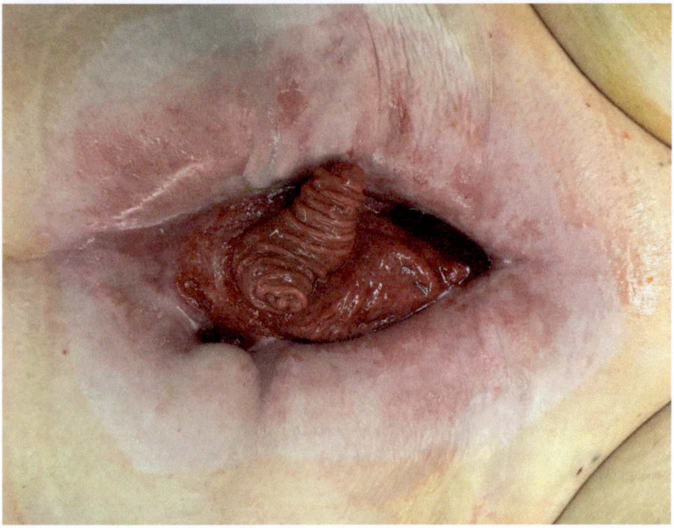

Fig. 7.8 Enteroatmospheric fistulas

sigmoid fistula which accounts for 15–30% [21, 22]. Most commonly the inflamed ileum is strictured, and a segment of the ileum proximal to the stricture fistulizes to other organs (Fig. 7.9). In the case of ileo-sigmoid fistula, although ileal resection with primary repair of the sigmoid is described, we recommend ileal resection along with sigmoid resection since the location of the fistula is usually on the mesenteric side of the colon and thus is difficult to repair primarily.

Perianal fistulas rarely drive inpatient admission, but sepsis from perirectal abscess and fistula can drive or be present during hospitalization especially in the setting of immunocompromise, diabetes, and/or obesity (Fig. 7.10). The American Society of Colon and Rectal Surgeons 2016 Clinical Practice Guidelines give a strong recommendation based on low-quality evidence that, like Crohn's abdominal fistulas, "asymptomatic [perianal] fistulas in patients with Crohn's disease do not require surgical treatment." [23] This is recommended because these fistulas can often remain asymptomatic for years. Symptomatic fistulas in

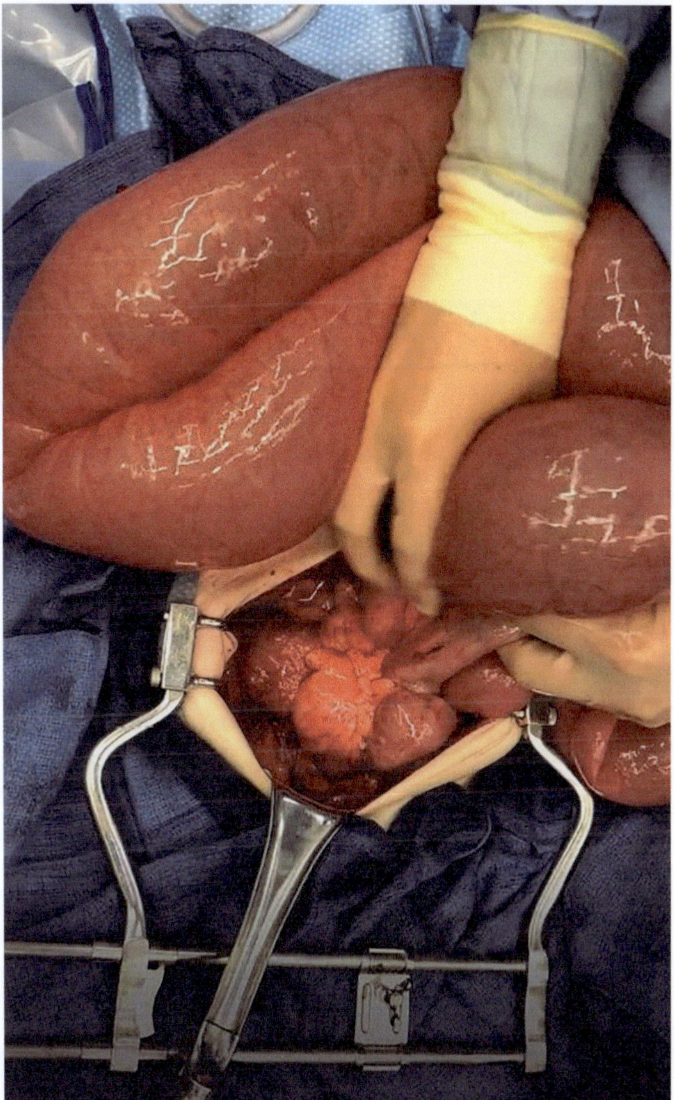

Fig. 7.9 Ileosigmoid fistula with small bowel obstruction caused by stricture

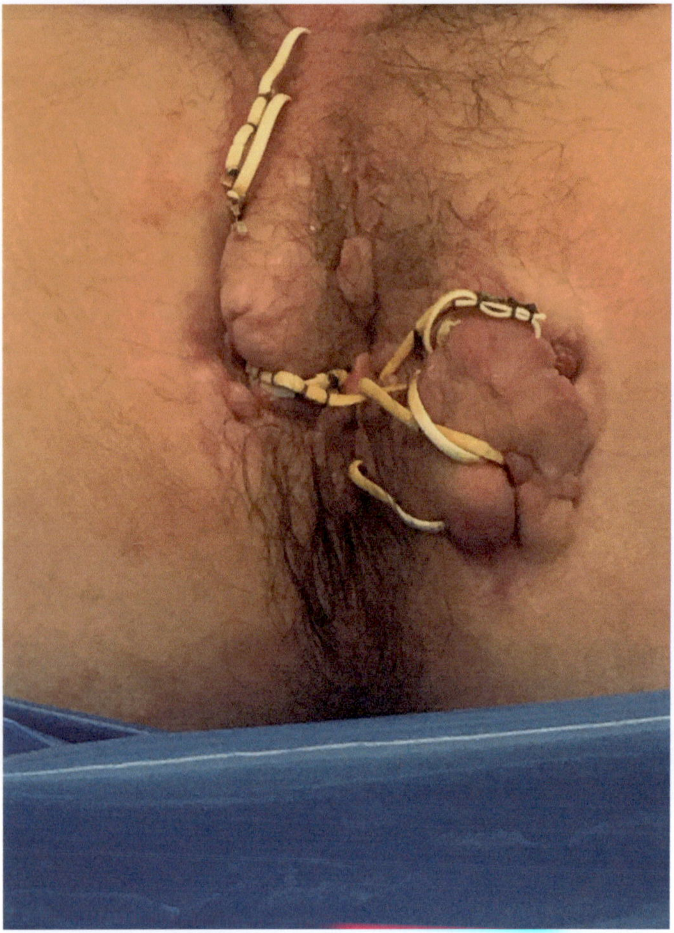

Fig. 7.10 Perianal fistulas with setons

hospitalized patients should be managed with loose draining setons and be coordinated with gastroenterology for starting biologic therapy. Patients with complex perianal disease who are persistently symptomatic despite maximal medical therapy should be counseled that although diversion is an option, remission of symptoms is only seen in under quarter of patients. In one series of 168 patients with severe perianal disease who underwent fecal diversion followed for a mean of 5.7 years, only 22% achieved stoma closure, 33% had stoma with the rectum in situ, and 45% underwent proctectomy [24].

Hemorrhage

Acute hemorrhage due to CD is uncommon. Most of the literature on the topic is small retrospective reviews like a retrospective series of 70 patients noted that the probability of bleeding after diagnosis of Crohn's disease was 1.7%, 3.6%, 6.5%, and 10.3% after 1, 5, 10, and 20 years [25]. In addition to the usual stabilization and resuscitation of GI hemorrhage, localization should first be attempted with institution's standard methods of evaluation including endoscopy, CT angiography, nuclear scan, and/or interventional angiography. Embolization is an option in the setting of limited disease. If a super-selective embolization of the bleeding vessel can't be done due to lack of visualization at the time of angiography, there is another option. One alternate method described by the authors in 2003 is the combined use of preoperative provocative angiography and highly selective methylene blue injection to localize an occult small bowel bleeding site in a patient with Crohn's disease. This methylene blue-guided approach is especially valuable in the setting of multiple small bowel resections and impending short bowel syndrome.

In this case, methylene blue was injected into the bleeding vessel which was identified in the jejunum, allowing a small bowel resection to be performed [26]. This technique was later reviewed by other investigators who used it in four patients preoperatively who also went on to have a limited small bowel resection. [27, 28]

Colitis

Toxic megacolon is a surgical emergency. Upon initial evaluation in the hospital, colitis patients should be divided into those that need emergent surgery and those that need urgent nonoperative management that may need surgery later in the admission. If a patient presents with instability from septic shock, severe hemorrhage, or intestinal perforation, then the management is resuscitation and emergency surgery for subtotal colectomy with end ileostomy. The diagnostic criterion for toxic megacolon is radiographic colonic dilation greater than 5 cm any place in the colon plus any three of the following: fever >38 C (100.4 F), heart rate > 120, neutrophilic leukocytosis >10.5 × 10 [9]/L, anemia, and at least one of the following: dehydration, altered consciousness, electrolyte disturbances, and hypotension [29]. Patients with toxic megacolon require close multidisciplinary care with a low threshold for resection.

In the setting of colitis in a hospitalized patient that has Crohn's disease, a broad differential of colitis should be considered including cytomegalovirus and *Clostridium difficile*; workup should include stool studies, biopsy by judicious flexible sigmoidoscopy, and testing of drug levels if the patient has been on biologic therapy. Coordination of multidisciplinary care is an important factor in medical management and the therapeutic relationship with the patient. Testing should include albumin and prealbumin to assess malnutrition, hemoglobin, C-reactive protein, and fecal calprotectin to establish a baseline and assess laboratory response to medical therapy during admission. If candidates have not seen biologic therapy, we test colitis patients on admission with QuantiFERON-TB gold to be aware of a tuberculosis infection that may affect their ability to be a candidate for biologic therapy. Initial evaluation should include at least an abdominal x-ray to assess for findings which on physical exam and history might be obscured by steroids or biologic therapy. It is important to establish expectation with the patient and the gastroenterology team of how long it is reasonable to pursue medical therapy. Although initial therapy for de novo colitis in a hospitalized patient is intravenous glucocorticoid, it should be understood that after definite window of nonresponse, we typically recommend 72 hours, a second-line therapy, such as a biologic therapy or cyclosporine, should be started. Ideally the patient, surgeon, and gastroenterologist are on the same page that after nonresponse to second-line therapy, surgical options will be more likely. In our institution, these patients are admitted to our IBD service where they are comanaged by IBD gastroenterologists and surgeons, which includes both rounding daily.

In the setting of colitis refractory to medical management in a hospitalized patient, we recommend a subtotal colectomy with end ileostomy leaving the rectosigmoid stump at the base of the line wound if open, or if minimally invasive surgery, then the specimen should be extracted via a low midline wound. Although some advocate minimally invasive total colectomy specimens being brought out of via the ileostomy site in some clinical settings, this is not a setting that we would recommend trans-trephine specimen extraction. Crohn's patients after total colectomy will have a permanent end ileostomy, and bringing a bulky specimen through the trephine incision can be assumed to hasten the formation of a parastomal hernia. The two main purposes of advocating for lower midline extraction with tacking of stump to fascia are to decrease the rate of pelvic sepsis at the index case and to decrease the case of fistula between rectal stump and other organs between the index and second-stage case. Lower midline wounds with tacked rectosigmoid stump act as an extraperitoneal escape valve for the contents of a rectosigmoid stump blowout to avoid pelvic sepsis. Even though the rate of pelvic sepsis in ulcerative colitis patients after subtotal colectomy with intraperitoneal stump is relatively low, the magnitude of insult to the those few patients that do suffer from pelvic sepsis is enough for us to advocate tacking the stump [30, 31]. If the stump does blow out via the extraction site, this can typically be managed with local wound care and potentially placing a stoma bag on the extraction site. The second reason is that it makes the second stage less fraught with complication. After the patient has recovered for 6 months from their index surgery, it will be time for either ileorectal anastomosis or completion proctectomy depending on the extent of rectal inflammation. The rectal stump being tacked to the anterior abdominal wall fascia drastically decreases the chance of it adhering to other bowel, ovaries, bladder, or uterus. It is also easier to enter an untouched presacral plane than one that has been entered during a partial proctectomy at the time of index surgery.

To accomplish fascial closure with tacking of the rectosigmoid stump, we use a series of interrupted figure-of-eight 1 polydioxanone sutures. We affix the stump to the base, by incorporating our figure-of-eight fascial suture closure with bites of the epiploica and fat of the rectosigmoid stump, taking care not to make full-thickness bites into the bowel. If the stump can't reach the abdominal wall well, then we recommend routine transanal placement of a 32 French mushroom catheter in rectal remnant at termination of the surgical procedure. Although there is a paucity of literature on the topic, a series of 41 patients with this routine transanal catheter approach showed an intra-abdominal sepsis rate of 0% [32]. An overly liberal clinical diagnosis of Crohn's disease in these settings can wrongfully eliminate the future option of intestinal continuity via ileal pouch-anal anastomosis. We caution patients being labeled as "Crohn's colitis" in these settings unless they have a preexisting perianal or small bowel involvement as the pathologic diagnosis can be hard to differentiate due to transmural inflammation in the acute setting.

Spontaneous Perforation

Spontaneous perforation is a potentially lethal but relatively rare sequela of CD. A retrospective review found that spontaneous perforation occurred in just 1.5% or 21 of 1415 patients admitted with CD at 1 institution over a 23-year period [33]. In that series 3.3 years was the mean duration from onset of CD symptoms to perforation. Perforations tend to occur in areas of the small or large bowel proximally to segments strictured by chronic disease. Index of suspicion should be high as steroids or biologics can mask typical physical exam finding. In our opinion, most of these perforations are secondary to untimely referral for surgical management. Free perforation requires urgent operative exploration and resection of perforated segment. A laparoscopic approach can be considered if the patient is stable and the extent of bowel dilation doesn't preclude safe entry into the peritoneum; conversion to open should be performed if visualization is inadequate. Although resection is the current standard of care, it should be noted that simple suturing of the perforation was historically attempted with disastrous consequences. In a series of 99 patients, the 3 patients who underwent nonoperative management had 100% mortality. The patients in the series who were treated with a simple suture of perforation suffered a 39% mortality which is 10 times higher than the 4% mortality of those treated with resection and anastomosis. Notably, those treated with resection with diversion had a mortality rate of 0% [34]. After resection is formed, the decision of undiverted primary anastomosis, diverted primary anastomosis, or diversion should be considered. Most patients in the authors' practice would receive primary anastomosis with proximal diversion, although at the extremes of clinical status, others can be considered. An otherwise healthy well-nourished stable patient with minimal contamination and preserved albumin and prealbumin, not on steroids, with healthy bowel, and who could well tolerate rescue from anastomotic leak could be considered for primary anastomosis without diversion. An unstable malnourished patient could be considered for a split ostomy or an end loop in which both open ends of the bowel are brought out via the same trephine incision.

Technical Approach

Surgical management benefits from perioperative coordination. Anesthesia team should be aware preoperatively of the increased risk of bleeding and have large-bore IVs and arterial lines appropriate to the task. This is especially true for patients who require pelvic surgery for which we have a universal policy of arterial line, two large-bore IVs, central line, and ureteral stents for reoperative pelvic surgery. Urologic or gynecologic teams involved in multivisceral disease should have the opportunity to evaluate nonemergent cases preoperatively. Gastroenterology team who will be managing steroids should advise on postoperative taper and planning for postoperative biologic therapy. For patients with severe jejunoileitis and nonsurgical disease remaining in situ, we support biologic therapy starting within 4 weeks after surgery.

The extent of bowel resection has been an area of significant investigation, but as a general principle, we recommend limited bowel resection. Fazio et al. showed in 1996 study of 152 CD patients undergoing resection that recurrence, defined as reoperation for recurrent pre-anastomotic disease, was not different in two randomly assigned groups in which the proximal line of resection was 2 cm (limited resection, pinch test as described above) or 12 cm (extended resection) with a median follow-up of 56 months. He also found that recurrence rates did not increase when microscopic CD was present at the resection margins [35]. This less extensive approach to resection margins is thought to be one of the factors that lead to the decrease in the rates of short bowel syndrome of CD patients [36]. Although more recent studies have shown that histologic positive margins are correlated with endoscopic recurrence of CD based on colonoscopy 6 months after ileocecal resection (56.5% versus 4.8%, $p < 0.001$), it should be appreciated that this is merely endoscopic recurrence which may not correlate with the need for future resection [37].

Distinct from the extent of small bowel resection is the consideration of the extent of mesenteric resection during ileocolic resection. Coffey et al. in 2018 published a study of recurrence in two cohorts: cohort A (n = 30) who underwent conventional ileocolic resections where the mesentery was divided flush with the intestine and cohort B (n = 34) who underwent resections which included excision of the mesentery. Coffey found that the reoperation rates were 40% and 2.9% in cohorts A and B ($P = 0.003$) [38]. While we recommend high ligation of ileocolic artery during ileocolic resection, we caution that high ligation in the setting of phlegmon risks abdominal catastrophe by causing irreparable injury to superior mesenteric artery and vein (Fig. 7.11).

Once the extent of resection is planned, the method of mesenteric division should be considered. The approach for the division of Crohn's mesentery during resection needs to be tailored to the individual segment of mesentery's characteristics. Thin relatively uninflamed mesentery can be divided with traditional approaches or the commonly used electrothermal bipolar tissue sealing systems. The mesentery that is thickened can be controlled by sequential clamping with Kocher clamps, and after it is divided,

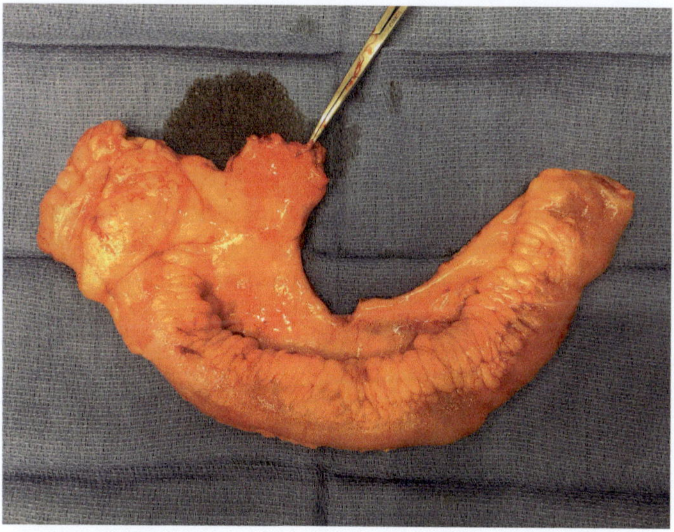

Fig. 7.11 Ileocolic resection specimen with high ligation of ileocolic

then the stumps can be stick-tied with 0 or 1-0 chromic suture in at least three knots. If a bipolar tissue-sealing device is being considered for intermediate tissue, the greatest width sealer available should be used.

Conclusion

Patients hospitalized for Crohn's disease exacerbations are at an increased risk for CD-associated complication than outpatients. Information about the patient's outside records and imaging should be sought if possible. The team should look for strategies that optimize the patient's recovery such as a percutaneous drainage of abscess as a bridge to a less morbid elective surgery. Planning multiple steps ahead can help the surgeon and the multidisciplinary team best construct a plan for the long-term goals of the patient in addition to addressing the issues that brought about hospitalization.

Clinical-Based Vignette and Question

A 35-year-old man with a 10-year history of Crohn's disease is hospitalized with a mid-ileal stricture that is 15 cm in length and angulated. He has been deemed refractory to medical management and reports no weight loss, CRP level is 0, and both albumin and prealbumin are normal. His past surgical history is notable for a resection of 110 cm of the small bowel 6 months ago. What is the most appropriate next step in management (choose one)?

A. Endoscopic dilation
B. Heineke-Mikulicz strictureplasty
C. Finney strictureplasty
D. Side-to-side isoperistaltic strictureplasty
E. Small bowel resection

Correct answer: C

Angulation of stricture and stricture length over 4 cm are contraindications to endoscopic dilation. Finney strictureplasty is recommended for strictures that are 10–20 cm in length, Heineke-Mikulicz strictureplasty is used for strictures under 10 cm, and side-to-side isoperistaltic strictureplasty is used for strictures over 20 cm. Strictureplasty rather than resection should be considered if the patient has a previous history of >100 cm small bowel resection or recurrence after recent resection within the preceding 12 months.

References

1. Molodecky NA, et al. Increasing incidence and prevalence of the inflammatory bowel diseases with time, based on systematic review. Gastroenterology. 2012;142(1):46–54.e42
2. Malarcher CA, Wheaton AG, Liu Y, et al. Hospitalization for Crohn's disease—United States, 2003–2013. MMWR. 2017;66(14):377–81.
3. Dietz DW, Fazio VW, Laureti S, Strong SA, Hull TL, Church J, Remzi FH, Lavery IC, Senagore AJ. Strictureplasty in diffuse Crohn's jejunoileitis: safe and durable. Dis Colon Rectum. 2002;45(6):764–70.

4. Louis E, Collard A, Oger AF, Degroote E, Aboul Nasr El Yafi FA, Belaiche J. Behaviour of Crohn's disease according to the Vienna classification: changing pattern over the course of the disease. Gut. 2001;49:777–82.
5. Broering DC, et al. Strictureplasty for large bowel stenosis in Crohn's disease: quality of life after surgical therapy. Int J Color Dis. 2001;16(2):81–7. https://doi.org/10.1007/s003840000278.
6. Kristo I, Riss S, Argeny S, Maschke S, Chitsabesan P, Stift A. Incidental adenocarcinoma in patients undergoing surgery for stricturing Crohn's disease. World J Gastroenterol. 2017;23(03):472–7.
7. Paine E, Shen B. Endoscopic therapy in inflammatory bowel diseases (with videos). Gastrointest Endosc. 2013;78:819–35.
8. Morar PS, et al. Crohn's stricture study (CroSS) group. Aliment Pharmacol Ther. 2015;42(10):1137–48.
9. Hirai F. Current status of endoscopic balloon dilation for Crohn's disease. Intest Res. 2017;15(2):166–73.
10. Alastruey CL, Murcia XA, Comas ME. The role of stents in the treatment of Crohn's disease strictures. Endosc Int Open. 2016;4(3):E301–8.
11. Laureti S, Fazio VW. Obstruction in Crohn's disease: strictureplasty versus resection. Curr Treat Options Gastroenterol. 2000;3:191–201.
12. Yamamoto T, Fazio VW, Tekkis PP. Safety and efficacy of strictureplasty for Crohn's disease: a systematic review and meta-analysis. Dis Colon Rectum. 2007;50(11):1968–86.
13. Ambe R, Campbell L, Cagir B. A comprehensive review of strictureplasty techniques in Crohn's disease: types, indications, comparisons, and safety. J Gastrointest Surg. 2012;16(1):209–17.
14. Fazio VW, Marchetti F, Church M, et al. Effect of resection margins on the recurrence of Crohn's disease in the small bowel. A randomized controlled trial. Ann Surg. 1996;224(4):563–73.
15. Ribeiro MB, Greenstein AJ, Yamazaki Y, Aufses AH Jr. Intra-abdominal abscess in regional enteritis. Ann Surg. 1991;213(1):32–6.
16. Clancy C, et al. A meta-analysis of percutaneous drainage versus surgery as the initial treatment of Crohn's disease-related intra-abdominal. Abscess J Crohns Colitis. 2016;10(2):202–8.
17. Poritz LS, Koltun WA. Percutaneous drainage and ileocolectomy for spontaneous intraabdominal abscess in Crohn's disease. J Gastrointest Surg. 2007;11(2):204–8.
18. Schwartz DA, Loftus EV Jr, Tremaine WJ, et al. The natural history of fistulizing Crohn's disease in Olmsted County, Minnesota. Gastroenterology. 2002;122:875–80.
19. Siegmund B, Feakins RM, Barmias G, et al. Results of the fifth scientific workshop of the ECCO (II): pathophysiology of perianal fistulizing disease. J Crohns Colitis. 2016;10:377–86.
20. Bell SJ, Williams AB, Wiesel P, et al. The clinical course of fistulating Crohn's disease. Aliment Pharmacol Ther. 2003;17:1145–51.

21. Farmer RG, Hawk WA, Turnbull RB Jr. Clinical patterns in Crohn's disease: a statistical study of 615 cases. Gastroenterology. 1975;68(4 Pt 1):627–35.
22. Broe PJ, Cameron JL. Surgical management of ileosigmoid fistulas in Crohn's disease. Am J Surg. 1982;143(5):611–3.
23. Vogel JD, et al. Clinical practice guideline for the management of anorectal abscess, fistula-in-ano, and rectovaginal fistula. Dis Colon Rectum. 2016;59(12):1117–33.
24. Gu J, Valente MA, Remzi FH, Stocchi L. Factors affecting the fate of faecal diversion in patients with perianal Crohn's disease. Color Dis. 2015;17(1):66–72.
25. Kim K-J, et al. Risk factors and outcome of acute severe lower gastrointestinal bleeding in Crohn's disease. Dig Liver Dis. 2012;44(9):723–8.
26. Remzi FH, et al. Combined use of preoperative provocative angiography and highly selective methylene blue injection to localize an occult small-bowel bleeding site in a patient with Crohn's disease: report of a case. Dis Colon Rectum. 2003;46(2):260–3.
27. Pai M, et al. Preoperative superselective mesenteric angiography and methylene blue injection for localization of obscure gastrointestinal bleeding. JAMA Surg. 2013;148(7):665–8.
28. Gifford SM, et al. Methylene blue enteric mapping for intraoperative localization in obscure small bowel hemorrhage: report of a new technique and literature review: combined intraoperative methylene blue mapping and enterectomy. J Gastrointest Surg. 2012;16(11):2177–81.
29. Jalan KN, et al. An experience of ulcerative colitis. Toxic dilation in 55 cases. Gastroenterology. 1969;57(1):68–82.
30. Carter FM, McLeod RS, Cohen Z. Subtotal colectomy for ulcerative colitis: complications related to the rectal remnant. Dis Colon Rectum. 1991;34(11):1005–9.
31. Jinyu G, et al. Intraperitoneal or subcutaneous: does location of the (colo) rectal stump influence outcomes after laparoscopic total abdominal colectomy for ulcerative colitis? Dis Colon Rectum. 2013;56(5):615–21.
32. Karch LA, et al. Subtotal colectomy with Hartmann's pouch for inflammatory bowel disease. Dis Colon Rectum. 1995;38(6):635–9.
33. Greenstein AJ, Sachar DB, Mann D, et al. Spontaneous free perforation and perforated abscess in 30 patients with Crohn's disease. Ann Surg. 1987;205:72–6.
34. Greenstein AJ, Mann D, Sachar DB, Aufses AH Jr. Free perforation in Crohn's disease: I. A survey of 99 cases. Am J Gastroenterol. 1985;80(9):682–9.
35. Fazio VW, et al. Effect of resection margins on the recurrence of Crohn's disease in the small bowel. A randomized controlled trial. Ann Surg. 1996;224(4):563–73.
36. Thompson JS. Short bowel syndrome and malabsorption – causes and prevention. Viszeralmedizin. 2014;30(3):174–8.

37. Poredska K, et al. The influence of microscopic inflammation at resection margins on early postoperative endoscopic recurrence after ileocaecal resection for Crohn's disease. J Crohn's Colitis. 2020;14(3):361–8.
38. Coffey CJ, et al. Inclusion of the mesentery in ileocolic resection for Crohn's disease is associated with reduced surgical recurrence. J Crohns Colitis. 2018;12(10):1139–50.

8 Management of Hospitalized Patients with Inflammatory Bowel Disease and CMV Infection or Clostridium Difficile Infection

Sara El Ouali and Jean-Paul Achkar

Introduction

Patients hospitalized with inflammatory bowel disease (IBD) can often have a superimposed infection as a contributing factor to their disease flare. In particular, *Clostridioides difficile* and cytomegalovirus infection can both complicate the course of IBD and are associated with adverse outcomes. Early recognition and treatment are key. In this chapter we will review risk factors and course for these infections and also discuss diagnosis and treatment approaches.

S. El Ouali
Digestive Disease Institute, Cleveland Clinic, Abu Dhabi, UAE
e-mail: ElOualS2@ClevelandClinicAbuDhabi.ae

J.-P. Achkar (✉)
Department of Gastroenterology, Hepatology and Nutrition, Cleveland Clinic, Cleveland, OH, USA
e-mail: achkarj@ccf.org

J. D. Feuerstein, A. S. Cheifetz (eds.), *Management of Inpatient Inflammatory Bowel Disease*,
https://doi.org/10.1007/978-1-0716-1987-2_8

Clostridioides difficile Infection

Clostridioides difficile (*C. difficile*) is a spore-forming, toxin-producing, gram-positive anaerobic bacillus which is transmitted via fecal-oral route [1]. Patients with IBD are at increased risk of *C. difficile* infection (CDI), which is associated with increased morbidity and mortality [2]. Symptoms of CDI and IBD flares are similar and often overlap including diarrhea, blood in the stool, fever, and abdominal pain [2]. Given the nonspecific presentation of CDI in IBD, all patients hospitalized with worsening symptoms should be tested for CDI [1]. Recent antibiotic use is not as common in patients with IBD compared to non-IBD patients [3] and should therefore not be a primary consideration when considering whether to test for *C. difficile* [1].

Epidemiology

CDI is a significant public health problem with 500,000 infections and up to 30,000 deaths in the United States every year [4]. In addition, *C. difficile* is common among inpatients. In one study, *C. difficile* was found in up to 10% of asymptomatic inpatients, and more than one third of them progressed to symptomatic CDI [5]. Patients with IBD are at particularly increased risk of CDI with an eight-time higher frequency in ulcerative colitis (UC) and a five-time higher frequency in Crohn's disease (CD) compared to the general population [6]. Among patients hospitalized with an IBD flare, the incidence of CDI is up to 12.9% [2, 7] and has continued to increase in recent years [6].

Risk Factors

Although IBD itself is a risk factor for CDI, other traditional risk factors for CDI may not be present in patients with IBD [1]. A recent meta-analysis of 24 retrospective studies found that colonic involvement and biologic and antibiotic use were associated with an increased risk of CDI in IBD [8]. Compared with the general population, CDI in IBD has several atypical features: it occurs at a younger age, is more often community acquired, and is less frequently associated with antibiotic use [1].

Outcomes

Patients with IBD complicated by CDI have an increased risk of complications and a worse prognosis compared to patients with IBD alone [9]. Inpatients with IBD and CDI have increased risks of readmission [10], colectomy [10–12], and postoperative complications [12] along with longer hospital stays [9, 10]. Hospitalized patients with IBD and CDI also have a four-time greater risk of mortality than patients with IBD alone or CDI alone [11].

In addition, patients with IBD are 33% more likely to have recurrent CDI compared with the general population [13].

Diagnosis

Stool-Based Diagnostic Tests

When assessing for CDI, it is important to differentiate between asymptomatic carriage and true infection. Therefore, only patients with active symptoms should be tested [1]. The optimal approach to diagnosing CDI relies on a two-step method. Initially, glutamate dehydrogenase (GDH) antigen testing using enzyme immunoassay (EIA) should be performed [1]. This is a highly sensitive test as GDH is present in all *C. difficile* strains and has a rapid turnaround time. If positive, this test should be followed by toxin A and B testing (using EIA) in order to detect toxin production indicating true infection [14]. If results are discordant, nucleic acid amplification test (NAAT), a highly sensitive test which detects toxigenic strains, can be used [1]. Although NAAT can be used alone, a two-step algorithm is generally preferred as NAAT does not test for toxin production and may lead to overdiagnosis of CDI [4]. NAAT can also be used as part of a two-step algorithm followed by toxin testing [4].

Other tests for CDI include toxigenic culture or cell culture cytotoxicity neutralization assay, but are cumbersome and slow and therefore not recommended for routine use [4].

Endoscopic Features

Endoscopic features of CDI are nonspecific in IBD. The classic finding of pseudomembranes (Fig. 8.1) is found in 31–50% of patients with CDI without concurrent IBD [15, 16] and is even less common in IBD [2]. In two retrospective studies of patients with CDI, pseudomembranes were found on lower endoscopy in none of the IBD patients in one study (compared to half of patients without IBD) and in 13% of IBD patients in the other study [17]. In another retrospective study, the most common endoscopic

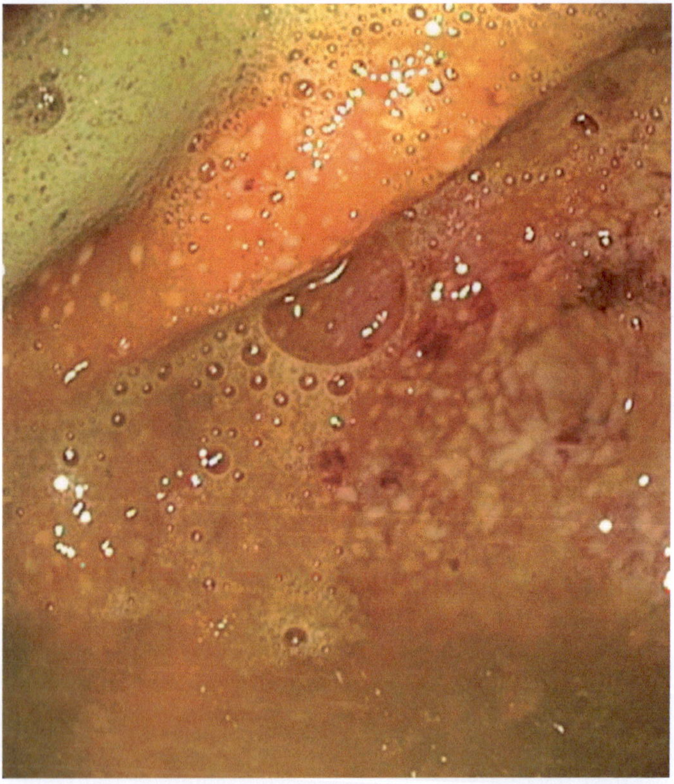

Fig. 8.1 Pseudomembranes seen on colonoscopy in a patient with ulcerative colitis complicated by *Clostridioides difficile* infection

finding of CDI-associated IBD was mucus and pus; pseudomembranes were not seen [14].

Histologic Features

Histologic findings are nonspecific, although the presence of microscopic pseudomembranes can be suggestive of CDI [15]. In a retrospective analysis of patients hospitalized with a UC exacerbation, 44.4% of patients with concurrent CDI had microscopic pseudomembranes compared with only 11% of patients without CDI. No other histopathologic features were found to be predictive of CDI in these patients [18].

Management

Treatment of *C. difficile* Infection

Management of CDI is tailored to the severity of the presentation. According to the 2017 Infectious Diseases Society of America (IDSA) practice guidelines, vancomycin 125 mg orally four times daily or fidaxomicin 200 mg twice daily for 10 days should be used for a first episode of CDI [4]. These agents are preferred over metronidazole, which is no longer listed as a first-line therapy due to recent randomized controlled data demonstrating the superiority of other agents in this setting [4, 19].

Specifically in patients with IBD, retrospective data have shown vancomycin to be superior to metronidazole in patients hospitalized with IBD and CDI, leading to reduced length of stay and fewer readmissions [1, 20]. The choice of vancomycin as first-line therapy in IBD is supported by recent IBD practice guidelines [1, 21]. The recommended duration of treatment is 10–14 days [4]. Interestingly, a recent retrospective study showed reduced rates of CDI recurrence among patients with IBD receiving a longer duration of vancomycin treatment (21–42 days) compared with a standard duration of treatment (10–14 days) [9].

In fulminant CDI (defined as CDI complicated by hypotension, shock, ileus, or megacolon), vancomycin 500 mg orally 4 times daily in addition to rectal vancomycin in the case of an ileus is recommended by the IDSA guidelines, despite the lack of high-quality evidence for both recommendations in this setting [4]. Intravenous metronidazole 500 mg 3 times daily should be added as well, especially in the setting of an ileus [4]. Colectomy may be necessary in fulminant CDI refractory to medical therapy in particular in patients with megacolon, acute abdomen, perforation, or shock [4]. Surgical management of hospitalized patients with IBD is further discussed in Chaps. 4 and 7.

Fecal Microbiota Transplantation (FMT) in Hospitalized Patients with Severe CDI

FMT has been evaluated in severe CDI and is associated with anywhere from 50 to 91% cure rates in the overall population [22–24]. However, data in patients with IBD are limited. Several studies assessing FMT in IBD included a small number of patients with severe CDI and have found success rates ranging from 75 to 79% [25–27].

Of note, FMT also appears to be less effective for recurrent CDI in the setting of IBD [2]. In a prospective study evaluating colonoscopy-delivered FMT in CDI, only 74.4% of patients with IBD cleared CDI as opposed to 92.1% of patients without IBD [21]. In addition, about a quarter of patients with IBD experienced a disease exacerbation after the procedure which has also been reported in other studies [3].

Managing Immunosuppression in the Setting of C. *difficile* Infection

Managing immunosuppression in a patient with IBD and CDI remains controversial with divergence in opinions and limited evidence to guide the optimal approach [28]. In a multicenter retrospective study, patients with IBD and CDI who were on immunomodulators and antibiotics had worse outcomes including increased risk of death and colectomy within 3 months compared to patients on antibiotics only [29]. However more recent data found no such association including a multicenter retrospective study, which showed that immunosuppressive therapies were not associated with increased mortality and colectomy rates, but other factors such as low serum albumin, high creatinine, and low hemoglobin were associated with adverse outcomes [30]. Furthermore, another study showed that escalation of therapy to biologics or corticosteroids within 90 days of an episode of CDI was not associated with worse outcomes [31]. Based on available data, an expert review panel on CDI in IBD does not recommend withholding immunosuppression in patients with severe IBD and considers escalation of immunosuppressive therapy to be reasonable after a few days of antibiotic therapy [1]. However, it is emphasized that management of immunosuppressive therapy in patients with IBD and concurrent CDI should be individualized [1].

Cytomegalovirus Infection

Cytomegalovirus (CMV) is a DNA virus and part of the *Herpesviridae* family. CMV colitis can occur in the setting of severe or steroid-refractory colitis and is associated with adverse outcomes in patients with IBD. Although several sensitive and specific tests are available to diagnose CMV, the challenge remains in distinguishing latent CMV infection from true CMV disease. Therefore, determining whether CMV is an "innocent bystander" or a true pathogen is still controversial, perhaps due to conflicting evidence given a lack of accepted definitions and diagnostic gold standard [41]. CMV colitis is associated with adverse outcomes including increased risks of medically refractory disease, hospitalization, and colectomy [21, 32, 33].

Epidemiology

CMV seroprevalence in the general population ranges from 40 to 100% [34]. Although the primary infection is often asymptomatic, it persists and leads to latent infection. It can therefore subsequently reactivate, especially in the setting of immunosuppression [35, 36].

CMV colitis occurs in about 14–21% of patients with IBD admitted with severe colitis with an even higher prevalence of 33–36% in steroid-refractory colitis [32, 37]. The prevalence of CMV infection appears to be higher in UC than in CD [38, 39].

Risk Factors

Corticosteroids, cyclosporine, and immunomodulators (including thiopurines and methotrexate) have all been found to increase the risk of CMV reactivation or infection. Antitumor necrosis factors, however, have not been found to increase the risk of CMV infection [33].

In addition, age older than 30 years, refractory disease, splenomegaly, absence of leukocytosis, and CMV DNA > 2000 copies per mL plasma have also been identified as possible risk factors for CMV colitis [39]. Given that IBD patients admitted to the hospital have multiple of these risk factors, a high degree of suspicion must be maintained.

Clinical Presentation

Although most primary CMV infections are asymptomatic, they can occasionally lead to a mononucleosis-like syndrome [36]. CMV reactivation (detection of CMV in a CMV-seropositive patient due to recurrent infection by the same strain) [40] appears to be common and is also often asymptomatic in patients with IBD on immunosuppressive therapy [35, 39, 41]. In a case-control study, CMV reactivation in patients with an IBD flare did not have an impact on the clinical course [41]. Antiviral therapy is not necessary for reactivation and immunosuppression can generally be continued [42]. In a prospective study of patients hospitalized with moderate to severe UC on immunosuppressive therapy, 70% were immunoglobulin G (IgG) positive at baseline and 52% of them reactivated over an 8-week period. None of them had evidence of CMV infection on colon biopsies. Colectomy and remission rates were the same regardless of CMV status or reactivation and despite not receiving antiviral therapy [35].

CMV reactivation has to be distinguished from CMV colitis, which is associated with a severe course and adverse outcomes [40, 43]. Clinical features often overlap with those of IBD, but in addition, systemic symptoms such as fever, cervical lymphadenopathy, and splenomegaly may be present. Leukopenia and thrombocytopenia appear to be more common in patients with documented CMV colitis [43–45].

Patients with IBD and CMV were also found to have more severe weight loss and higher C-reactive protein (CRP) levels than patients without CMV [45].

Diagnosis

Who Should Be Tested?

The American College of Gastroenterology (ACG) UC guidelines recommend that all patients hospitalized with acute severe UC undergo a sigmoidoscopy with biopsies to rule out CMV within 72 hours of admission [21]. In order to help identify patients with IBD at increased risk for CMV colitis, a model was developed using variables that were found to be independently associated with CMV disease including immunomodulator therapy, refractory disease, and age older than 30 years [46]. The model allows calculation of a CMV risk score which had moderate accuracy in distinguishing IBD patients with CMV from those without infection.

Diagnostic Tests

Although multiple modalities are available to test for the presence of CMV, the challenge in diagnosing CMV remains in distinguishing true CMV colitis from latent CMV.

CMV culture can be done on blood and tissue, including colon biopsies. Although highly specific, it is not helpful in identifying patients with CMV colitis given a long incubation period and lower sensitivity than other modalities [43].

Serology can diagnose latent or active infection (through IgG or IgM status) but cannot help identify patients with CMV colitis [39]. Although a positive IgG means a patient with IBD can potentially be susceptible to CMV reactivation, this is not clinically relevant and should not impact the choice of immunosuppressive therapy in patients with IBD [42].

CMV DNA can be measured through PCR testing and can be done in blood or colonic tissue with rapidly available results. Studies report different ranges of accuracy given no accepted gold standard [47]. However, a recent study which defined the gold standard as antiviral responsive CMV colitis (as a marker of true disease instead of latent CMV) found a sensitivity of 100% and specificity of 94% for blood-based CMV PCR in diagnosing CMV colitis. This is especially helpful as a negative result can help rule out CMV colitis in this setting [45]. However, the optimal cutoff value for quantitative tissue PCR has not yet been determined [36, 48]. The CMV DNA load in colon biopsies has been found to correlate with clinical response to immunosuppressive treatments [39]. In two prospective studies assessing patients with moderate to severe UC flares complicated by CMV, a CMV DNA load in colon biopsies higher than 250 copies/milligram of tissue was predictive of a medically refractory course [49, 50]. In contrast, a retrospective study did not find a correlation between CMV DNA load and colectomy rates [51].

Endoscopic examination and biopsies are an essential part of the diagnostic algorithm [39]. Ulcers have been found to be a predictor of CMV colitis in several studies [52–54]. Endoscopic findings such as irregular ulcerations, wide mucosal defects, punched out ulcerations, and longitudinal ulcerations may be suggestive of CMV infection in patients with UC [55]. Punched out or longitudinal ulcers were found to have a sensitivity and specificity above 70% for the diagnosis of CMV colitis in this setting [55]. Interestingly, in a small prospective study, patients with UC and CMV without large ulcers on endoscopy did well without antiviral therapy, as opposed to patients with deep ulcers, who, despite antiviral therapy, eventually had worsening of their UC course [54]. Multiple biopsies are recommended as the distribution of CMV disease may be patchy [39, 53]. In addition, biopsies from the ulcer base appear to have a higher yield [21].

Histopathology appears to be the most useful modality in diagnosing CMV colitis, through hematoxylin and eosin (H&E) staining and immunohistochemistry (IHC) [39]. H&E staining may show intranuclear eosinophilic inclusions surrounded by clear cytoplasm within enlarged cells, giving it the typical “owl’s eye” appearance [36] (Figure 8.2a). The sensitivity of H&E is

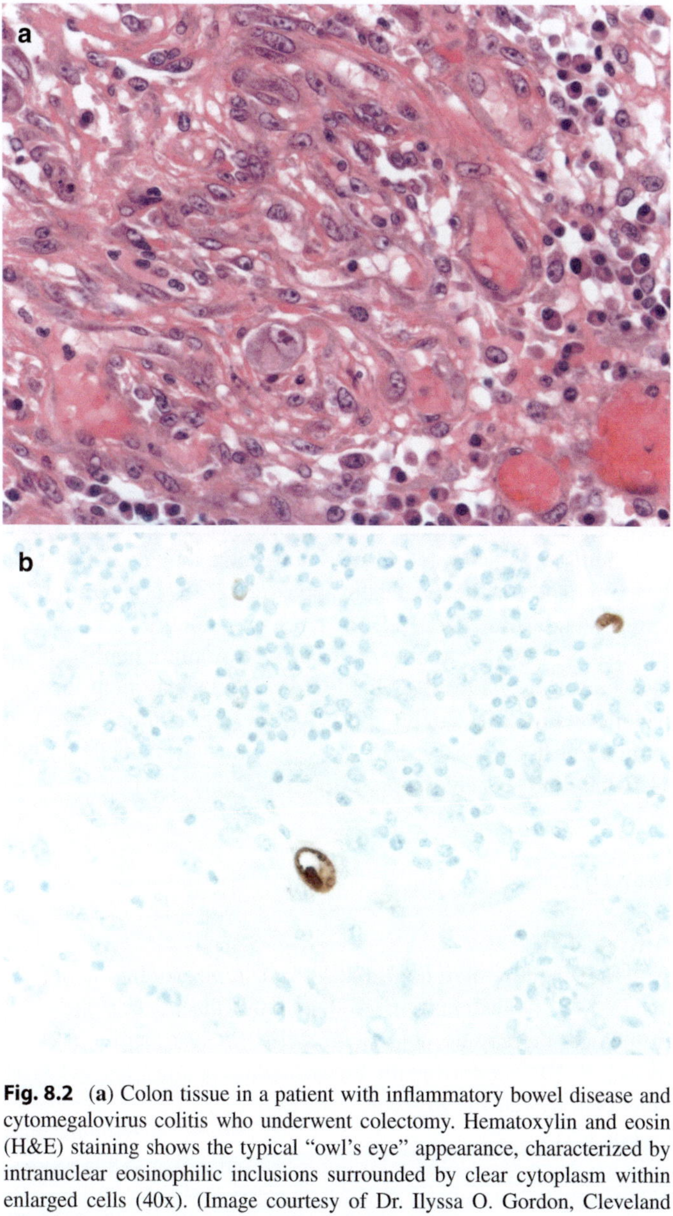

Fig. 8.2 (**a**) Colon tissue in a patient with inflammatory bowel disease and cytomegalovirus colitis who underwent colectomy. Hematoxylin and eosin (H&E) staining shows the typical "owl's eye" appearance, characterized by intranuclear eosinophilic inclusions surrounded by clear cytoplasm within enlarged cells (40x). (Image courtesy of Dr. Ilyssa O. Gordon, Cleveland Clinic) (**b**) Immunohistochemistry confirms cytomegalovirus (40x). (Image courtesy of Dr. Ilyssa O. Gordon, Cleveland Clinic)

low [52] but can be increased with IHC which uses antibodies against the CMV antigen pp65 [36] (Figure 8.2b). The sensitivity and specificity of immunohistochemistry are 67% and 98%, respectively [39].

The density of CMV cells on colon biopsies appears to be associated with clinical outcomes. Having five or more CMV-positive cells by IHC on colon biopsies was found to be associated with an increased risk of colectomy [47]. In another study, a higher density of inclusion bodies in biopsies was associated with improved response to antiviral therapy [56].

Approach to Diagnosis

Overall, although multiple tests are available, the most useful approach still relies on the identification of CMV in colonic tissue [39]. Biopsies for histopathology and IHC can be combined with CMV PCR testing in the blood or colonic tissue [42, 43]. Although societal guidelines emphasize the importance of ruling out CMV in patients with acute steroid-resistant colitis, they do not provide clear guidance on the diagnostic approach [21, 57]. The European Crohn's and Colitis Organisation (ECCO) guidelines recommend ruling out CMV "preferably by tissue PCR or immunohistochemistry" and suggest testing blood CMV DNA "may help identify patients with CMV colitis" [42]. ACG UC guidelines state that "immunohistochemistry staining, rapid viral culture methods, and PCR-based assays are the preferred modalities" [21].

Management

Antiviral Therapy

Antiviral therapy may not be necessary in all patients with IBD and CMV [21]. Patients with IBD with mild disease or responding to medical therapy do not appear to benefit from antiviral treatment [58–60], supporting the theory that CMV may also act as an "innocent bystander" in some cases [39].

For CMV colitis however, antiviral therapy in patients with IBD has been associated with improved outcomes and is recommended by ECCO and ACG guidelines [21, 42].

Recent evidence appears to support the importance of antiviral therapy in patients with IBD complicated by CMV colitis. A meta-analysis which stratified for disease severity found antiviral therapy to be associated with lower rates of colectomy specifically in patients with steroid-refractory disease [60]. In a case-control study, antiviral therapy in patients with IBD and concomitant CMV disease reduced the rate of colectomy, especially in patients with five or more viral inclusions in each biopsy specimen [56]. Antiviral treatment with ganciclovir has also been associated with increased rates of clinical remission at 6 months [50].

Intravenous ganciclovir is the treatment of choice for CMV colitis, although this is supported by limited retrospective data in IBD [21, 42]. It is given at a dose of 5 mg/kg twice a day, over 2–3 weeks. Intravenous ganciclovir can be transitioned to oral valganciclovir after 3–5 days depending on the patient's response [42].

Oral valganciclovir has been evaluated for CMV disease in patients with solid organ transplants and appears to be equivalent to intravenous ganciclovir [61, 62]. Although there are no data supporting this in IBD, oral valganciclovir may be an option in some selected patients [21, 39].

However, in a small retrospective study in patients with IBD and CMV colitis, a 2-week treatment with oral valganciclovir was associated with more colectomies and decreased clinical response than 2-week intravenous ganciclovir [63].

Ganciclovir may lead to side effects such as myelosuppression in up to 40% of patients, as well as nausea, vomiting, rash, and headaches [43]. Foscarnet can be used in case of intolerance or suspected resistance to ganciclovir [36]. However, colectomy should not be delayed in patients with medically refractory severe disease based on the presence of CMV in the colon [21].

Although 70–79% of patients with IBD and CMV colitis respond to ganciclovir therapy [21, 32, 64]recurrence rates can be as high as 57% [32].

Immunosuppression in the Setting of CMV

Whether immunosuppression should be held during treatment for CMV colitis remains controversial and is guided by limited evidence [39]. In a small prospective study of patients with IBD and CMV infection (as diagnosed by positive serology or CMV DNA in colon tissue), CMV infection did not progress despite the administration of infliximab [65]. In a multicenter retrospective study of patients hospitalized with UC and CMV colitis, no difference in colectomy rates was found between patients receiving antivirals only and patients receiving antivirals with immunosuppressive therapy, including infliximab and/or cyclosporine [57]. However, ECCO guidelines do recommend discontinuation of immunosuppressive therapy in patients with severe steroid-refractory colitis until "colitis symptoms improve."

Conclusion

C. difficile and CMV can both complicate the course of IBD and are associated with adverse outcomes. In the right clinical context, it is essential to test for the presence of a superimposed infection and initiate adequate treatment. The management of immunosuppressive therapy in this setting has to be individualized, but both the infection and underlying IBD have to be aggressively treated.

Disclosure The authors declared no financial conflict of interest.

References

1. Khanna S, Shin A, Kelly CP. Management of Clostridium difficile infection in inflammatory bowel disease: expert review from the clinical practice updates committee of the AGA Institute. Clin Gastroenterol Hepatol. 2017;15(2):166–74.
2. D'Aoust J, Battat R, Bessissow T. Management of inflammatory bowel disease with Clostridium difficile infection. World J Gastroenterol. 2017;23(27):4986–5003.
3. Bossuyt P, Verhaegen J, Van Assche G, Rutgeerts P, Vermeire S. Increasing incidence of Clostridium difficile-associated diarrhea in inflammatory bowel disease. J Crohns Colitis. 2009;3(1):4–7.

4. McDonald LC, Gerding DN, Johnson S, Bakken JS, Carroll KC, Coffin SE, et al. Clinical practice guidelines for Clostridium difficile infection in adults and children: 2017 update by the Infectious Diseases Society of America (IDSA) and Society for Healthcare Epidemiology of America (SHEA). Clin Infect Dis. 2018;66(7):e1–e48.
5. Baron SW, Ostrowsky BE, Nori P, Drory DY, Levi MH, Szymczak WA, et al. Screening of Clostridioides difficile carriers in an urban academic medical center: understanding implications of disease. Infect Control Hosp Epidemiol. 2020;41(2):149–53.
6. Ricciardi R, Ogilvie JW Jr, Roberts PL, Marcello PW, Concannon TW, Baxter NN. Epidemiology of Clostridium difficile colitis in hospitalized patients with inflammatory bowel diseases. Dis Colon Rectum. 2009;52(1):40–5.
7. Axelrad JE, Joelson A, Nobel YR, Lawlor G, Green PHR, Lichtiger S, et al. Enteric infection in relapse of inflammatory bowel disease: the utility of stool microbial PCR testing. Inflamm Bowel Dis. 2017;23(6):1034–9.
8. Balram B, Battat R, Al-Khoury A, D'Aoust J, Afif W, Bitton A, et al. Risk factors associated with Clostridium difficile infection in inflammatory bowel disease: a systematic review and meta-analysis. J Crohns Colitis. 2019;13(1):27–38.
9. Lei DK, Ollech JE, Andersen M, Weisshof R, Zmeter N, Sossenheimer P, et al. Long-duration Oral vancomycin to treat Clostridioides difficile in patients with inflammatory bowel disease is associated with a low rate of recurrence. Am J Gastroenterol. 2019;114(12):1904–8.
10. Chen XL, Deng J, Chen X, Wan SS, Wang Y, Cao Q. High incidence and morbidity of Clostridium difficile infection among hospitalized patients with inflammatory bowel disease: a prospective observational cohort study. J Dig Dis. 2019;20(9):460–6.
11. Ananthakrishnan AN, McGinley EL, Binion DG. Excess hospitalisation burden associated with Clostridium difficile in patients with inflammatory bowel disease. Gut. 2008;57(2):205–10.
12. Negrón ME, Rezaie A, Barkema HW, Rioux K, De Buck J, Checkley S, et al. Ulcerative colitis patients with Clostridium difficile are at increased risk of death, colectomy, and postoperative complications: a population-based inception cohort study. Am J Gastroenterol. 2016;111(5):691–704.
13. Razik R, Rumman A, Bahreini Z, McGeer A, Nguyen GC. Recurrence of Clostridium difficile infection in patients with inflammatory bowel disease: the RECIDIVISM study. Am J Gastroenterol. 2016;111(8):1141–6.
14. Surawicz CM, Brandt LJ, Binion DG, Ananthakrishnan AN, Curry SR, Gilligan PH, et al. Guidelines for diagnosis, treatment, and prevention of Clostridium difficile infections. Am J Gastroenterol. 2013;108(4):478–98.
15. Issa M, Ananthakrishnan AN, Binion DG. Clostridium difficile and inflammatory bowel disease. Inflamm Bowel Dis. 2008;14(10):1432–42.

16. Seppälä K, Hjelt L, Sipponen P. Colonoscopy in the diagnosis of antibiotic-associated colitis. A prospective study. Scand J Gastroenterol. 1981;16(4):465–8.
17. Ben-Horin S, Margalit M, Bossuyt P, Maul J, Shapira Y, Bojic D, et al. Prevalence and clinical impact of endoscopic pseudomembranes in patients with inflammatory bowel disease and Clostridium difficile infection. J Crohns Colitis. 2010;4(2):194–8.
18. Wang T, Matukas L, Streutker CJ. Histologic findings and clinical characteristics in acutely symptomatic ulcerative colitis patients with superimposed Clostridium difficile infection. Am J Clin Pathol. 2013;140(6):831–7.
19. Johnson S, Louie TJ, Gerding DN, Cornely OA, Chasan-Taber S, Fitts D, et al. Vancomycin, metronidazole, or tolevamer for Clostridium difficile infection: results from two multinational, randomized, controlled trials. Clin Infect Dis. 2014;59(3):345–54.
20. Horton HA, Dezfoli S, Berel D, Hirsch J, Ippoliti A, McGovern D, et al. Antibiotics for treatment of Clostridium difficile infection in hospitalized patients with inflammatory bowel disease. Antimicrob Agents Chemother. 2014;58(9):5054–9.
21. Rubin DT, Ananthakrishnan AN, Siegel CA, Sauer BG, Long MD. ACG clinical guideline: ulcerative colitis in adults. Am J Gastroenterol. 2019;114(3):384–413.
22. Fischer M, Sipe B, Cheng Y-W, Phelps E, Rogers N, Sagi S, et al. Fecal microbiota transplant in severe and severe-complicated Clostridium difficile: a promising treatment approach. Gut Microbes. 2017;8(3):289–302.
23. Ianiro G, Masucci L, Quaranta G, Simonelli C, Lopetuso LR, Sanguinetti M, et al. Randomised clinical trial: faecal microbiota transplantation by colonoscopy plus vancomycin for the treatment of severe refractory Clostridium difficile infection—single versus multiple infusions. Aliment Pharmacol Ther. 2018;48(2):152–9.
24. Agrawal M, Aroniadis OC, Brandt LJ, Kelly C, Freeman S, Surawicz C, et al. The Long-term efficacy and safety of fecal microbiota transplant for recurrent, severe, and complicated Clostridium difficile infection in 146 elderly individuals. J Clin Gastroenterol. 2016;50(5):403–7.
25. Fischer M, Kao D, Kelly C, Kuchipudi A, Jafri S-M, Blumenkehl M, et al. Fecal microbiota transplantation is safe and efficacious for recurrent or refractory Clostridium difficile infection in patients with inflammatory bowel disease. Inflamm Bowel Dis. 2016;22(10):2402–9.
26. Meighani A, Hart BR, Bourgi K, Miller N, John A, Ramesh M. Outcomes of fecal microbiota transplantation for Clostridium difficile infection in patients with inflammatory bowel disease. Dig Dis Sci. 2017;62(10):2870–5.
27. Hirten RP, Grinspan A, Fu S-C, Luo Y, Suarez-Farinas M, Rowland J, et al. Microbial engraftment and efficacy of fecal microbiota transplant

for clostridium difficile in patients with and without inflammatory bowel disease. Inflamm Bowel Dis. 2019;25(6):969–79.
28. Yanai H, Nguyen GC, Yun L, Lebwohl O, Navaneethan U, Stone CD, et al. Practice of gastroenterologists in treating flaring inflammatory bowel disease patients with clostridium difficile: antibiotics alone or combined antibiotics/immunomodulators? Inflamm Bowel Dis. 2010;17(7):1540–6.
29. Ben-Horin S, Margalit M, Bossuyt P, Maul J, Shapira Y, Bojic D, et al. Combination immunomodulator and antibiotic treatment in patients with inflammatory bowel disease and Clostridium difficile infection. Clin Gastroenterol Hepatol. 2009;7(9):981–7.
30. Ananthakrishnan AN, Guzman-Perez R, Gainer V, Cai T, Churchill S, Kohane I, et al. Predictors of severe outcomes associated with Clostridium difficile infection in patients with inflammatory bowel disease. Aliment Pharmacol Ther. 2012;35(7):789–95.
31. Lukin DJ, Lawlor G, Hudesman DP, Durbin L, Axelrad JE, Passi M, et al. Escalation of immunosuppressive therapy for inflammatory bowel disease is not associated with adverse outcomes after infection with Clostridium difficile. Inflamm Bowel Dis. 2019;25(4):775–81.
32. Oh SJ, Lee CK, Kim Y-W, Jeong SJ, Park YM, Oh CH, et al. True cytomegalovirus colitis is a poor prognostic indicator in patients with ulcerative colitis flares: the 10-year experience of an academic referral inflammatory bowel disease center. Scand J Gastroenterol. 2019;54(8):976–83.
33. Pillet S, Pozzetto B, Roblin X. Cytomegalovirus and ulcerative colitis: place of antiviral therapy. World J Gastroenterol. 2016;22(6):2030–45.
34. Krech U. Complement-fixing antibodies against cytomegalovirus in different parts of the world. Bull World Health Organ. 1973;49(1):103–6.
35. Matsuoka K, Iwao Y, Mori T, Sakuraba A, Yajima T, Hisamatsu T, et al. Cytomegalovirus is frequently reactivated and disappears without antiviral agents in ulcerative colitis patients. Am J Gastroenterol. 2007;102(2):331–7.
36. Sager K, Alam S, Bond A, Chinnappan L, Probert CS. Review article: cytomegalovirus and inflammatory bowel disease. Aliment Pharmacol Ther. 2015;41(8):725–33.
37. Criscuoli V, Casà A, Orlando A, Pecoraro G, Oliva L, Traina M, et al. Severe acute colitis associated with CMV: a prevalence study. Dig Liver Dis. 2004;36(12).818–20.
38. Roblin X, Pillet S, Berthelot P, Del Tedesco E, Phelip J-M, Chambonnière M-L, et al. Prevalence of cytomegalovirus infection in steroid-refractory Crohn's disease. Inflamm Bowel Dis. 2012;18(7):E1396–E7.
39. Siegmund B. Cytomegalovirus infection associated with inflammatory bowel disease. Lancet Gastroenterol Hepatol. 2017;2(5):369–76.
40. Ljungman P, Boeckh M, Hirsch HH, Josephson F, Lundgren J, Nichols G, et al. Definitions of cytomegalovirus infection and disease in transplant patients for use in clinical trials. Clin Infect Dis. 2017;64(1):87–91.

41. Delvincourt M, Lopez A, Pillet S, Bourrier A, Seksik P, Cosnes J, et al. The impact of cytomegalovirus reactivation and its treatment on the course of inflammatory bowel disease. Aliment Pharmacol Ther. 2014;39(7):712–20.
42. Rahier JF, Magro F, Abreu C, Armuzzi A, Ben-Horin S, Chowers Y, et al. Second European evidence-based consensus on the prevention, diagnosis and management of opportunistic infections in inflammatory bowel disease. J Crohn's Colitis. 2014;8(6):443–68.
43. Kandiel A, Lashner B. Cytomegalovirus colitis complicating inflammatory bowel disease. Am J Gastroenterol. 2006;101(12):2857–65.
44. Maher MM, Nassar MI. Acute cytomegalovirus infection is a risk factor in refractory and complicated inflammatory bowel disease. Dig Dis Sci. 2009;54(11):2456–62.
45. Kredel LI, Mundt P, van Riesen L, Jöhrens K, Hofmann J, Loddenkemper C, et al. Accuracy of diagnostic tests and a new algorithm for diagnosing cytomegalovirus colitis in inflammatory bowel diseases: a diagnostic study. Int J Color Dis. 2019;34(2):229–37.
46. McCurdy JD, Jones A, Enders FT, Killian JM, Loftus EV Jr, Smyrk TC, et al. A model for identifying cytomegalovirus in patients with inflammatory bowel disease. Clin Gastroenterol Hepatol. 2015;13(1):131–7; quiz e7
47. Zagórowicz E, Bugajski M, Wieszczy P, Pietrzak A, Magdziak A, Mróz A. Cytomegalovirus infection in ulcerative colitis is related to severe inflammation and a high count of cytomegalovirus-positive cells in biopsy is a risk factor for colectomy. J Crohns Colitis. 2016;10(10):1205–11.
48. Römkens TEH, Bulte GJ, Nissen LHC, Drenth JPH. Cytomegalovirus in inflammatory bowel disease: a systematic review. World J Gastroenterol. 2016;22(3):1321–30.
49. Pillet S, Williet N, Pouvaret A, Del Tedesco E, Saint-Sardos P, Pozzetto B, et al. Distribution of cytomegalovirus DNA load in the inflamed colon of ulcerative colitis patients. Am J Gastroenterol. 2016;111(3):439–41.
50. Roblin X, Pillet S, Oussalah A, Berthelot P, Del Tedesco E, Phelip J-M, et al. Cytomegalovirus load in inflamed intestinal tissue is predictive of resistance to immunosuppressive therapy in ulcerative colitis. Am J Gastroenterol. 2011;106(11):2001–8.
51. Long MD, Onyiah JC, Miller M, Herfarth HH. Cytomegalovirus viral load in the colon and risk of colectomy in hospitalized patients with inflammatory bowel diseases. Inflamm Bowel Dis. 2016;22(6):E21–E2.
52. Mavropoulou E, Ternes K, Mechie N-C, Bremer SCB, Kunsch S, Ellenrieder V, et al. Cytomegalovirus colitis in inflammatory bowel disease and after haematopoietic stem cell transplantation: diagnostic accuracy, predictors, risk factors and disease outcome. BMJ Open Gastroenterol. 2019;6(1):e000258.

53. McCurdy JD, Enders FT, Jones A, Killian JM, Loftus EV Jr, Bruining DH, et al. Detection of cytomegalovirus in patients with inflammatory bowel disease: where to biopsy and how many biopsies? Inflamm Bowel Dis. 2015;21(12):2833–8.
54. Omiya M, Matsushita M, Tanaka T, Kawamata S, Okazaki K. The absence of large ulcer predicts latent cytomegalovirus infection in ulcerative colitis with positive mucosal viral assay. Intern Med. 2010;49(21):2277–82.
55. Suzuki H, Kato J, Kuriyama M, Hiraoka S, Kuwaki K, Yamamoto K. Specific endoscopic features of ulcerative colitis complicated by cytomegalovirus infection. World J Gastroenterol. 2010;16(10):1245–51.
56. Jones A, McCurdy JD, Loftus EV Jr, Bruining DH, Enders FT, Killian JM, et al. Effects of antiviral therapy for patients with inflammatory bowel disease and a positive intestinal biopsy for cytomegalovirus. Clin Gastroenterol Hepatol. 2015;13(5):949–55.
57. Kopylov U, Papamichael K, Katsanos K, Waterman M, Bar-Gil Shitrit A, Boysen T, et al. Impact of infliximab and cyclosporine on the risk of colectomy in hospitalized patients with ulcerative colitis complicated by cytomegalovirus-a multicenter retrospective study. Inflamm Bowel Dis. 2017;23(9):1605–13.
58. Kopylov U, Sasson G, Geyshis B, Oikawa MT, Barshack I, Eliakim R, et al. Cytomegalovirus positive ulcerative colitis: a single center experience and literature review. World J Gastrointest Pathophysiol. 2013;4(1):18–23.
59. Kim YS, Kim Y-H, Kim JS, Cheon JH, Ye BD, Jung S-A, et al. The prevalence and efficacy of ganciclovir on steroid-refractory ulcerative colitis with cytomegalovirus infection: a prospective multicenter study. J Clin Gastroenterol. 2012;46(1):51–6.
60. Shukla T, Singh S, Loftus EV Jr, Bruining DH, McCurdy JD. Antiviral therapy in steroid-refractory ulcerative colitis with cytomegalovirus: systematic review and meta-analysis. Inflamm Bowel Dis. 2015;21(11):2718–25.
61. Baradhi KM, Aure RL, El-Amm JM. High-dose valganciclovir treatment for resistant cytomegalovirus colitis due to UL97 and UL54 mutations. Transplant Proc. 2018;50(1):142–4.
62. Åsberg A, Humar A, Rollag H, Jardine AG, Mouas H, Pescovitz MD, et al. Oral valganciclovir is noninferior to intravenous ganciclovir for the treatment of cytomegalovirus disease in solid organ transplant recipients. Am J Transplant. 2007;7(9):2106–13.
63. Ahmed I, Kassem W, Salam Y, Furnari M, Mehta T. Outcome of cytomegalovirus colitis in inflammatory bowel disease with different regimes of ganciclovir. Middle East J Dig Dis. 2018;10(4):219–27.
64. Kim YS, Kim YH, Kim JS, Cheon JH, Ye BD, Jung SA, et al. The prevalence and efficacy of ganciclovir on steroid-refractory ulcerative colitis

with cytomegalovirus infection: a prospective multicenter study. J Clin Gastroenterol. 2012;46(1):51–6.

65. D'Ovidio V, Vernia P, Gentile G, Capobianchi A, Marcheggiano A, Viscido A, et al. Cytomegalovirus infection in inflammatory bowel disease patients undergoing anti-TNFα therapy. J Clin Virol. 2008;43(2):180–3.

Nutrition Management in Patients Hospitalized with Inflammatory Bowel Disease

9

Trusha Patel, Natalie L. Stoner, and Andrew B. Grossman

Introduction

Diet and nutrition have long been acknowledged to play a role in both the pathogenesis and treatment of inflammatory bowel disease (IBD) [1–3]. In particular, malnutrition and growth impairment (in the pediatric population) are complications of IBD that are often most prominent at diagnosis and during times of increased disease activity. Thus, nutritional management is of particular importance at the time of inpatient hospitalization. While assessment of nutritional status and management of malnutrition are routine components of pediatric IBD care, identification and

T. Patel (✉) · A. B. Grossman
Department of Pediatrics, Division of Gastroenterology, Hepatology and Nutrition, Children's Hospital of Philadelphia, Philadelphia, PA, USA
e-mail: PatelT3@email.chop.edu; GROSSMANAN@email.chop.edu

N. L. Stoner
Center for Pediatric Inflammatory Bowel Disease, Children's Hospital of Philadelphia, Philadelphia, PA, USA
e-mail: STONERN@email.chop.edu

J. D. Feuerstein, A. S. Cheifetz (eds.), *Management of Inpatient Inflammatory Bowel Disease*,
https://doi.org/10.1007/978-1-0716-1987-2_9

management of malnutrition are also imperative in adult IBD care. Indeed, a 2017 study of adult IBD patients attending routine outpatient visits demonstrated that 16% of these patients were malnourished [4]. This incidence is further increased in adults with active IBD, and a recent study demonstrated that, depending on the criteria used to determine undernutrition, between 25 and 69.7% of adults with active IBD were undernourished in the setting of active disease [5]. Thus, as malnutrition is prevalent not only in children with IBD, but in adults as well, both pediatric and adult IBD providers must be adept at appropriate evaluation and management. However, a 2016 survey of adult gastroenterologists demonstrated that less than 50% consider themselves to have "very good" knowledge of nutrition in IBD or perceive nutrition to be "very important" in IBD care. Only 68% reported screening all IBD patients for malnutrition, thus providing evidence of a practice and knowledge gap [6].

In this chapter, we review strategies to accurately assess the nutritional status of an inpatient with IBD, develop a plan for the provision of appropriate nutrition, and monitor for appropriate response to the nutrition interventions implemented. Furthermore, we briefly discuss special considerations for patients at risk for refeeding syndrome, undergoing surgery, and with comorbid obesity. While collaboration with a registered dietician (RD) is invaluable in the care of patients with IBD and should be incorporated whenever possible, this chapter is meant to serve as a resource for clinicians to be well-versed in the basics of optimal nutritional evaluation and support for patients with IBD even when a registered dietician is not immediately available for collaboration.

Given the clinical expertise of the authors, as well as the abundance of literature discussing nutrition in pediatric IBD, some of the information in this chapter will focus on the nutritional management of children and adolescents hospitalized with IBD, but the majority of this information can also be extrapolated to adults with IBD, and adult-specific information is included when appropriate and available. Specific nutritional considerations for geriatric patients are not discussed here. Furthermore, specialized diets proposed for the treatment of inflammatory bowel disease are not addressed, as they are largely outpatient interventions, but we refer readers to other sources that have covered these in detail [1, 7–11].

We utilize the Nutrition Care Process (NCP) as a framework to guide the nutritional management of patients hospitalized with IBD. The NCP is a systematic method that is used to provide high-quality nutrition care and to facilitate the gathering of the best evidence to guide nutrition support [12]. The NCP is comprised of four basic steps: nutrition assessment and reassessment, diagnosis, intervention, and monitoring/evaluation [12].

Nutrition Assessment and Diagnosis

Timely execution of nutrition support plays an important role in the management of IBD. By performing a nutritional risk assessment at the time of hospital admission, IBD patients at higher risk for nutrition-related complications can be identified and readily referred to a RD or expert clinician if they are not already a standard part of the care team [13]. A nutrition assessment is a comprehensive approach to identifying nutrition-related problems, comprising areas such as medical, nutrition, and medication histories; nutrition-focused physical examination; anthropometric measurements; and biomedical data/medical diagnostic tests and procedures [14]. The purpose of an in-depth nutrition assessment is to estimate nutritional needs, evaluate the appropriateness of the nutrition regimen, and identify those at risk for developing malnutrition, which is a devastating and key complication of IBD. We suggest an initial nutrition assessment should be completed and documented for all IBD patients within 24 hours from admission. Follow-up reassessment should be completed within 7 days of the initial assessment (or sooner if warranted by a change in clinical status) for patients with special diets, tube feeds, and parenteral nutrition orders [15].

Many clinicians utilize screening tools to standardize the initial components of this nutrition assessment. Most screening tools, including the Nutritional Risk Screening (NRS) 2002 tool, utilize screening questions to target dynamic parameters such as recent weight loss, recent food intake, current body mass index, and disease severity to discern patients who would benefit from nutrition intervention. The European Society for Clinical Nutrition and Metabolism (ESPEN) recommends using the NRS 2002 for inpatients, as this tool uses a score system to identify patients at risk for malnutrition or who are already malnourished to help determine need for nutrition intervention [13]. With this tool, patients are evaluated with four pre-screening questions to assess for low BMI, weight loss, reduced food intake, and critical illness. If any questions are answered positively, a screening proceeds with additional questions to identify nutritional status and the severity of the disease. For each criterion, a score of 0–3 points can result. Patients that receive a total score ≥3 points are considered at risk of malnutrition or already malnourished, and nutrition intervention is recommended [13]. Similarly, the Malnutrition Universal Screening Tool (MUST) was developed to identify malnourished patients in all care settings, although ESPEN recommends this be used in ambulatory settings [13]. There are more than 30 additional screening and nutrition assessment tools to assess nutritional status, including the Mini Nutritional Assessment, the Short Nutritional Assessment Questionnaire, the Malnutrition Screening Tool, and the Subjective Global Assessment [16]. Currently, there is no universal gold standard for the assessment of nutritional status, and the existing nutrition assessment tools (NAT) and nutrition screen tests (NST) lack specificity for the IBD patient population, creating potential gaps in treatment [17]. Thus, clinicians must select screening and assessment tools with an understanding of their limitations and should supplement these tools with their clinical judgment. We recommend using the NRS 2002 when screening inpatients with IBD for malnutrition.

The five main domains of nutrition assessment as they relate to IBD patients are summarized in Table 9.1. In practice, the nutrition assessment begins as the dietitian gathers data from patient interview, nutrition-focused physical findings, observations and measurements, and the medical record. Obtaining a detailed diet history is an important step of the nutrition assessment. Methods of obtaining a diet history in hospitalized patients include 24-hour

Table 9.1 Five domains of a nutrition assessment with examples related to IBD patients [18, 43–46]

Anthropometric measurements	Height, weight, weight history, body mass index (BMI), growth chart z-scores[a], percentile ranks[a], mid-parenteral height[a], skinfold measurements, DEXA, and any available objective measures of body composition or changes in any of these parameters
Patient history	Age, gender, review of clinical diagnoses/surgical history/medical history/family medical history, activity patterns, ethnicity, religion, social history
Food/nutrition-related history	Food record/diary, medication and complementary alternative medicine use, recent starvation, risk for refeeding syndrome, food allergy/intolerances, foods that cause an increase in gastrointestinal symptoms, food insecurity, strict adherence to selective diet, past or present needs for enteral/parenteral nutrition
Biochemical data, medical tests, and procedures	Urea nitrogen or urine sodium, prealbumin, albumin, c-reactive protein, erythrocyte sedimentation rate, calcium, phosphorus, alkaline phosphatase, ferritin, serum iron, total iron binding capacity, zinc, magnesium, complete blood count (CBC), basic metabolic panel (BMP), vitamin labs (A, E, D), PT/INR, folate, and methylmalonic acid. Stool studies including fecal calprotectin, fecal lactoferrin, and *C. difficile* infection. Results of recent procedures/imaging studies if available
Nutrition- focused physical findings	Skin integrity, fluid accumulation or deficit, muscle and subcutaneous fat wasting, functional status, nutritional deficiencies, oral health, aspiration risk, developmental status[a]

[a]Recommended in pediatrics

dietary recall or inpatient calorie counts, both well-suited for inpatients to measure energy, protein, micronutrient deficiencies, and excesses. However, both of these methods do have limitations, as a 24-hour dietary recall requires good respondent memory and inpatient calorie counts can often be derailed by NPO status and do not accurately represent the well state [18]. A more accurate method to obtain diet history is a 3- to 7-day food record which can be analyzed for macronutrients (fat, carbohydrates, and protein) and micronutrients (vitamins, trace elements) [19]. However, this can be challenging for patients to record, and there is an increasing demand for more accurate dietary assessment methods. Various innovative approaches have been proposed, such as a manual dietary assessment, dietitian-supported assessment, wearable devices monitoring food intake, and computer-aided assessment [13, 19].

Once a dietary history is obtained by one of the previously discussed means, the next step in the nutrition assessment is to complete a physical examination, which can provide insight into conditions such as malnutrition, obesity, edema, dehydration, and vitamin deficiencies and excesses [18]. Assessing for disease-related symptoms such as nausea, bloating, diarrhea, ostomy output, constipation, abdominal discomfort, hematochezia, pain, and reflux, particularly in relation to specific foods or meal timing, can help clinicians anticipate additional factors that may impact a patient's ability to receive and tolerate adequate nutrition. Symptoms such as these, along with disease-specific alterations in nutrient absorption and metabolic demands, contribute to the high frequency of underweight status and alterations of anthropometric parameters in body composition of fat and muscle mass in IBD patients [20].

Understanding body mass index (BMI) and BMI-for-age z-scores (in pediatrics) can help classify a patient as underweight, normal weight, overweight, or obese (refer to Table 9.2 for BMI classifications). The Academy of Nutrition and Dietetics and the

Table 9.2 Body mass index classifications [18, 47]

BMI: kg/m^2	2–20 years	Adults
Underweight	Less than 5th percentile	<18.5
Normal	5th–85th percentile	18.5–24.9
Overweight	85th–95th percentile	25.0–29.9
Obese	≥95th percentile	>30 Class I: 30.0–34.9 Class II: 35.0–39.90 Class III: ≥40

American Society for Parenteral and Enteral Nutrition (ASPEN) recommend separate standardized sets of diagnostic indicators for pediatric malnutrition and adult malnutrition. For pediatric patients, the indicators for diagnosing malnutrition when one single data point is available include z-score for weight-for-height/length, BMI-for-age, length/height-for-age, and mid-upper arm circumference. Additional indicators when two or more data points are available include: weight gain velocity (<2 years of age), weight loss (2–20 years of age), deceleration in weight-for-length z-score, and inadequate nutrient intake [21]. The specific criteria for determining whether a child meets criteria for mild, moderate, or severe malnutrition are well-defined in Table 9.3 (using a single data point) and Table 9.4 (using two or more data points) in the 2015 Consensus Statement of the Academy of Nutrition and Dietetics/ASPEN regarding indicators for the identification and documentation of pediatric malnutrition [21]. For adult patients, the identification of two or more of the following six characteristics is recommended for malnutrition diagnosis: insufficient energy intake, weight loss, loss of muscle mass, loss of subcutaneous fat, edema, and diminished hand grip strength [22]. Specific parameters for using these characteristics to diagnose moderate or severe malnutrition in various contexts (including acute illness, chronic illness, and specific social or environmental circumstances) are summarized in Table 9.1 of the 2012 consensus criteria released by the Academy of Nutrition and Dietetics/ASPEN regarding the identification and documentation of adult malnutrition [22].

While a nutrition assessment can help define a patient's nutritional status and dietary intake, accurately determining energy output can help determine a patient's caloric needs and guide the development of a plan for nutrition intervention. Indirect calorimetry (IC) is a clinical tool that uses respiratory gas exchange to approximate a patient's basal metabolic rate and provides the most accurate measures of resting energy expenditure (REE) [23]. While IC can provide an accurate estimation of caloric needs and is particularly helpful in determining the caloric needs of extremely young, frail, already malnourished, and critically ill patients, it is not widely utilized in an inpatient setting due to cost

Table 9.3 Guidelines for estimating nutritional needs in adults and pediatrics [16, 25, 48–57]

Adults	
Calories	IC is desirable. In the absence of IC, consider weight-based equations or predictive equations *Examples:* Weight-based equations: 25–30 kcal/kg/d for BMI <30 Mifflin-St. Jeor: Men: RMR = 9.99 × weight (kg) + 6.25 × height (cm) – 4.92 × age (y) + 5 Women: RMR = 9.99 × weight (kg) + 6.25 × height (cm) – 4.92 × age (y) – 161 Harris-Benedict: Men: energy expenditure = 66 + 13.75 (wt in kg) + 5.0 × height (cm) – 6.75 × age (y) Women: energy expenditure = 665 + 9.6 (wt in kg) + 1.8 × height (cm) – 4.67 × age (y) WHO/FAO/UNU: Ages 18–30: 15.3 × wt + 679 (males), 14.7 × wt + 496 (females) Ages 31–60: 11.6 × wt + 879 (males), 8.7 × wt + 829 (females) Ages >60: 13.5 × wt + 487 (males), 10.5 × wt + 596 (females) RDA: Ages 19–24: 40 kcal/kg (males) and 38 kcal/kg (females) Stress factors for hospitalized adult: Resting (lying or sitting): 1.0–1.4 × BMR/RMR Sedentary/light activity: 1.4–1.6 × BMR/RMR Moderate activity: 1.6–1.8 × BMR/RMR Medical (e.g., inflammatory bowel disease): 1.1–1.2 × BMR/RMR
Protein	1.2–2.0 g/kg/actual body weight. Protein needs may be increased in patients with burns, multi-trauma, or active disease

Table 9.3 (continued)

Children	
Calories	In the absence of IC, initial estimates of energy expenditure may be based on published formulas with attention to imbalance between energy intake and expenditure *Examples:* WHO/FAO/UNU equations: REE × stress factor Ages 0–3: 60.9 × wt − 54 (males), 61 × wt − 51 (females) Ages 3–10: 22.7 × wt + 495 (males), 22.5 × wt + 499 (females) Ages 10–18: 17.5 × wt + 651 (males), 12.2 × wt + 746 (females) Stress factors for WHO/FAO/UNU: REE × 1.3: For a well-nourished child at bedrest with mild to moderate stress REE × 1.5: For a normally active child with mild to moderate stress, an inactive child with severe stress, or a child with minimal activity and malnutrition requiring catch-up growth REE × 1.7: For an active child requiring catch-up growth or an active child with severe stress RDA: 0–6 months: 108 kcal/kg 6–12 months: 98 kcal/kg 1–3 years: 102 kcal/kg 4–6 years: 90 kcal/kg 7–10 years: 70 kcal/kg 11–14 years: 55 kcal/kg (males), 47 kcal/kg (females) 15–18 years: 45 kcal/kg (males), 40 kcal/kg (females)
Protein	Clinical conditions should be considered when estimating protein requirements DRI: 1–3 years: 1.05 g/kg 4–13 years: 0.95 g/kg 11–18 years: 0.85 g/kg For critically ill children: 0–2 years: 2–3 g/kg/day 2–13 years: 1.5 g/kg/day 13–18 years: 1.5 g/kg/day

BMR basal metabolic rate, *FAO/WHO/UNU* Food and Agriculture Organization/World Health Organization/United Nations University, *IC* indirect calorimetry, *kcal* kilocalorie, *lb* pound, *mL* milliliter, *RDA* recommended dietary allowance, *RMR* resting metabolic rate, *Wt* weight in kilograms, *DRI* dietary reference intakes, *y* year

Table 9.4 Indications for nutrition therapy in IBD patients [15]

Oral nutrition supplements	Enteral nutrition	Parenteral nutrition
Consumed orally	*Provided via nasogastric/nasoenteric tube, gastrostomy tube, or jejunostomy tube*	*Central or peripheral route may be selected according to duration. Peripheral route is not preferred due to the risk of infiltration*
If unable to meet nutritional needs through diet Insufficient oral intake prior to surgery Patients at mild, moderate, or severe nutritional risk (significant weight loss or BMI z-score) Candidates for enteral nutrition therapy	If oral feeding is not possible or tolerated Functional GI tract, but unable to swallow safely CD patients with a distal (low ileal or colonic) fistula and low output If patient is anticipated to be unable to eat for more than 7 days perioperatively Cannot maintain oral intake above 60–75% of recommended intake for a prolonged period Patient at moderate or severe nutritional risk Candidates for enteral nutrition therapy	Patients who are intolerant of or in whom enteral nutrition is not feasible GI tract is dysfunctional Short bowel disease with severe malabsorption and/or fluid/electrolyte loss Postoperative nutrition support for patients with contraindications to enteral nutrition Bowel obstruction or ileus with no possibility of placing feeding tube beyond the obstruction Anastomotic leak High-output intestinal fistula Severe shock Intestinal ischemia Severe intestinal hemorrhage Prolonged inability to tolerate goal enteral nutrition rate

and training required [23]. Over 200 predictive equations to estimate a patient's energy expenditure while at rest have been cited in the literature, yet accuracy rates of these equations range from 40% to 75% when compared with IC [16]. Nonetheless, given their convenience and ease, predictive equations have replaced IC to estimate REE in clinical practice.

Accurate estimation of an individual's daily caloric needs can prevent over- and underfeeding. Table 9.3 serves as a reference for age- and gender-specific predictive equations to estimate energy needs for both adults and children. The equations listed in this table account for differences in body composition among age groups. When IC is not available (as in most clinical settings), clinicians should select the appropriate published equation to use based on patient demographics and clinical context. In our practice, for pediatric patients weighing <10 kg, calorie requirements are calculated using the appropriate age-specific RDA equations. For children >10 kg, we recommend using the Food and Agriculture (FAO)/World Health Organization (WHO) equation to calculate REE (with the appropriate activity/stress adjustment factor, explained in the following paragraph and Table 9.3), which is widely used in hospital settings [19]. For adults, simple weight-based equations (25–30 kcal/kg actual body weight/day) are the most widely utilized method to calculate caloric needs and are what we recommend using in practice for nonobese adult patients. For obese adult patients, we recommend the Mifflin-St. Jeor equation (using actual body weight) to predict RMR [24]. However, a variety of other equations are also available for more detailed calculation of caloric needs (Tables 9.3 and 9.6) and may be utilized when initial calculations are suspected to be inaccurate due to increased metabolic needs or losses [16]. For example, equations such as the Mifflin-St. Jeor and Harris-Benedict were created using healthy adult subjects but can be adapted to specific disease states that increase resting energy expenditure as well as energy expended in activity [25] (Table 9.3).

To demonstrate the practical application of these predictive equations in the management of IBD patients in the inpatient setting, we consider the case of a 13-year-old girl with ileocolonic Crohn's disease (CD) who is exclusively tube fed and is admitted to the hospital for restaging of IBD in the setting of progressive symptoms. Her biggest active issues are bloody diarrhea, growth failure, and moderate malnutrition. Using the pediatric equation for REE based on the patient's age in the range of 10–18 years in

Table 9.3 and her current weight of 33.0 kg, the patient's REE is estimated to be about 1150 calories. However, this is then multiplied by an activity factor of 1.7 (for an active child requiring catch-up growth or an active child with severe stress; in this case, severe, active IBD) for a total recommended caloric intake of 1950 calories. Her current tube feeding regimen provides approximately 1500 calories or an REE × 1.30, which is below her recommended intake to support caloric needs for catch-up growth and weight gain. She would thus require an additional 450 calories to meet her nutritional needs. By using REE as a foundation to assess this patient's caloric needs, her care team could adjust her feeding regimen to provide adequate calories and optimize her nutritional status.

In addition to considering a patient's caloric needs, clinicians will also need to consider the composition of a patient's diet. While the recommended distribution of macronutrients (fat, carbohydrate, protein) in the diet is similar to that of the general population, patients with IBD may have increased protein requirements in particular settings. For example, increased protein intake may be recommended in adult patients in the postoperative setting or those with short bowel syndrome. Poor nutritional status, active disease, weight loss, and growth failure may also necessitate an increased protein requirement in children [15].

Nutrition Intervention

Ultimately, once a patient's caloric, micronutrient, and macronutrient needs are determined, the patient and care team will need to choose the best route of nutrition delivery. Selecting the appropriate feeding method for a patient hospitalized with IBD is a highly individualized decision. Methods of appropriate nutrient delivery may include full age-appropriate oral diets, total enteral nutrition via feeding tube, total parenteral nutrition (PN), or various combinations of these. In general, oral nutrition is always preferred when not precluded by patient- or disease-specific factors. However, when a patient is unable to meet his or her nutritional needs with oral intake alone, often due to lack of appetite or increased abdominal pain, nausea, vomiting, or diarrhea with a regular diet in the setting of active IBD, then enteral nutrition and parenteral nutrition should be considered. When possible, enteral nutrition is preferred to parenteral nutrition due to a favorable risk profile and maintenance of physiologic activities of digestion. However, oral or enteral nutrition may not be feasible in all patients. For example, patients with high-grade bowel obstructions, those with short bowel syndrome resulting from multiple bowel resections, or those with high-output fistulas may not be candidates for enteral nutrition in the short term. Table 9.4 reviews considerations that may guide clinicians to choose various routes of supplemental nutrition in inpatients with inflammatory bowel disease. Ultimately, the decision to provide nutrition via oral, enteral, or parenteral routes is highly individualized, and clinicians must take into account many variables.

Nutrition Reassessment

Once a nutrition assessment is completed, caloric needs are determined, and the appropriate nutrition intervention is implemented, the patient's nutritional status and care plan should be reassessed on a continual basis, as needs may change throughout the hospitalization. For example, patients with ongoing active disease may experience a decline in oral intake due to persistent or worsening symptoms, periods of fasting prior to imaging or other interventions, or increased metabolic demands due to the stress of surgical procedures [13]. For adults, in whom simple weight-based equations are typically used to calculate caloric needs, further calculations which account for basal metabolic rate, as well as an activity/stress factor based on disease state, may be useful when the initially estimated caloric needs do not result in appropriate nutrition. Furthermore, even the calculated REE with the activity factor above may not always adequately determine nutritional needs for IBD patients, due to associated factors including increased caloric demand due to intestinal losses associated with malabsorption and significant systemic inflammation, with resultant inadequate caloric goals set by the formulas [23]. Thus, ongoing reevaluation and adjustment of goals and interventions is critical to achieve optimal nutrition.

Nutrition Monitoring and Evaluation

The focus of nutrition monitoring and evaluation is to monitor progress toward a patient's nutritional goals by evaluating key nutrition care indicators, which may include weight, nutrient intake, biochemical parameters, functional capabilities, and quality of life. Depending on patient age, nutritional state at admission, and the mode of feeding that is selected, various clinical and biochemical parameters will need to be monitored at different frequencies. Generally, if a patient is well-nourished at the time of hospitalization without any signs or symptoms of specific macro- or micronutrient deficiencies (reviewed below) and will be receiving oral nutrition, additional monitoring beyond age-appropriate tracking of weight is not indicated. In our experience, this typically includes daily weights in infants, twice-weekly weights in toddlers and school-aged children, and weekly weights in hospitalized adults. However, if a patient is malnourished at the onset of hospitalization, clinicians must assess nutritional status, including weight trend, more frequently. Additionally, for malnourished patients who may be at risk for refeeding syndrome (discussed below), close monitoring of electrolytes (with special attention to potassium, magnesium, and phosphorus) is recommended.

For patients receiving PN, close monitoring of electrolytes is indicated regardless of nutritional status. The following biochemical indices should be assessed prior to initiation of parenteral nutrition: basic metabolic panel, calcium, magnesium, phosphorus, hepatic function panel, prealbumin, and triglycerides [19]. After the initiation of PN, regular biochemical monitoring is required, initially daily and subsequently at reduced frequencies, guided by the stability of the patient's electrolytes and any changes that are made to the PN, but at a minimum frequency of once weekly [26]. As patients on long-term PN are at risk for specific nutritional deficiencies due to a subtle mismatch between nutrient needs and PN content, monitoring of specific nutritional deficiencies, including vitamins A, D, E, selenium, zinc and copper, ceruloplasmin, and fatty acid profile, is indicated in patients on long-term PN [26]. Although no clear guidelines exist regarding the timing of these laboratory studies, in our practice, we screen for these deficiencies 4–6 weeks after initiation in patients who remain on PN at that time.

Even for patients who are not receiving PN, several vitamin and mineral deficiencies have been reported with increased frequency in IBD patients, regardless of nutritional status, in comparison to the general population. Inadequate dietary intake, increased intestinal loss, malabsorption, drug interactions, hypermetabolic state, and long-term parenteral nutrition are contributing mechanisms of micronutrient deficits identified in IBD patients [27]. Since more than 95% of vitamins and minerals from foods are absorbed in the proximal small bowel, micronutrient deficiencies are particularly seen in CD patients with active small bowel disease or multiple resections [27]. In our practice, we consider measuring micronutrients with primary absorption in the jejunum (thiamine, vitamin B2, vitamin B12) approximately once every 6 months (or more frequently if warranted) for patients with active small bowel disease or previous resections. Furthermore, certain medications are found to affect nutrient utilization. Common drug-nutrient interactions for IBD patients include glucocorticoids associated with bone alteration, sulfasalazine as a folic acid antagonist, and cholestyramine associated with malabsorption of fat-soluble vitamins, iron, and vitamin B12 [20]. Other major micronutrient deficits are linked to bone health (calcium, vitamin D, and possibly vitamin K), anemia (iron, folate, and vitamin B12), wound healing (zinc, vitamin A, and vitamin C), thrombophilia (folate, vitamin 6, and vitamin B12), and colorectal cancer risk [28]. All IBD patients, regardless of age, should be screened for anemia as it is reported more frequently in hospitalized patients with IBD [15]. Additionally, inadequate screening and management for iron deficiency and iron deficiency anemia in patients with IBD is well reported [29, 30]. Left untreated, anemia can complicate the course in both CD and ulcerative colitis (UC) [15]. Table 9.5 summarizes micronutrient deficiencies that should be considered in IBD patients and provides recommendations

Table 9.5 Micronutrient deficiencies in inflammatory bowel disease

Micronutrient	Signs of deficiency	Biochemical assessment	Contributing factors	Repletion dose for deficiency	Dietary sources
Vitamin A	Xerophthalmia, poor bone growth, hyperkeratosis [58]	Serum retinol levels <20 micrograms/dL [18, 59]	Steatorrhea, inadequate intake, increased disease activity, decreased bile acids, cholestyramine [46]	Age-specific dosage	Carrots, sweet potatoes, liver
Vitamin B6/ pyridoxine	Microcytic anemia, weight loss, depression, glossitis, cheilosis [18]	Low mean plasma PLP (pyridoxal-5-phosphate)	Malabsorption, inadequate dietary intake, malnutrition, corticosteroids, isoniazid [27]	50–100 mg orally once daily in adults [27, 60]	Meats, whole grains, vegetables, nuts
Vitamin B12/ cobalamin	Megaloblastic anemia with macrocytosis, cognitive decline [27, 59]	Elevated serum methylmalonic acid (MMA) (>270 μM) and homocysteine (>15 μM), low serum vitamin B12 levels (<150 pmol/L), elevated MCV [61]	Ileal/ileocolonic resection >20 cm, SIBO, gastritis, pernicious anemia, vegan diet [27, 62]	1000 μg vitamin B12 intramuscularly, ileal resection >60 cm requires lifelong supplementation [27, 63]	Organ meats, beef, fortified cereals, clam, crab, oyster

Micronutrient	Signs of deficiency	Biochemical assessment	Contributing factors	Repletion dose for deficiency	Dietary sources
Calcium	Muscle spasm, decreased bone density, hypoparathyroidism, hypertension [18]	Serum calcium not reflective of intake, DEXA scan	Inadequate dietary intake, malabsorption, hypomagnesemia (diarrhea), vitamin D deficiency, ileal resection, glucocorticoids [18, 59]	Age and gender specific depending on DRI for age	Milk, yogurt, cheese
Vitamin D	Abnormal bone metabolism [18, 27]	Serum 25 (OH)D3 concentrations below 50 nmol/l or 20 ng/ml [63]	Decreased sunlight exposure, malabsorption, glucocorticoids, anorexia [27]	Titration of oral supplements as appropriate [27]	Fatty fish, fortified milk, cod liver
Vitamin B9/ folate	Macrocytic megaloblastic anemia [18]	Low serum or RBC folate, elevated homocysteine and MCV [27]	Sulfasalazine/methotrexate, inadequate diet intake, malabsorption, active ileal disease, ileal resection [46, 63]	Folate supplementation of 1 mg/day [63]	Spinach, fortified cereals

(continued)

Table 9.5 (continued)

Micronutrient	Signs of deficiency	Biochemical assessment	Contributing factors	Repletion dose for deficiency	Dietary sources
Iron	Anemia [27, 46]	Universal screening for iron deficiency and anemia, including CBC, ferritin, TSAT, reticulocyte count (assess for anemia, assess for iron deficiency in relation to disease activity) [62]	Occult/overt blood loss, gastrointestinal bleeding, proton pump inhibitors and antacids, impaired iron metabolism [27, 46]	Oral iron in patients with mild anemia (>10 g/dl) and negative inflammatory markers as initial trial, IV iron therapy (ferric carboxymaltose) preferred for active disease (pediatric and adult) [15, 62]	Meats, beans, fortified cereals, lentils, green leafy vegetables
Vitamin K	Bleeding, easy bruisability [18]	Prolonged PT/INR	Liver disease, inadequate diet intake, bile salt deficiency, steatorrhea, biliary obstruction, use of coumarin anticoagulants, and antibiotic use [18, 27, 46]	Orally, intravenously, subcutaneously, or intramuscularly [27]. Common doses include 1–10 mg orally and 0.5–10 mg intravenously	Dark leafy greens (vitamin K1)

Micronutrient	Signs of deficiency	Biochemical assessment	Contributing factors	Repletion dose for deficiency	Dietary sources
Magnesium	Muscle cramps, fatigue, hypocalcemia, hypophosphatemia [46]	Urine or low serum magnesium [27]	Inadequate diet intake, chronic diarrhea, malabsorption, refeeding syndrome [27, 46, 63]	Rate and dose repletion should be based on severity of clinical manifestations or degree of hypomagnesemia [27]	Peanuts, bran, legumes, bean sprouts
Selenium	Cardiomyopathy, skeletal muscle dysfunction [46]	Glutathione peroxidase, serum selenium <70 μg/mL [18]	Inadequate dietary intake, long-term PN, severe intestinal disorders, kidney dialysis [27, 46]	100mcg/day orally [27]	Meat, Brazil nuts, lobster, tuna, shrimp
Zinc	Scaly eczematous plaques, impaired growth velocity, poor taste acuity, poor wound healing [27]	Serum zinc, low alkaline phosphatase [46]	Inadequate dietary intake, prolonged diarrheal episodes >4 weeks, fistula output [27, 46]	2–4 weeks of oral zinc as prolonged intake can interfere with iron and copper absorption [18, 27, 63]	Chicken, nuts, lentils, fortified cereals

PT/INR prothrombin time, *INR* international normalized ratio, *DRI* dietary reference intake regarding contributing factors (which clinicians can use to guide the need for screening), signs of deficiency, biochemical assessment, repletion dose (where applicable), and dietary sources of specific nutrients. Repletion doses should be adjusted based on response. As always, clinicians must use clinical judgment to guide the need for screening and treatment of macro- and micronutrient deficiencies.

Special Consideration: Refeeding Syndrome

All patients who are malnourished at the time of hospital admission should be evaluated to determine the risk of refeeding syndrome with increased nutrition delivery. Refeeding syndrome was recently defined by ASPEN as "a measurable reduction in levels of 1 or any combination of phosphorus, potassium, and/or magnesium, or the manifestation of thiamin deficiency, developing shortly (hours to days) after initiation of calorie provision to an individual who has been exposed to a substantial period of undernourishment" [31]. Although exact guidelines regarding what qualifies as a substantial period of undernourishment do not exist, it is clear that many patients with inflammatory bowel disease (in whom poor appetite, malabsorption, and increased gastrointestinal losses are common) are at risk. Indeed, CD is acknowledged by ASPEN as a clinical condition with increased risk of refeeding syndrome. Furthermore, ASPEN consensus criteria indicate that low weight-for-length or BMI; recent weight loss; decreased energy intake (<75% of estimated needs) over the prior 3–7 days; low pre-feeding serum potassium, phosphorus, or magnesium concentrations; higher-risk comorbidities (including CD); and evidence of loss of subcutaneous fat or muscle mass all place patients at higher risk for refeeding syndrome. The detailed criteria utilized to determine whether both adult and pediatric patients are at mild, moderate, or significant risk for developing refeeding syndrome are outlined in these consensus recommendations published in April 2020 and are summarized in Table 9.3 and Table 9.5

of that document [31]. In children at significant risk for refeeding syndrome, nutrition should be initiated with 40–50% of the goal intake, typically starting with a glucose infusion rate around 4–6 mg/kg/min. Generally, for adults, 100–150 grams of dextrose or 10–20 kcal/kg is provided in the first 24 hours, followed by an advance of 33% of the goal every 1–2 days [31]. Serum potassium, magnesium, and phosphorus should be monitored prior to initiation of nutrition and every 12 hours for the first 3 days, with plan to replete electrolytes as needed and consider decreasing nutrition provision if electrolytes become difficult to correct. In high-risk patients, thiamin supplementation (2 mg/kg, up to 100 mg) prior to initiation of feeding is also recommended, with continued supplementation daily for up to 5–7 days in patients with severe starvation, alcoholism, or clinical signs/symptoms of thiamin deficiency [31].

Special Consideration: Perioperative Nutrition

While nutritional management is important in all hospitalized patients with IBD, optimization of nutritional status is of particular importance for patients undergoing surgery. Numerous prior studies have demonstrated that malnutrition is associated with increased perioperative complications in a variety of conditions [32–34]. Similarly, preoperative weight loss and sarcopenia have been associated with adverse surgical outcomes in patients with IBD [35–38]. Preoperative interventions that optimize nutritional status, including supplemental enteral and parenteral nutrition, have been associated with improved perioperative outcomes in patients undergoing surgery for IBD [39–41]. In this context, the 2017 guidelines of the European Society for Clinical Nutrition and Metabolism (ESPEN) provide recommendations regarding perioperative nutritional management in IBD patients [15].

While emergency surgery should not be delayed for nutritional optimization, supplemental nutrition (enteral or parenteral) should be initiated in patients who are malnourished at the time of surgery or if an oral diet cannot be started within 7 days after surgery. The authors acknowledge that oral nutrition is preferred to enteral nutrition and that parenteral nutrition should be used only when needs cannot be met with oral intake, including nutrition supplements, or supplemental enteral nutrition. In cases of non-emergent or elective surgery, ESPEN guidelines suggest delaying surgery for 7–14 days if possible to provide intensive nutrition support to decrease the risk of perioperative complications [15]. Postoperatively, early enteral nutrition should be considered when feasible.

Special Consideration: Obesity

While malnutrition is common in patients with IBD and often manifests with low BMI, clinicians must remember that not all IBD patients are malnourished and not all patients who are undernourished at a particular point in time will have a low BMI. Indeed, 5–40% of adult patients with IBD are considered obese [42]. Among hospitalized adult IBD patients with BMI >25, 57% show evidence of malnutrition [17]. Thus, it is crucial for clinicians to look beyond BMI and provide a thorough nutrition assessment to identify obese patients who are at nutritional risk.

The nutrition assessment for an obese patient should include actual body weight, usual body weight, ideal body weight, BMI and obesity category, waist circumference measurement (>35 inches in nonpregnant women and >40 inches for men are associated with higher risk of developing obesity-related conditions), as well as preexisting and emerging comorbidities [16]. Guidelines for calculating energy requirements for obese adults are outlined in Table 9.6. Once a nutrition assessment is complete and energy requirements are calculated, clinicians can then use an interdisciplinary approach to safely achieve weight loss and reduce other health risks without further contributing to malnutrition in patients with obesity.

Table 9.6 Guidelines for estimating energy requirements for obese adult patients [16, 18, 24]

Calories	Indirect calorimetry, use of a predictive equation (i.e., Mifflin-St. Jeor equation), or weight-based equations 1. Mifflin-St. Jeor (using actual body weight; appropriate for all obese adults) Men (kcal/day): 5 + 10 × wt (kg) + 6.25 × Ht (cm) – 5 × age (y) Women (kcal/day): −161 + 10 × wt (kg) + 6.25 × Ht (cm) – 5 × age (y) 2. Weight-based equations (for critically ill obese adults) 11–14 kcal/kg ABW/day for BMI 30–50 22–25 kcal/kg IBW/day for BMI >50
Protein	2.0 g/kg IBW/d with a BMI 30–39.9 kg/m^2 2.5 g/kg IBW/d with a BMI ≥40 kg/m^2

ABW actual body weight, *IBW* ideal body weight, *Ht* height, *Y* year, *Wt* weight

Practical Application: 17-Year-Old Boy with Crohn's Disease

In order to demonstrate the practical applications of the concepts, equations, and clinical considerations previously discussed in this chapter, we now examine the case of a 17-year-old boy who presents for 4 months of intermittent abdominal pain and diarrhea which have acutely worsened in the week prior to admission. At presentation, the patient is noted to have microcytic anemia (hemoglobin 9.8, MCV 71), mild hypoalbuminemia (albumin 3.6), and elevated inflammatory markers (ESR 42, CRP 24 with upper limit of normal 4.9). Stool infectious studies are negative. Diagnostic evaluation including upper endoscopy, ileocolonoscopy, and MR enterography is completed and is consistent with severe ileocecal CD without evidence of stricture or abscess. The patient is admitted for initiation of medical therapy.

At the time of admission, a nutrition assessment is completed. He is 57 kg and has lost 9 kg since the last visit at the pediatrician 3 months earlier. His BMI is approximately 16 kg/m^2 (Z-score −3.0) which, along with his weight loss of 13.7%

of his usual body weight, is consistent with severe malnutrition. Diet history is notable to decreased appetite and oral intake due to abdominal pain and diarrhea. Limited exam shows a thin and chronically ill-appearing teenage boy. Despite improvement in symptoms with initiation of medical therapy during his hospitalization, he continues to have poor oral intake. His calorie counts during the first 3 days of admission demonstrate an average daily caloric intake of 1500 calories per day. His calculated REE is 1648, and, given his severe disease, with an activity factor of 1.7–2.0, he would require 2800 to 3300 calories per day for adequate nutrition and recovery of his weight gain. Given ongoing poor intake despite medical therapy and oral supplementation, the patient is unable to increase his caloric intake, and the decision is made to place a nasogastric tube (NG) for supplemental nutrition. Prior to initiation of supplemental nutrition, his electrolytes, including potassium, magnesium, and phosphorus, are all within normal limits. Based on BMI-for-age z-score (−3 or greater) that is a change from baseline, he is determined to be at risk for refeeding syndrome [31]. Given this, the decision is made to gradually increase his caloric intake. Based on a goal caloric intake of 3000 calories, the patient will require an additional 1000 ml of 1.5 calorie-per-ml formula to meet his goal caloric intake. Given his risk for refeeding syndrome, he is started on 40% of his additional caloric needs, with a regimen of 400 ml of formula run overnight at 50 ml/hour over 8 hours. Electrolytes are checked daily and potassium, magnesium, and phosphorus remain stable. Thus, rate is increased by 20% per night (25 ml/hour increase per night) to an ultimate regimen of 125 ml/hour for 8 hours overnight, with persistently stable electrolytes. Upon reaching his goal feeds, his symptoms are also well-controlled with medical therapy. Thus, the patient will be discharged on this supplemental feeding regimen, with the plan to wean supplemental feeds as weight and appetite improve. Ideally, he will follow up with both his gastroenterologist and a registered dietician as an outpatient.

Conclusions

As reviewed here, there are many factors that must be considered to allow clinicians to provide high-quality nutritional management for patients with IBD in the inpatient setting. Optimization of nutrition plays an important role not only in a patient's overall health but also more specifically in a patient's ability to overcome inflammation and/or recover from any invasive interventions that may be required. While collaboration with a registered dietician is always ideal to help achieve optimal nutrition in hospitalized patients with IBD, this may not always be feasible, and the information reviewed in this chapter may serve as a guide to help clinicians manage hospitalized patients with IBD and help these patients meet their nutritional needs.

References

1. Stein R, Baldassano RN. Dietary therapies for inflammatory bowel disease. In: Mamula PGA, Baldassano RN, Kelsen JR, Markowitz JE, editors. Pediatric inflammatory bowel disease. Cham: Springer International Publishing; 2017. p. 473–83.
2. Lee D, Albenberg L, Compher C, Baldassano R, Piccoli D, Lewis JD, et al. Diet in the pathogenesis and treatment of inflammatory bowel diseases. Gastroenterology. 2015;148(6):1087–106.
3. Kleinman RE, Baldassano RN, Caplan A, Griffiths AM, Heyman MB, Issenman RM, et al. Nutrition support for pediatric patients with inflammatory bowel disease: a clinical report of the North American Society for Pediatric Gastroenterology, Hepatology and Nutrition. J Pediatr Gastroenterol Nutr. 2004;39(1):15–27.
4. Casanova MJ, Chaparro M, Molina B, Merino O, Batanero R, Duenas-Sadornil C, et al. Prevalence of malnutrition and nutritional characteristics of patients with inflammatory bowel disease. J Crohns Colitis. 2017;11(12):1430–9.
5. Mijac DD, Jankovic GL, Jorga J, Krstic MN. Nutritional status in patients with active inflammatory bowel disease: prevalence of malnutrition and methods for routine nutritional assessment. Eur J Intern Med. 2010;21(4):315–9.

6. Tinsley A, Ehrlich OG, Hwang C, Issokson K, Zapala S, Weaver A, et al. Knowledge, attitudes, and beliefs regarding the role of nutrition in IBD among patients and providers. Inflamm Bowel Dis. 2016;22(10):2474–81.
7. Suskind DL, Cohen SA, Brittnacher MJ, Wahbeh G, Lee D, Shaffer ML, et al. Clinical and fecal microbial changes with diet therapy in active inflammatory bowel disease. J Clin Gastroenterol. 2018;52(2):155–63.
8. Cohen SA, Gold BD, Oliva S, Lewis J, Stallworth A, Koch B, et al. Clinical and mucosal improvement with specific carbohydrate diet in pediatric Crohn disease. J Pediatr Gastroenterol Nutr. 2014;59(4):516–21.
9. Svolos V, Hansen R, Nichols B, Quince C, Ijaz UZ, Papadopoulou RT, et al. Treatment of active Crohn's disease with an ordinary food-based diet that replicates exclusive enteral nutrition. Gastroenterology. 2019;156(5):1354–67. e6
10. Sigall-Boneh R, Pfeffer-Gik T, Segal I, Zangen T, Boaz M, Levine A. Partial enteral nutrition with a Crohn's disease exclusion diet is effective for induction of remission in children and young adults with Crohn's disease. Inflamm Bowel Dis. 2014;20(8):1353–60.
11. Levine A, Wine E, Assa A, Sigall Boneh R, Shaoul R, Kori M, et al. Crohn's disease exclusion diet plus partial enteral nutrition induces sustained remission in a randomized controlled trial. Gastroenterology. 2019;157(2):440–50.e8
12. Swan WI, Vivanti A, Hakel-Smith NA, Hotson B, Orrevall Y, Trostler N, et al. Nutrition care process and model update: toward realizing people-centered care and outcomes management. J Acad Nutr Diet. 2017;117(12):2003–14.
13. Reber EGF, Vasiloglou MF, Schuetz P, Stanga Z. Nutritional risk screening and assessment. J Clin Med. 2019;8(7):1065.
14. Teitelbaum D, Guenter P, Howell WH, Kochevar ME, Roth J, Seidner DL. Definition of terms, style, and conventions used in A.S.P.E.N. guidelines and standards. Nutr Clin Pract. 2005;20(2):281–5.
15. Forbes A, Escher J, Hebuterne X, Klek S, Krznaric Z, Schneider S, et al. ESPEN guideline: clinical nutrition in inflammatory bowel disease. Clin Nutr. 2017;36(2):321–47.
16. McClave SA, Taylor BE, Martindale RG, Warren MM, Johnson DR, Braunschweig C, et al. Guidelines for the provision and assessment of nutrition support therapy in the adult critically ill patient: Society of Critical Care Medicine (SCCM) and American Society for Parenteral and Enteral Nutrition (A.S.P.E.N.). JPEN J Parenter Enteral Nutr. 2016;40(2):159–211.
17. Li S, Ney M, Eslamparast T, Vandermeer B, Ismond KP, Kroeker K, et al. Systematic review of nutrition screening and assessment in inflammatory bowel disease. World J Gastroenterol. 2019;25(28):3823–37.

18. The ASPEN adult nutrition support core curriculum. 3rd ed. American Society for Parenteral and Enteral Nutrition; 2017.
19. Carney LN, Nepa A, Cohen SS, Dean A, Yanni C, Markowitz G. Parenteral and enteral nutrition support: determining the best way to feed. In: Corkins MR, editor. The A.S.P.E.N. pediatric nutrition support core curriculum. 2010. p. 433–48.
20. Scaldaferri F, Pizzoferrato M, Lopetuso LR, Musca T, Ingravalle F, Sicignano LL, et al. Nutrition and IBD: malnutrition and/or sarcopenia? A practical guide. Gastroenterol Res Pract. 2017;2017:8646495. https://doi.org/10.1155/2017/8646495.
21. Becker P, Carney LN, Corkins MR, Monczka J, Smith E, Smith SE, et al. Consensus statement of the Academy of Nutrition and Dietetics/American Society for Parenteral and Enteral Nutrition: indicators recommended for the identification and documentation of pediatric malnutrition (undernutrition). Nutr Clin Pract. 2015;30(1):147–61.
22. White JV, Guenter P, Jensen G, Malone A, Schofield M, Academy Malnutrition Work Group, et al. Consensus statement: Academy of Nutrition and Dietetics and American Society for Parenteral and Enteral Nutrition: characteristics recommended for the identification and documentation of adult malnutrition (undernutrition). JPEN J Parenter Enteral Nutr. 2012;36(3):275–83.
23. Carpenter A, Pencharz P, Mouzaki M. Accurate estimation of energy requirements of young patients. J Pediatr Gastroenterol Nutr. 2015;60(1):4–10.
24. Dickerson RN, Patel JJ, McClain CJ. Protein and calorie requirements associated with the presence of obesity. Nutr Clin Pract. 2017;32(1_suppl):86S–93S.
25. Ferrie S, Ward M. Back to basics: estimating energy requirements for adult hospital patients. Nutr Diet. 2007;64(3):192–9.
26. Mirtallo JM. Overview of parenteral nutrition. In: Gottschlich MM, editor. The ASPEN nutrition support core curriculum: a cased based approach – the adult patient. American Society for Parenteral and Enteral Nutrition; 2007. p. 264–76.
27. Hwang C, Ross V, Mahadevan U. Micronutrient deficiencies in inflammatory bowel disease: from A to zinc. Inflamm Bowel Dis. 2012;18(10):1961–81.
28. Yoon SM. Micronutrient deficiencies in inflammatory bowel disease: trivial or crucial? Intest Res. 2016;14(2):109–10.
29. Sjoberg D, Holmstrom T, Larsson M, Nielsen AL, Holmquist L, Ronnblom A. Anemia in a population-based IBD cohort (ICURE): still high prevalence after 1 year, especially among pediatric patients. Inflamm Bowel Dis. 2014;20(12):2266–70.
30. Goodhand JR, Kamperidis N, Rao A, Laskaratos F, McDermott A, Wahed M, et al. Prevalence and management of anemia in children, adolescents,

and adults with inflammatory bowel disease. Inflamm Bowel Dis. 2012;18(3):513–9.
31. da Silva JSV, Seres DS, Sabino K, Adams SC, Berdahl GJ, Citty SW, et al. ASPEN consensus recommendations for refeeding syndrome. Nutr Clin Pract. 2020;35(2):178–95.
32. Engelman DT, Adams DH, Byrne JG, Aranki SF, Collins JJ Jr, Couper GS, et al. Impact of body mass index and albumin on morbidity and mortality after cardiac surgery. J Thorac Cardiovasc Surg. 1999;118(5):866–73.
33. Dannhauser A, Van Zyl JM, Nel CJ. Preoperative nutritional status and prognostic nutritional index in patients with benign disease undergoing abdominal operations – part I. J Am Coll Nutr. 1995;14(1):80–90.
34. Garth AK, Newsome CM, Simmance N, Crowe TC. Nutritional status, nutrition practices and post-operative complications in patients with gastrointestinal cancer. J Hum Nutr Diet. 2010;23(4):393–401.
35. Maeda K, Nagahara H, Shibutani M, Otani H, Sakurai K, Toyokawa T, et al. A preoperative low nutritional prognostic index correlates with the incidence of incisional surgical site infections after bowel resection in patients with Crohn's disease. Surg Today. 2015;45(11):1366–72.
36. Alves A, Panis Y, Bouhnik Y, Pocard M, Vicaut E, Valleur P. Risk factors for intra-abdominal septic complications after a first ileocecal resection for Crohn's disease: a multivariate analysis in 161 consecutive patients. Dis Colon Rectum. 2007;50(3):331–6.
37. Fujikawa H, Araki T, Okita Y, Kondo S, Kawamura M, Hiro J, et al. Impact of sarcopenia on surgical site infection after restorative proctocolectomy for ulcerative colitis. Surg Today. 2017;47(1):92–8.
38. Pedersen M, Cromwell J, Nau P. Sarcopenia is a predictor of surgical morbidity in inflammatory bowel disease. Inflamm Bowel Dis. 2017;23(10):1867–72.
39. Guo Z, Guo D, Gong J, Zhu W, Zuo L, Sun J, et al. Preoperative nutritional therapy reduces the risk of anastomotic leakage in patients with Crohn's disease requiring resections. Gastroenterol Res Pract. 2016;2016:5017856.
40. Wang H, Zuo L, Zhao J, Dong J, Li Y, Gu L, et al. Impact of preoperative exclusive enteral nutrition on postoperative complications and recurrence after bowel resection in patients with active Crohn's disease. World J Surg. 2016;40(8):1993–2000.
41. Jacobson S. Early postoperative complications in patients with Crohn's disease given and not given preoperative total parenteral nutrition. Scand J Gastroenterol. 2012;47(2):170–7.
42. Singh S, Dulai PS, Zarrinpar A, Ramamoorthy S, Sandborn WJ. Obesity in IBD: epidemiology, pathogenesis, disease course and treatment outcomes. Nat Rev Gastroenterol Hepatol. 2017;14(2):110–21.
43. Boullata JI, Carrera AL, Harvey L, Escuro AA, Hudson L, Mays A, et al. ASPEN safe practices for enteral nutrition therapy [formula: see text]. JPEN J Parenter Enteral Nutr. 2017;41(1):15–103.

44. Nutrition Care Process. Academy of Nutrition and Dietetics. 2020. https://www.eatrightpro.org/practice/practice-resources/nutrition-care-process. Accessed 6 Feb 2020.
45. Kleinman R, Greer FR, editors. Pediatric nutrition. 7th ed. Elk Grove Village: American Academy of Pediatrics; 2014.
46. Kleinman RE, Baldassano, RN, Caplan A, Griffits A, Heyman MB, Issenmen RM, et al. Nutrition Support for Pediatric Patients With Inflammatory Bowel Disease: A Clinical Report of the North American Society for Pediatric Gastroenterology, Hepatology and Nutrition, Journal of Pediatric Gastroenterology and Nutrition. 2004;39(1):15–27.
47. Barlow SE, The Expert Committee. Expert committee recommendations regarding the prevention, assessment, and treatment of child and adolescent overweight and obesity: summary report. Pediatrics. 2007;120(Supplement December 2007):S164–92.
48. Mehta NM, Bechard LJ, Cahill N, Wang M, Day A, Duggan CP, et al. Nutritional practices and their relationship to clinical outcomes in critically ill children – an international multicenter cohort study*. Crit Care Med. 2012;40(7):2204–11.
49. Academy of Nutrition and Dietetics (A.N.D), Evidence Analysis Library. EE Predictive Formula Equations (2005). 2020. https://www.andeal.org/topic.cfm?menu=5299&pcat=1071&cat=3209. Accessed 4 Feb 2020.
50. Academy of Nutrition and Dietetics (A.N.D), Evidence Analysis Library. HYD: Estimating Fluid Needs (2007). 2020. https://www.andeal.org/topic.cfm?menu=2820&cat=3217. Accessed 25 Feb 2020.
51. Holliday MA, Segar WE. The maintenance need for water in parenteral fluid therapy. Pediatrics. 1957;19(5):823–32.
52. Manual of Clinical Nutrition Management. Compass Group. 2013. https://morrisondining.compass-usa.com/tmc/Documents/Manual%20of%20Clinical%20Nutrition%20(new).pdf. Accessed 20 Feb 2020.
53. World Health Organization. Energy and protein requirements. Report of joint FAO/WHO/UNU expert consultation. Technical report series 724. Geneva: World Health Organization.
54. Recommended Dietary Allowances te, National Academy of Sciences, National Academy Press 1989; 33–36.
55. Pediatric Nutrition Helpful Hints. Nestle Health Science. 2016. p. 1–32. https://www.nestlehealthscience.us/asset-library/documents/resources/pediatric%20helpful%20hints.pdf. Accessed 3 Feb 2020
56. Nutrition Assessment of Adults. Manual of clinical dietetics. 6th ed. Chicago: American Dietetic Association; 2000.
57. Critch J, et al. Enteral nutrition as first-line therapy in treat children and adolescents with Crohn's disease. North American Society for Pediatric Gastroenterology Hepatology, and Nutrition (NASPGHAN) and the NASPGHAN Foundation for Children's Digestive Health and Nutrition. 2013. https://www.naspghan.org/files/documents/pdfs/cme/podcasts/EN%20Newsltr_WEB.pdf. Accessed 2 Feb 2020.

58. Wolf G. A History of Vitamin A and Retinoids. FASEB J. 1996;10(9):1102–7.
59. Issokson K. Common micronutrient deficiencies in IBD. Crohn's & Colitis Foundation. 2017. https://www.crohnscolitisfoundation.org/sites/default/files/legacy/science-and-professionals/nutrition-resource-/micronutrient-deficiency-fact.pdf. Accessed 20 Jan 2020.
60. Johnson L. Vitamin B6 deficiency and dependency. 2019. https://www.merckmanuals.com/professional/nutritional-disorders/vitamin-deficiency-d,-and-toxicity/vitamin-b6-deficiency-and-dependency. Accessed 3 Feb 2020.
61. Dibb M, Subramanian S. Anaemia in inflammatory bowel disease. Frontline Gastroenterol. 2014;5(3):190–6.
62. Breton J GA, Stevenson J, Scwab E, McDermott J, Law C, et al. CHOP clinical pathway for evaluation and treatment of iron deficiency and anemia in patients with inflammatory bowel disease (IBD). 2019. https://www.chop.edu/clinical-pathway/iron-deficiency-anemia-inflammatory-bowel-disease-ibd-clinical-pathway. Accessed 3 Mar 2020.
63. Miele E, Shamir R, Aloi M, Assa A, Braegger C, Bronsky J, et al. Nutrition in pediatric inflammatory bowel disease: a position paper on behalf of the Porto Inflammatory Bowel Disease Group of the European Society of Pediatric Gastroenterology, Hepatology and Nutrition. J Pediatr Gastroenterol Nutr. 2018;66(4):687–708.

Quality of Care in the Management of Hospitalized Patients with Inflammatory Bowel Disease

10

Joshua L. Hudson and Edward L. Barnes

Introduction

Delivering high-quality care to inpatients with inflammatory bowel disease (IBD) is critical to improving short- and long-term outcomes for individual patients and decreasing the significant costs associated with the management of IBD. When combined, Crohn's disease (CD) and ulcerative colitis (UC) represent the

J. L. Hudson
Department of Medicine, University of North Carolina School of Medicine, Chapel Hill, NC, USA
e-mail: Joshua.Hudson@unchealth.unc.edu

E. L. Barnes (✉)
Division of Gastroenterology and Hepatology, University of North Carolina at Chapel Hill, Chapel Hill, NC, USA

Multidisciplinary Center for Inflammatory Bowel Diseases, University of North Carolina at Chapel Hill, Chapel Hill, NC, USA

Center for Gastrointestinal Biology and Disease, University of North Carolina at Chapel Hill, Chapel Hill, NC, USA
e-mail: edward_barnes@med.unc.edu

J. D. Feuerstein, A. S. Cheifetz (eds.), *Management of Inpatient Inflammatory Bowel Disease*,
https://doi.org/10.1007/978-1-0716-1987-2_10

fifth most expensive condition managed by gastroenterologists in the United States [1]. In addition to the costs associated with the initial hospitalization, patients with CD and UC remain at risk for readmission and other complications after discharge, including venous thromboembolism (VTE) and infection. Simple measures taken in the hospital can decrease the morbidity/mortality and length of stay, prevent further complications in IBD patients, and significantly improve outcomes in this population. In this chapter, we will employ an evidence-based methodology to review fundamental interventions for hospitalized IBD patients. We will also explore novel approaches for enhancing the quality of care delivered to inpatients with CD and UC.

Venous Thromboembolism Prophylaxis

The need to assess for prophylaxis for VTE is well recognized among practitioners when admitting nonsurgical patients to the hospital. Numerous studies have examined the risk of VTE, which includes deep vein thrombosis and pulmonary embolism, in patients with IBD and have found it to be elevated when compared with the standard patient population. A consensus statement from the American College of Chest Physicians (ACCP) offers tools for assessing both the risk of VTE and the risk of clinically significant bleeding developing while hospitalized in order to allow practitioners to make informed decisions about VTE prophylaxis on admission [2]. Unfortunately, the ACCP guidelines and the most widely used prediction tools for VTE, the Geneva score and Padua prediction score, do not comment on patients with IBD [3, 4].

In general, patients with IBD are at a two- to threefold increase of VTE events while hospitalized as compared to patients without IBD [5, 6]. This risk is further increased, up to six- to eightfold, in the setting of an acute IBD flare [5–7]. Despite the plethora of data on the increased risk of VTE in patients with IBD, rates of VTE prophylaxis in this patient population are poor, particularly on nonsurgical services. In one study by Papa et al., rates of VTE prophylaxis administration to IBD patients on

Table 10.1 Recommended VTE prophylaxis

IBD patient type	VTE prophylaxis recommendation
Hospitalized for reason(s) unrelated to IBD or in clinical remission	Pharmacological VTE prophylaxis[a]
Hospitalized for moderate-to-severe IBD flare without severe bleeding[b]	Pharmacological VTE prophylaxis
Hospitalized for moderate-to-severe IBD flare with severe bleeding	Mechanical VTE prophylaxis with intermittent pneumatic compression
Undergoing general or abdominal surgery	Pharmacological VTE prophylaxis
Presenting in the outpatient setting with IBD flare not requiring admission	No VTE prophylaxis

[a]Pharmacological VTE prophylaxis should be with low-molecular-weight heparin, low-dose unfractionated heparin, or fondaparinux
[b]Severe bleeding is clinically apparent bleeding with hemodynamic compromise

medical services (gastroenterology, general medicine, or hospital medicine) varied from 37% to 57%, which was significantly below that of surgical services (93–96%) [8]. The most commonly cited reason for withholding VTE prophylaxis in the IBD patient population is concern for hematochezia, with one study demonstrating a fourfold decrease in the likelihood of VTE prophylaxis prescription in the presence of hematochezia [9]. This concern is unfounded, however. There is a minimal risk for severe bleeding due to VTE prophylaxis, even in the setting of an acute flare of UC or CD [10].

Two recently published guidelines have specifically addressed VTE prophylaxis in IBD patients [7, 11]. In general, pharmacological prophylaxis against VTE is recommended for patients with IBD admitted for reasons not associated with IBD, those admitted for non-severe gastrointestinal bleeding, and those patients admitted for a moderate-to-severe flare of IBD with non-severe gastrointestinal bleeding (Table 10.1). In patients with IBD and severe gastrointestinal bleeding, mechanical VTE prophylaxis is recommended initially, with conversion to pharmacological prophylaxis after severe bleeding has been stabilized [7, 11]. Given the significantly increased risk for thromboembolic events among hospitalized patients with IBD, VTE prophylaxis remains a critical issue.

Testing for *Clostridioides difficile* Infection

Clostridioides difficile [(*C. difficile*) formerly *Clostridium difficile*] is a serious gastrointestinal infection that is most often associated with use of antibiotics. Additional risk factors include age >65, extended stays in hospitals or nursing homes, and prior infection with *C. difficile* [12]. IBD patients have an increased prevalence of *C. difficile* infection as well. Patients with UC seem to be at the greatest risk for *C. difficile* infection; however patients with CD also have an increased risk of infection [13]. One study that analyzed data from the Nationwide Inpatient Sample noted an eight-time greater prevalence of *C. difficile* infection in UC patients as compared to non-IBD patients and all-hospital discharges [14]. In the same analysis, CD was associated with a two-time greater prevalence of *C. difficile infection* compared to non-IBD patients [14]. With this increased prevalence of disease also come numerous adverse outcomes including a higher mortality in IBD patients with *C. difficile* infection as well as increased healthcare costs, lengths of stay, and surgery rates and a decreased responsiveness to medical therapy for IBD [15].

Given the increased prevalence of *C. difficile* infections in IBD patients, numerous organizations have published guidelines that strongly encourage routine testing for *C. difficile* in all IBD patients presenting to the hospital with an acute flare of IBD or flare-like symptoms [11, 13, 16]. First-line treatment of *C. difficile* in IBD patients should be with oral vancomycin-based therapy [16]. The use of metronidazole was previously favored as first-line therapy for mild-to-moderate IBD flares, but this therapy is no longer recommended based on numerous publications, including recently published guidelines from the Infectious Diseases Society of America [16–18]. Studies have suggested that IBD-directed immunosuppressive therapy should be held for the first 48–72 hours of pathogen-directed therapy and then cautiously resumed [19]. While close monitoring of the patient during the resumption of immunosuppressive therapy is recommended, continued treatment of IBD is critical. In a retrospective multi-center cohort study of 207 patients with IBD and documented *C. difficile* infection, 62 patients underwent escalation to a biologic or corticosteroid therapy. Severe outcomes (death, sepsis, and/or colectomy) occurred in 15.6% of non-escalated patients compared to 1.8% of therapy-escalated patients, indicating that therapy escalation for IBD within 90 days of *C. difficile* infection may be necessary in carefully selected patients [20].

Pain Management

Both acute and chronic abdominal pain are common symptoms in patients with IBD. Despite a lack of evidence for efficacy, opioid analgesics are often used for pain management in IBD patients, particularly in the inpatient setting. Several studies have shown the deleterious effects of opioids on IBD patients including increased length of hospital stays, higher risk to become a chronic opioid user, and higher mortality [21, 22]. In addition, a prior cohort study from a longitudinal registry demonstrated that opioid analgesics do not improve pain or quality-of-life scores in this patient population [23]. This is particularly problematic when noting that in retrospective evaluations, the use of opioid pain medications among patients admitted for UC or CD was not significantly associated with the presence of active disease on cross-sectional imaging or endoscopy [24]. Despite these factors, inpatients with IBD who receive opioids are significantly more likely to receive opioids at discharge, with dose-response relationships noted in a retrospective evaluation of over 800 inpatients from 1 academic medical center [25]. Furthermore, a chronic pain syndrome has been associated with an increased risk for readmission among patients with IBD [26].

There are also concerns that opioid therapies may mask warning signs of progressive disease, particularly when serial abdominal examinations and other physical exam findings are being utilized. Unfortunately, the optimal pain management strategies for inpatients with IBD have not been identified to this point. There is some limited evidence for the low fermentable carbohydrate (FODMAP) diet as well as limited evidence for referral to psychotherapy services for assistance with IBD-associated abdominal pain [27, 28]. While the most efficacious method of pain management remains to be determined, several important steps can be taken to limit the use of opioid therapy for inpatients with IBD. In the development of enhanced recovery protocols and enhanced recovery after surgery (ERAS) algorithms, IBD surgeons have placed an emphasis on utilizing non-opioid analgesics [29]. A similar multidisciplinary approach focusing on the factors associated with pain control among nonsurgical inpatients with IBD may yield important benefits.

Methods to Improve Quality of Care

High-Volume IBD Centers and IBD-Focused Inpatient Service

High-volume, large, and often academic medical centers tend to offer more specialized care than is available at community hospital settings. There are several studies examining surgical outcomes of IBD patients that receive care at high-volume centers versus community hospitals. These studies have found lower postoperative mortality and higher likelihood to proceed to surgery without increased length of stay or associated hospitalization costs when IBD patients undergo their surgery at a high-volume IBD center [30, 31]. Prior studies have also examined the impact of early specialized care on the outcomes of IBD patients and found that referral to a gastroenterologist within 1 year of diagnosis of IBD is associated with a decreased risk of surgery [32]. More recently, studies have examined the impact of IBD patients receiving care directly from a gastroenterologist while hospitalized. In a population-based cohort study of hospitalized patients with UC from Ontario, Canada, those patients admitted under a gastroenterologist demonstrated reduced in-hospital and 1-year mortality when compared to a group of patients admitted under non-gastroenterologists. However, in-hospital colectomy rates and UC-specific readmissions rates were similar between the two groups [33].

Law et al. examined the impact of specific changes in care delivery on outcomes among inpatients with IBD [34]. The authors utilized a unique study design where a control population was accumulated over a 1-year period during which all IBD patients were managed in consultation with or were primarily under the care of a general gastroenterologist. The population from this control period was compared to a population admitted after the implementation of a specialized IBD inpatient service. In a comparison of the two groups, the authors noted significant differences in the rate of C-reactive protein (CRP) testing, use of high-dose biologic therapy, and a shorter time to IBD-related surgical procedures. In evaluating post-discharge outcomes, those patients treated on the IBD specialty inpatient service demonstrated higher rates of remission at 90 days after discharge when compared to those patients in the control population. Given the growing complexity of IBD care and the diverse needs of IBD patients, high-volume centers and direct involvement by IBD specialists may drive improved outcomes in this patient population. Further demonstration of these trends in other populations is necessary and may lead to wider implementation.

Admission Order Sets

Since the broad adoption of the electronic health record (EHR), admission order sets have also become widely available as a tool to assist clinicians in more efficiently admitting patients to the hospital. They include basic orders needed by all hospitalized patients and over time have come to incorporate quality measures to allow healthcare systems to improve their compliance with such measures and better standardize patient care. Whether it is pediatric respiratory illness or sepsis care in the emergency department, there are numerous studies showing improved guideline adherence, lower cost of care, decreased length of stay, and more efficient delivery of care when admission order sets are used [35–37]. Only one study thus far has evaluated the impact of implementation of a standardized inpatient protocol for UC care. Authors from the University of California San Francisco designed a study aimed to address three key evidence-based care metrics (VTE prophylaxis, *C. difficile* testing, and opioid avoidance). While their hospital system already had above-average *C. difficile* testing rates, the authors demonstrated a significant increase in the rate of pharmacological VTE prophylaxis administration as well as significant decreases in both the rate of overall opioid use and the median daily morphine equivalents administered [38]. Further studies are needed to assess the impact of order sets on the quality of care delivered to IBD patients, but their success in other disease processes suggests they would be beneficial in the inpatient management of CD and UC.

The Cost of Inpatient Care and Factors Driving Readmission

The care for patients with IBD in the United States is associated with a significant cost burden, both to the individual patient and the healthcare system [39]. Although the drivers of cost in the care of patients with IBD are shifting, as many costs are now attributable to specific therapies or the use of healthcare services for comorbidities, hospital admissions and particularly hospital readmissions represent significant expenditures [39]. Multiple studies in both pediatric and adult patient populations have shown a hospital readmission rate in excess of 20% in IBD patients within 90 days of hospital discharge with associated costs of over $600 million [26, 40]. While some hospital readmissions are unavoidable, several associations or risk factors for higher rates of readmission in IBD patients have been demonstrated. In a systematic review and meta-analysis that included 17 cohort studies, Nguyen et al. identified multiple common reasons for readmission including a flare of IBD, infection, and complications from an unplanned surgery [41]. Additionally, comorbid psychiatric conditions (including anxiety and depression), chronic pain syndromes, and having Medicaid insurance have all been associated with an increased risk of readmission (Table 10.2) [26, 42].

Given the significant costs associated with readmission among patients with CD and UC, future efforts may focus on preventing readmission via an increased emphasis on those modifiable risk factors. In a prospective study of over 300 patients from Australia, the integration of a psychological care model was associated with a significant decrease in emergency department visits and overall costs [43]. By focusing on the role that these potentially modifiable risk factors have on the disease course and specifically the risk of hospital readmission, we may be able to identify those patients at greatest risk for readmission or other complications during their initial hospitalization and thus tailor interventions early in the hospitalization to improve both short- and long-term outcomes in this particularly vulnerable population.

Table 10.2 Risk factors associated with readmission at 30 and 90 days among patients with Crohn's disease and ulcerative colitis

Risk factor	OR for 30-day readmission (95% CI)	OR for 90-day readmission (95% CI) [26]
Anxiety		CD: 1.31 (1.21–1.43) [26] UC: 1.28 (1.14–1.45) [26]
Depression	UC: 1.40 (1.16–1.66) [44]	CD: 1.27 (1.07–1.50) [26] UC: 1.35 (1.07–1.70) [26]
Chronic pain		CD: 1.31 (1.18–1.46) [26] UC: 1.44 (1.21–1.73) [26]
Tobacco abuse		CD: 1.13 (1.06–1.22) [26]
Admission for pain control	IBD: 2.27 (1.69–3.03) [41]	
Total parenteral nutrition	IBD: 2.13 (1.36–3.35) [41]	
Prior or unplanned surgery	IBD: 3.11 (2.27–4.25) [41]	

CI confidence interval, *CD* Crohn's disease, *IBD* inflammatory bowel disease, *OR* odds ratio, *UC* ulcerative colitis

Conclusions

The management of inpatients with CD and UC continues to expand in complexity given an increasing number of potential therapies and the need for multidisciplinary management strategies. However, the implementation of several measures focused on improving the quality of care for inpatients with IBD can significantly improve outcomes related to the initial hospitalization and on follow-up after discharge. Special attention should be given to VTE prophylaxis, *C. difficile* testing, and pain management strategies. Several novel strategies to improve care in this population are emerging to improve the quality of care and optimize care delivery for inpatients with IBD. While each of these strategies will require further validation in other populations, these should inspire us to re-evaluate the care of each inpatient admitted with CD or UC, as these are potentially the most critical moments of an individual patient's disease course.

References

1. Peery AF, Crockett SD, Murphy CC, Lund JL, Dellon ES, Williams JL, et al. Burden and cost of gastrointestinal, liver, and pancreatic diseases in the United States: update 2018. Gastroenterology. 2019;156(1):254–72.e11
2. Kahn SR, Lim W, Dunn AS, Cushman M, Dentali F, Akl EA, et al. Prevention of VTE in nonsurgical patients: antithrombotic therapy and prevention of thrombosis, 9th ed: American College of Chest Physicians evidence-based clinical practice guidelines. Chest. 2012;141(2 Suppl):e195S–226S.
3. Chopard P, Spirk D, Bounameaux H. Identifying acutely ill medical patients requiring thromboprophylaxis. J Thromb Haemost. 2006;4(4):915–6.
4. Barbar S, Noventa F, Rossetto V, Ferrari A, Brandolin B, Perlati M, et al. A risk assessment model for the identification of hospitalized medical patients at risk for venous thromboembolism: the Padua Prediction Score. J Thromb Haemost. 2010;8(11):2450–7.
5. Kaddourah O, Numan L, Jeepalyam S, Abughanimeh O, Ghanimeh MA, Abuamr K. Venous thromboembolism prophylaxis in inflammatory bowel disease flare-ups. Ann Gastroenterol. 2019;32(6):578–83.

6. Yuhara H, Steinmaus C, Corley D, Koike J, Igarashi M, Suzuki T, et al. Meta-analysis: the risk of venous thromboembolism in patients with inflammatory bowel disease. Aliment Pharmacol Ther. 2013;37(10):953–62.
7. Nguyen GC, Bernstein CN, Bitton A, Chan AK, Griffiths AM, Leontiadis GI, et al. Consensus statements on the risk, prevention, and treatment of venous thromboembolism in inflammatory bowel disease: Canadian Association of Gastroenterology. Gastroenterology. 2014;146(3):835–48.e6
8. Papa A, Papa V, Marzo M, Scaldaferri F, Sofo L, Rapaccini GL, et al. Prevention and treatment of venous thromboembolism in patients with IBD: a trail still climbing. Inflamm Bowel Dis. 2015;21(5):1204–13.
9. Faye AS, Hung KW, Cheng K, Blackett JW, Mckenney AS, Pont AR, et al. Minor hematochezia decreases use of venous thromboembolism prophylaxis in patients with inflammatory bowel disease. Inflamm Bowel Dis. 2020;26:1394–400.
10. Ra G, Thanabalan R, Ratneswaran S, Nguyen GC. Predictors and safety of venous thromboembolism prophylaxis among hospitalized inflammatory bowel disease patients. J Crohns Colitis. 2013;7(10):e479–85.
11. Rubin DT, Ananthakrishnan AN, Siegel CA, Sauer BG, Long MD. ACG clinical guideline: ulcerative colitis in adults. Am J Gastroenterol. 2019;114(3):384–413.
12. Czepiel J, Dróżdż M, Pituch H, Kuijper EJ, Perucki W, Mielimonka A, et al. Clostridium difficile infection: review. Eur J Clin Microbiol Infect Dis. 2019;38(7):1211–21.
13. Khanna S, Shin A, Kelly CP. Management of Clostridium difficile infection in inflammatory bowel disease: expert review from the clinical practice updates committee of the AGA Institute. Clin Gastroenterol Hepatol. 2017;15(2):166–74.
14. Nguyen GC, Kaplan GG, Harris ML, Brant SR. A national survey of the prevalence and impact of Clostridium difficile infection among hospitalized inflammatory bowel disease patients. Am J Gastroenterol. 2008;103(6):1443–50.
15. Issa M, Vijayapal A, Graham MB, Beaulieu DB, Otterson MF, Lundeen S, et al. Impact of Clostridium difficile on inflammatory bowel disease. Clin Gastroenterol Hepatol. 2007;5(3):345–51.
16. McDonald LC, Gerding DN, Johnson S, Bakken JS, Carroll KC, Coffin SE, et al. Clinical practice guidelines for Clostridium difficile infection in adults and children: 2017 update by the Infectious Diseases Society of America (IDSA) and Society for Healthcare Epidemiology of America (SHEA). Clin Infect Dis. 2018;66(7):e1–e48.
17. Johnson S, Louie TJ, Gerding DN, Cornely OA, Chasan-Taber S, Fitts D, et al. Vancomycin, metronidazole, or tolevamer for Clostridium difficile infection: results from two multinational, randomized, controlled trials. Clin Infect Dis. 2014;59(3):345–54.

18. Fu N, Wong T. Clostridium difficile infection in patients with inflammatory bowel disease. Curr Infect Dis Rep. 2016;18(6):19.
19. D'Aoust J, Battat R, Bessissow T. Management of inflammatory bowel disease with Clostridium difficile infection. World J Gastroenterol. 2017;23(27):4986–5003.
20. Lukin DJ, Lawlor G, Hudesman DP, Durbin L, Axelrad JE, Passi M, et al. Escalation of immunosuppressive therapy for inflammatory bowel disease is not associated with adverse outcomes after infection with Clostridium difficile. Inflamm Bowel Dis. 2019;25(4):775–81.
21. Targownik LE, Nugent Z, Singh H, Bugden S, Bernstein CN. The prevalence and predictors of opioid use in inflammatory bowel disease: a population-based analysis. Am J Gastroenterol. 2014;109(10):1613–20.
22. Cohen-Mekelburg S, Rosenblatt R, Gold S, Burakoff R, Waljee A, Saini S, et al. The impact of opioid epidemic trends on hospitalized inflammatory bowel disease patients. J Crohns Colitis. 2018;12(9):1030–5.
23. Coates MD, Seth N, Clarke K, Abdul-Baki H, Mahoney N, Walter V, et al. Opioid analgesics do not improve abdominal pain or quality of life in Crohn's disease. Dig Dis Sci. 2020;65:2379–87.
24. Long MD, Barnes EL, Herfarth HH, Drossman DA. Narcotic use for inflammatory bowel disease and risk factors during hospitalization. Inflamm Bowel Dis. 2012;18(5):869–76.
25. Dalal RS, Palchaudhuri S, Snider CK, Lewis JD, Mehta SJ, Lichtenstein GR. Exposure to intravenous opioids is associated with future exposure to opioids in hospitalized patients with inflammatory bowel diseases. Clin Gastroenterol Hepatol. 2020;18:2269–78.e3
26. Barnes EL, Kochar B, Long MD, Kappelman MD, Martin CF, Korzenik JR, et al. Modifiable risk factors for hospital readmission among patients with inflammatory bowel disease in a nationwide database. Inflamm Bowel Dis. 2017;23(6):875–81.
27. Norton C, Czuber-Dochan W, Artom M, Sweeney L, Hart A. Systematic review: interventions for abdominal pain management in inflammatory bowel disease. Aliment Pharmacol Ther. 2017;46(2):115–25.
28. Durchschein F, Petritsch W, Hammer HF. Diet therapy for inflammatory bowel diseases: the established and the new. World J Gastroenterol. 2016;22(7):2179–94.
29. Barnes EL, Lightner AL, Regueiro M. Peri-operative and post-operative management of patients with Crohn's disease and ulcerative colitis. Clin Gastroenterol Hepatol. 2020;18:1356–66.
30. Ananthakrishnan AN, McGinley EL, Binion DG. Does it matter where you are hospitalized for inflammatory bowel disease? A nationwide analysis of hospital volume. Am J Gastroenterol. 2008;103(11):2789–98.
31. Kaplan GG, McCarthy EP, Ayanian JZ, Korzenik J, Hodin R, Sands BE. Impact of hospital volume on postoperative morbidity and mortality following a colectomy for ulcerative colitis. Gastroenterology. 2008;134(3):680–7.

32. Nguyen GC, Nugent Z, Shaw S, Bernstein CN. Outcomes of patients with Crohn's disease improved from 1988 to 2008 and were associated with increased specialist care. Gastroenterology. 2011;141(1):90–7.
33. Murthy SK, Steinhart AH, Tinmouth J, Austin PC, Nguyen GC. Impact of gastroenterologist care on health outcomes of hospitalised ulcerative colitis patients. Gut. 2012;61(10):1410–6.
34. Law CCY, Sasidharan S, Rodrigues R, Nguyen DD, Sauk J, Garber J, et al. Impact of specialized inpatient IBD care on outcomes of IBD hospitalizations: a cohort study. Inflamm Bowel Dis. 2016;22(9):2149–57.
35. Chan AJ, Chan J, Cafazzo JA, Rossos PG, Tripp T, Shojania K, et al. Order sets in health care: a systematic review of their effects. Int J Technol Assess Health Care. 2012;28(3):235–40.
36. Gatewood MO, Wemple M, Greco S, Kritek PA, Durvasula R. A quality improvement project to improve early sepsis care in the emergency department. BMJ Qual Saf. 2015;24(12):787–95.
37. Dayal A, Alvarez F. The effect of implementation of standardized, evidence-based order sets on efficiency and quality measures for pediatric respiratory illnesses in a community hospital. Hosp Pediatr. 2015;5(12):624–9.
38. Lewin SM, McConnell RA, Patel R, Sharpton SR, Velayos F, Mahadevan U. Improving the quality of inpatient ulcerative colitis management: promoting evidence-based practice and reducing care variation with an inpatient protocol. Inflamm Bowel Dis. 2019;25(11):1822–7.
39. Park KT, Ehrlich OG, Allen JI, Meadows P, Szigethy EM, Henrichsen K, et al. The cost of inflammatory bowel disease: an initiative from the Crohn's & Colitis Foundation. Inflamm Bowel Dis. 2020;26(1):1–10.
40. Barnes EL, Kochar B, Long MD, Martin CF, Crockett SD, Korzenik JR, et al. The burden of hospital readmissions among pediatric patients with inflammatory bowel disease. J Pediatr. 2017;191:184–9.e1
41. Nguyen NH, Koola J, Dulai PS, Prokop LJ, Sandborn WJ, Singh S. Rate of risk factors for and interventions to reduce hospital readmission in patients with inflammatory bowel diseases. Clin Gastroenterol Hepatol. 2020;18(9):1939–48.e7
42. Axelrad JE, Sharma R, Laszkowska M, Packey C, Rosenberg R, Lebwohl B. Increased healthcare utilization by patients with inflammatory bowel disease covered by Medicaid at a tertiary care center. Inflamm Bowel Dis. 2019;25(10):1711–7.
43. Lores T, Goess C, Mikocka-Walus A, Collins KL, ALJ B, Chur-Hansen A, et al. Integrated psychological care reduces healthcare costs at a hospital-based inflammatory bowel disease service. Clin Gastroenterol Hepatol. 2021;19(1):96–103.e3
44. Poojary P, Saha A, Chauhan K, Simoes P, Sands BE, Cho J, et al. Predictors of hospital readmissions for ulcerative colitis in the United States: a national database study. Inflamm Bowel Dis. 2017;23(3):347–56.

Management of Pediatric Patients Hospitalized with Ulcerative

11

Athos Bousvaros

Introduction

Pediatric inflammatory bowel disease has significantly increased in incidence in childhood over the last 30 years, with the most rapid rate of increase noted in very young children. While most children can be managed as outpatients and may never require hospitalization, a significant proportion of children have more severe disease. Some of these children present with severe colitis at disease onset and require immediate hospitalization. Others will have a worsening of their condition over time, leading to one or many hospitalizations, until their disease can be stabilized either surgically or medically.

This chapter will initially give an overview of the management of pediatric ulcerative colitis (UC) and then focus on the complexities of managing inpatients with the disease. For additional

A. Bousvaros (✉)
Professor of Pediatrics, Harvard Medical School, Inflammatory Bowel Disease Center, Boston Children's Hospital, Boston, MA, USA
e-mail: athos.bousvaros@childrens.harvard.edu

J. D. Feuerstein, A. S. Cheifetz (eds.), *Management of Inpatient Inflammatory Bowel Disease*,
https://doi.org/10.1007/978-1-0716-1987-2_11

information, the reader is referred to the outstanding consensus guidelines by the European Society for Pediatric Gastroenterology, Hepatology, and Nutrition [1, 2].

Overview of Pediatric Ulcerative Colitis

Studies suggest that children with ulcerative colitis (UC) have a different phenotype than adults with ulcerative colitis. Specifically, a greater proportion of children with UC have more extensive disease (disease that involves the entire colon), compared to adults, where left-sided disease and proctitis are more common. As in adults, the most common presenting symptoms of pediatric ulcerative colitis include rectal bleeding, abdominal cramping around the time of bowel movements, and loose or watery diarrhea. Extraintestinal manifestations that occur include oligoarticular arthritis, erythema nodosum, or pyoderma gangrenosum. Skin manifestations rarely occur at disease presentation [3].

Assuming ulcerative colitis is suspected, the diagnostic evaluation includes laboratory studies (complete blood count, sedimentation rate, C-reactive protein, chemistries, albumin, and liver function tests). Fecal studies are done to exclude infection, particularly common enteric pathogens (*Salmonella*, *Shigella*, *Yersinia*, *Campylobacter*, *E. coli*) and *C. difficile*. Depending on geographic location where a patient is being assessed and their travel history, additional fecal studies (e.g., to exclude amoebiasis) may be indicated. Many clinicians will also order fecal calprotectin or lactoferrin, though the utility of these tests in a patient with known bloody diarrhea is questionable. The more definitive diagnostic evaluation of ulcerative colitis involves ileocolonoscopy, combined with upper endoscopy and biopsy in children. During colonoscopy, we recommend biopsies taken both in the terminal ileum and in different regions of the colon, including the ascending colon, transverse, descending, sigmoid, and rectum. As with adult ulcerative colitis, the pathologist will usually identify chronic active colitis. Granulomas should be absent, and their presence suggests Crohn's disease. However, nonspecific microscopic ileitis may be seen in pediatric patients with ulcerative colitis approximately 15% of the time. This does not warrant changing the diagnosis to Crohn's disease. Upper endoscopy is recommended by current pediatric guidelines because of the high prevalence of upper GI tract disease in children with ulcerative colitis and the potential for identifying features that might change the diagnosis to Crohn's disease [4, 5].

Milder cases of ulcerative colitis can often be treated initially with aminosalicylate therapy. In mild to moderate cases, a course of oral corticosteroid therapy may help induce remission and allow transition to aminosalicylates. In patients who cannot be maintained on aminosalicylates, there are many potential options for therapy. Thiopurines, while once a mainstay of long-term UC maintenance therapy in children and adults, are generally being less utilized in the pediatric population [6, 7]. Clinicians are transitioning instead to newer agents, including anti-TNF therapy, vedolizumab, and other newer medications. The reason for the transition away from thiopurines includes concerns about the small risk of lymphoma, particularly in adolescent males, as well as the emerging data on the new agents that suggests a favorable safety profile in adults [8–10]. However, the biologics are significantly more expensive than thiopurines, and under certain circumstances, it may be appropriate to continue to consider thiopurines. In contrast, methotrexate monotherapy, which was once thought to be a potential option in patients with ulcerative colitis, has now been demonstrated in two large clinical trials to be no superior to placebo [11, 12].

Management of Inpatient Severe Colitis

Initial Assessment and Evaluation

The determination of whether colitis is severe enough to warrant hospitalization in a child is ultimately the judgment of the treating clinician, whether a gastroenterologist seeing the patient in the clinic or an emergency department physician. However, a formal scale, the pediatric ulcerative colitis activity index (PUCAI) is a useful tool to confirm clinical judgment. The PUCAI, developed by Dan Turner in 2007, has been extensively validated and correlates with endoscopic disease severity and likelihood of hospitalization (Table 11.1) [13–15]. The PUCAI is also a useful measure in the hospital to assess response to therapy, as it has been utilized

Table 11.1 Pediatric ulcerative colitis activity index

Item	Points
1. Abdominal pain	
No pain	0 point
Pain can be ignored	5
Pain cannot be ignored	10
2. Rectal bleeding	
None	0
Small amount only, in less than 50% of stools	10
Small amount with most stools	20
Large amount (>50% of the stool content)	30
3. Stool consistency of most stools	
Formed	0
Partially formed	5
Completely unformed	10
4. Number of stools per 24 hours	
0–2	0
3–5	5
6–8	10
>8	15
5. Nocturnal stools (any episode causing wakening)	
No	0
Yes	10
6. Activity level	
No limitation of activity	0
Occasional limitation of activity	5
Severe restricted activity	10

The PUCAI score ranges from 0 to 85. A PUCAI score of 0–9 indicates disease remission, PUCAI of 10–34 indicates mild disease, 35–64 indicates moderate disease, over 65 indicates severe disease in many clinical trials. A hospitalized patient who has been treated for 5 days with intravenous corticosteroids, and has not had a significant decline in his PUCAI index, is likely to require additional medical rescue therapy [16].

The initial assessment of a child hospitalized with ulcerative colitis depends on whether this is a new-onset case or a patient with known disease. Initial stabilization of the patient involves laboratory assessment, including CBC, electrolytes, and albumin. Intravenous hydration is provided, usually at maintenance therapy or a little over maintenance therapy, as many of these children have difficulty taking in adequate amounts of fluid, and dehydration could in turn lead to other complications such as thrombosis. The American Academy of Pediatrics recommends normal saline, supplemented with potassium as a primary intravenous fluid (IVF) in children, because more hypotonic fluids have been associated with hyponatremia [17]. Our usual IVF is normal saline with 20 mEq/L potassium, given either at maintenance or 1.25 times maintenance.

In a new-onset case, diagnostic evaluation should proceed, ideally before beginning medical treatment. An ill child with a new diagnosis should undergo an abdominal plain film to exclude toxic megacolon. Even in the absence of toxic megacolon, findings on the abdominal plain film may have some value in predicting response to medication [18]. Once a hospitalized patient has been stabilized, stool studies as outlined above should occur. The patient should then undergo a cleanout and have the endoscopic studies performed (Fig. 11.1). Depending on disease severity, as well as the skill and comfort of the endoscopist, a complete colonoscopy may not be able to be performed. However, if the disease is not too severe, a full colonoscopy and ileoscopy should be attempted, because this may be the best opportunity to try to distinguish between ulcerative colitis and Crohn's disease. Over time, medical treatment may change the macroscopic and histologic findings, resulting in patchier inflammation and making it more difficult to differentiate between CD and UC [19]. During the procedure, the endoscopist should clearly identify the location of disease, as well as grade disease severity utilizing a formal scoring system such as the Mayo score [5, 20]. In addition to stan-

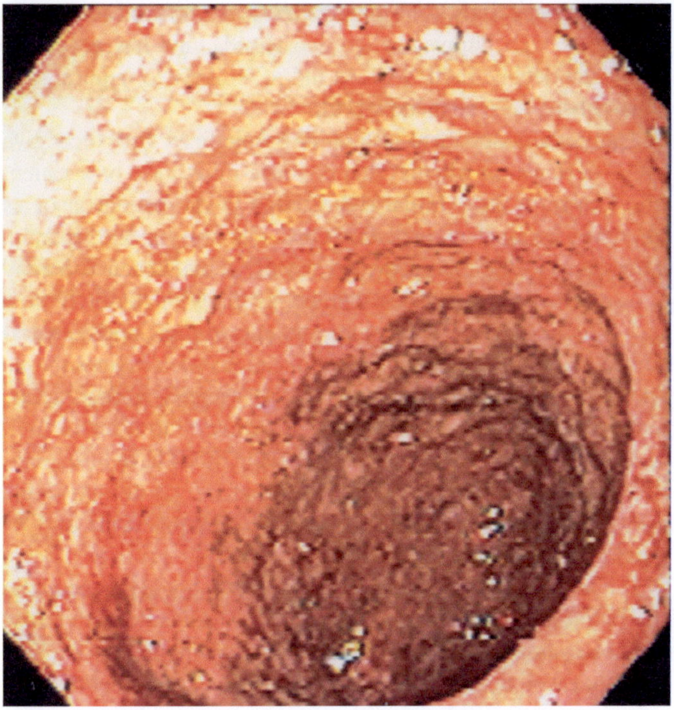

Fig. 11.1 Colonoscopic examination of severe colitis in a child (descending colon). Note the loss of vascular pattern, diffuse and continuous involvement, and significant ulceration

dard biopsies from the colon sent for histology, the pathologist should also assess for cytomegalovirus, both by looking for enlarged epithelial cells and also utilizing CMV immunostaining.

In contrast, in a patient with known ulcerative colitis, an immediate colonoscopy is usually not necessary. Review of the last colonoscopy can potentially characterize the extent and severity of disease. If the history is most consistent with a colitis flare (aka a patient with poorly controlled disease being readmitted), treatment (e.g., corticosteroids) can be started even before one has the results of stool cultures. If an infectious pathogen (most commonly *C. difficile*) is identified on stool cultures, the pathogen can be treated simultaneously with the colitis. However, if there is an acute deterioration in a patient with a long history of stable well-controlled disease, the clinician may decide to wait for infectious studies to come back before beginning empiric therapy with anti-inflammatory or immune suppressive medications. In all children with severe colitis, the possibility of new-onset cytomegalovirus infection needs to be considered, particularly before starting biologic therapy [21].

Supportive Care

Once the pediatric IBD patient has been admitted and stabilized, supportive care should focus on six primary areas: intravenous hydration, nutrition, treatment of anemia, prevention of thrombosis, pain control, and psychosocial support. Initially we provide intravenous fluids with 5% dextrose (D5) normal saline and 20 mEq/L of potassium, given at maintenance. Depending on the patient's age, weight, and ability to take in oral fluids, the amount of intravenous hydration may be reduced over time. In most patients with colitis, who are relatively pain-free and do not have ileus, there is no contraindication to oral nutrition, and we generally allow them to eat. The same approach is recommended in the European guidelines [1, 2]. In spite of some anecdotal reports that suggest restrictive diet such as the specific carbohydrate diet may be beneficial in inflammatory bowel disease, we do not impose a specific diet on hospitalized IBD patients [22]. Instead, we take a detailed history from the patient, identifying any potential dietary triggers, and advise the patient to avoid those foods that make them worse.

Patients who are unwilling or unable to eat may require parenteral nutrition during their hospital stay [23]. This involves placement of central access, usually through a peripherally inserted central catheter (PICC line), the tip of which should be placed at the superior vena cava near the right atrium. Placement of the PICC line allows the infusion of more concentrated forms of dextrose (above 10%), as well as lipids. However, as with any central line, there is an increased risk of infection and thrombosis.

Anemia in a patient with severe ulcerative colitis is likely to be a combination of active blood loss superimposed on anemia of chronic disease (in which iron absorption and utilization is impaired due to inflammation). While pediatric recommendations suggest a more restrictive approach to transfusion in children, these recommendations are largely based on experience from hematology and nephrology patients, as well as perioperative management of transfusion [24]. In addition, while the European Crohn's and Colitis Organization has published a recommendation on the management of anemia in patients with Crohn's and colitis, the management primarily focuses on patients with anemia from chronic illness rather than active bleeding. The ECCO panel recommends transfusion be considered in patients with hemoglobins under 7, but again this refers to stable patients without active bleeding [25]. According to this expert panel, "the decision to administer blood transfusions is not solely based on the hemoglobin level, but takes comorbidity and symptoms into account." Therefore, there are no specific evidence-based guidelines in children with active bleeding from severe colitis as to when and how to transfuse. Our practice has been to consider transfusion in patients with severe colitis and active bleeding who are either symptomatic (e.g., tachycardia or orthostasis) or have hemoglobins under 9. The decision to transfuse is a complex one and depends on the patient's symptoms, the degree of active bleeding, and also parental preferences. Some religions (e.g., Jehovah's Witnesses) explicitly forbid blood transfusions, and clinicians make every effort to avoid transfusions except in life-threatening situations [26].

In patients who are anemic but have low-volume GI bleeding, intravenous (IV) iron is a reasonable alternative to transfusion, though there may be a lag of days to weeks before an iron infusion raises his hemoglobin. The dose of iron needed to raise hemoglobin to normal levels in children over 40 kg can be calculated utilizing the Ganzoni formula ((body weight in kg × [target hemoglobin-actual hemoglobin in g/dL] × 0.24 + 500)0.58) = mg of iron) [25]. Many different iron preparations exist that can treat iron deficiency anemia. Iron dextran is our standard preparation, and the advantage of that preparation is that the entire dose of iron can be given during one infusion. However, iron dextran is associated with an increased risk of allergic reactions including anaphylaxis. Therefore, alternative IV iron preparations do exist which may carry a slightly lower risk, including ferric carboxymaltose and ferric gluconate [27, 28]. The amount of iron that can be given with these newer preparations more limited, and multiple doses may be needed.

Thrombosis prevention is an important component of supportive medical care in patients with inflammatory bowel disease. Retrospective and prospective studies have found an increased prevalence of thrombosis in children with IBD, both related and unrelated to the utilization of central catheters. As in adults, some of these thrombotic complications may be severe, including central nervous system venous thrombosis, pulmonary emboli, and clots of large vessels, including the inferior vena cava [29]. Fortunately, thrombosis in children is less common than in adults. At Boston children's, we utilize a thrombophilia screen which aids into our decision-making as to whether or not to administer prophylaxis. The screen includes questions about family history, assessment of physical findings (particularly body mass index), and also review of any medications that could potentially predispose to clotting [29, 30]. The most commonly utilized method of prophylaxis currently is with enoxaparin, 1 IU/kg/SQ administered twice daily. In contrast, current ESPGHAN guidelines suggest a dose of 1 IU/kg given daily, up to 100 units [1]. In some children who are "needle phobic" and at low risk for thrombosis, we discussed with the family in more detail the risks and benefits of prophylaxis. We hold prophylaxis in patients who are going to undergo surgery and also discontinue prophylaxis at the time of hospital discharge.

Pain control is another important aspect of supportive care. Once again, in this area, there are no formal guidelines as to what the best agent is or how often to dose medication for pain. Generally speaking, pain in patients with colitis tends to occur around the time of bowel movement and often resolves after the bowel movement is completed. Because bowel movements tend to occur suddenly and resolve quickly, the utilization of on-demand agents to treat this peri-defecatory pain is often ineffective. However, patients with severe colitis often have a period of time between 4 AM and 8 AM when they tend to have more frequent bowel movements, and in this situation a dose of pain medication may be helpful. We tend to avoid ketorolac, because of some reports that nonsteroidal medications may worsen colitis. A European consensus expert panel on the management of pain in children with IBD recommended a detailed assessment of patients with severe pain (to exclude toxic megacolon and perforation), utilization of hot packs and oral Tylenol as the preferred initial therapy, and consideration of low-dose morphine (up to 0.1 mg/kg per dose) [2]. We try to minimize morphine use out of the concern that we may precipitate an ileus but do utilize it on occasion. As with other chronic illnesses, long-term opioid use should be avoided to reduce the likelihood of future dependency [31]. In patients with significant pain-related anxiety, pharmacologic or psychologic anxiety management techniques may be helpful [32].

Lastly, but perhaps most importantly, psychosocial support is absolutely essential for children and families admitted with severe ulcerative colitis. Approximately 25% of children with IBD have anxiety and depression at any given time, and cognitive behavioral therapy has been shown to be effective at treating the psychosocial symptoms [33]. In the hospital, the psychosocial symptoms are often exacerbated, in part due to the lack of sleep that the hospital setting provides, in part due to disease severity, and in part due to medications we used to treat IBD (e.g., corticosteroids). Early involvement by psychology or social work may help identify risk factors and allow for interventions that may improve overall well-being [34]. In addition, given that outpatient adherence with medication regimens is quite challenging for patients and families, our social workers will often identify barriers to care (e.g., transportation or insurance issues) that the medical team may not identify.

Medical Therapy for Severe Colitis

While the clinician aims to stabilize the patient and treat complications of the underlying disease, the most important part of hospital-based therapy involves getting the inflammatory bowel disease itself under control. Once acute bacterial or viral infection has been excluded, the primary mode of therapy involves immune suppressive medications to control inflammation. There is also a limited role for antibiotic therapy. Medical therapies for ulcerative colitis are summarized in Table 11.2.

Intravenous corticosteroids are the time-honored treatment for pediatric and adult severe colitis and are generally the first agent utilized. The European expert panel recommends intravenous methylprednisolone, at a dose of 1–1.5 mg/kg, either once a day or in two divided doses, with a maximum dose of 60 mg/day. There are some relative contraindications to corticosteroid use, most notably in patients with behavioral disorders and a history of corticosteroid-induced psychosis. The pediatric ulcerative colitis activity index is utilized to assess response to corticosteroid ther-

Table 11.2 Medical therapies utilized in pediatric severe colitis

Medication	Dosage
Intravenous methylprednisolone	1.5 mg/kg/day, up to maximum of 60 mg
Antibiotics (per PRASCO trial)	
Vancomycin	250 mg/dose, given 4×/day,
	125 mg 4×/day in children under 8 years
Amoxicillin	50 mg/kg/day in three divided doses (up to 500 mg tid)
Metronidazole	5 mg/kg/dose given tid (up to 350 mg tid)
Doxycycline (children over 7)	2 mg/kg/dose bid, up to 100 mg bid
Ciprofloxacin (children under 7)	10 mg/kg/dose bid, up to 250 mg bid
Rescue agents	
Infliximab	5–10 mg/kg/dose (consider "intensified induction" by redosing in 3–5 days if no improvement)
Cyclosporine IV	Initial dose 2 mg/kg/day IV in two divided doses, aim for level of 150–400 ng/ml
Tacrolimus PO	0.2 mg/kg/day PO in two divided doses, aim for level of 10–15 ng/ml

References: [1–3, 36, 40]

apy, and the patient who does not have significant improvement (decrease in pediatric ulcerative colitis activity index by at least 20 points or decrease in clinical condition from moderate/severe to mild) after 3 to 5 days should be considered for rescue therapy with second-line agents. Approximately 50% of patients will not respond to intravenous corticosteroids and will require rescue therapy [16].

The role of antibiotic treatment in ulcerative colitis remains controversial. The 2011 European working group did not recommend empiric antibiotic use except in the case of toxic megacolon. However, more recent work suggests that an antibiotic cocktail may be of some benefit in acute severe colitis. An initial study by Turner and colleagues of 15 children treated with an antibiotic cocktail utilizing metronidazole, amoxicillin, vancomycin, and doxycycline resulted in a response rate of approximately 50% [35]. Based on this initial promising information, the investigators conducted a randomized control trial of these for antibiotics plus intravenous corticosteroids, compared to intravenous corticosteroids only. In children younger than 7 years of age, ciprofloxacin was utilized rather than metronidazole. The group treated with antibiotics had lower PUCAI scores at day 5 and also exhibited significant alterations in their microbiome. However, response rates at discharge, the utilization of infliximab, and the long-term colectomy rates did not vary between the two cohorts. The investigators concluded that "antibiotics cannot be routinely recommended until larger studies demonstrate a reduced need for second line treatment or colectomy" [36].

Rescue therapy in the child with acute severe colitis primarily involves treatment with either antitumor necrosis factor antibody or calcineurin inhibitors. Currently, intravenous infliximab is the most commonly utilized agent and acute severe colitis unresponsive to corticosteroid therapy. One study of children data suggested up to 70% of patients who do not respond to corticosteroid therapy may respond to infliximab [37]. However, this study was an open-label study, and 19% of patients treated underwent surgery within a year [37]. The standard FDA dosing of infliximab recommends 5 mg/kg, at 0, 2, and 6 weeks. However, both adult and pediatric clinicians tend to give higher doses to those with severe colitis, based on some pharmacokinetic data that suggest patients with severe colitis will lose infliximab in their stool, and tend to run lower serum levels of the medication. Lower serum levels correlate with worse outcomes in severe colitis, but it remains unclear as to whether this is simply an association or if this reflects causation (i.e., underdosing of infliximab results in less effective treatment of IBD). A study by Ananthakrishnan and colleagues in adults suggests that 10 mg/kg infliximab dosing might initially result in a lower rate of colectomy but that long-term outcomes were comparable in hospitalized patients that received high-dose versus low-dose infliximab [38]. In contrast, a pediatric study suggested improved outcomes and reduction in colectomy rates [39]. Given the absence of evidence-based recommendations, we tend to utilize standard dose (5 mg/kg), in hospitalized patients with mild to moderate steroid-unresponsive disease, and reevaluate in 3–5 days, and if no response, we then provide 10 mg/kg as a second dose. In severe colitis (Mayo score of 3 or PUCAI greater than 65), we will utilize 10 mg/kg as our initial dose and once again reevaluate in 3–5 days. Patients who respond to infliximab usually do so within 10 days, most commonly within the first week. In those who do not respond after two doses, we consider giving a third dose about 5–7 days after the second. Simultaneously, we obtain drug levels prior to the third dose to determine if the patient is indeed consuming infliximab. Children who do not respond to two doses of 10 mg/kg of infliximab are unlikely to respond.

The other alternative agents that have been in use for 30 years to treat severe colitis are the calcineurin inhibitor family. Both cyclosporine and tacrolimus have been successfully utilized to induce remission in children. One potential advantage of these agents is that they are small molecules, and their pharmacokinetics may be more reliable in a patient with severe colitis than infliximab. However, treatment with calcineurin inhibitors requires close monitoring to prevent toxicity. Our routine clinical practice when we utilize calcineurin inhibitors involves beginning at a tacrolimus dose of 0.1 mg/kg per dose, given orally twice daily (0.2 mg/kg/day). We assess all patients for cytomegalovirus and Epstein-Barr virus prior to or at the time of starting medication, and we monitor laboratory studies on an every other day basis. Monitoring includes complete blood count, sedimentation rate, chemistries, liver enzymes, BUN, creatinine, glucose, and tacrolimus levels. Based on randomized control trials from Japan, as well as our own clinical experience, a tacrolimus level of between 10 and 15 ng/mL correlates with a higher probability of remission [40, 41]. Toxicities of calcineurin inhibitors include hypertension, hyperglycemia, rising creatinine, and hypomagnesemia. While headaches and (rarely) seizures can occur from these medications, most neurologic side effects tend to be associated with high levels of medication. Alternatively, intravenous cyclosporine can be utilized; the recommended dose of cyclosporine by the European expert consensus panel is 2 mg/kg/day, but some older studies utilized the higher dose of 4 mg/kg/day [42, 43]. Cyclosporine can be given in two divided doses. *Pneumocystis jirovecii* prophylaxis should be utilized in all patients receiving calcineurin inhibitors.

When we utilize a second-line agent for treatment of severe colitis, we continue the corticosteroids until we are comfortable that a patient has exhibited significant improvement, i.e., has mild disease or has entered remission. At that time, corticosteroids can be tapered, and the second-line agent continued. Infliximab can be utilized for both induction and maintenance, while calcineurin inhibitors are generally considered induction agents. If the patient responds to a calcineurin inhibitor, that agent can be continued for a few months, but the aim should be to transition to some other maintenance agent. Maintenance agents that have been utilized historically include thiopurines and anti-TNF agents. More recently, utilization of tacrolimus as a bridge to vedolizumab is increasingly being utilized in clinical practice [44].

Hospital discharge should not be considered until a UC patient is deemed to be quite stable by the clinical team, on a drug regimen that can be managed as an outpatient. As mentioned above, mental health support and social support to ensure adherence with the outpatient drug regimen is essential. Readmission rates for adults with ulcerative colitis are high. In one study of pediatric IBD from a database, approximately 22% of patients were readmitted within 90 days of diagnosis, and the risk factor most consistently associated with readmission was history of anxiety and depression. However, the study did not focus exclusively on severe colitis [45].

There is limited published data on newer agents (vedolizumab, ustekinumab, or tofacitinib) in the treatment of IBD in children, and we do not know if they are effective in severe colitis [46–48]. None of these drugs have yet been approved by the FDA for treatment of ulcerative colitis, but pediatricians utilize them as rescue therapies if other medications have not been effective. However, limited data suggest that either vedolizumab or possibly tofacitinib in combination with a biologic may have some utility in the situation. Combination therapy with azathioprine and infliximab has also been shown to be more effective than infliximab alone in adults with severe colitis. However, pediatric clinicians in the United States infrequently utilize this approach in children anymore because of the concerns about hepatosplenic T-cell lymphoma [9].

Surgical Considerations

Approximately 20% of children with ulcerative colitis will require surgery within 10 years of diagnosis [49]. In children, a multicenter inception cohort of approximately 400 new-onset UC patients demonstrated that 25 patients (6%) underwent colectomy during the approximately 1-year period of follow-up [50]. Given that the primary indication for surgery is active disease despite medication, a child with ulcerative colitis who does not respond rapidly to hospital management is a potential surgical candidate.

The discussion of performing a colectomy with a child often involves a difficult conversation with the family. This is particularly true in a newly diagnosed patient, who has not yet had time to acclimate to their disease, let alone the possibility that surgery may be necessary. Given the potential necessity of surgery in such patients however, we tend to have the conversation early, typically after about 5 days of lack of response to intravenous corticosteroids, before the utilization of second-line therapy. We mention that surgery is always an option in a patient with active ulcerative colitis, and we review the benefits and risks of the surgical approach versus the medical approach. At that point, assuming the family is ready, we recommend a formal consultation with one of our IBD surgeons, so that they can review the benefits and risks of surgery in more detail.

Early in the course of disease, more families will opt for medical therapy rather than proceeding directly to colectomy. However, in a patient that does not respond to intravenous corticosteroids and at least one second-line agent, families may become more interested in the option of surgery. In patients with severe colitis who decide on surgery, we usually perform a colectomy and ileostomy, as a start to a "three-stage procedure" [51]. However, in some patients who desire a two-stage procedure, we may attempt to induce remission with a short-term agent such as a calcineurin inhibitor before proceeding to surgery [52]. In a patient that is being considered for surgery, we carefully review the prior data, the nutritional status, and the current medications and then have a "structured handoff" to our surgical colleague, providing them with the pertinent data that they may require (see Table 11.3).

Summary

The inpatient treatment of the child with ulcerative colitis is complex and involves both medical and psychosocial considerations. The first priority is to assess colitis severity, treat any emergent issues such as dehydration thrombosis or toxic megacolon, and exclude intercurrent infections. Supportive care involves intravenous hydration, treatment of anemia, prevention of thrombosis, adequate nutrition, pain control, and management of psychosocial considerations. Intravenous corticosteroids are generally the first-line of medical therapy. Antibiotics can be considered as an adjunct treatment. In a patient that does not respond to first-line therapy, infliximab or calcineurin inhibitors can be utilized. We recommend early discussion of the surgical alternative, because even if a family is not prepared for this consideration, education about this possibility will help prepare the patient and parents for the future.

Table 11.3 IBD surgical handoff checklist

Patient	
MR	
Primary gastroenterologist	
Primary attending surgeon	
Disease (CD, UC)	
Has small bowel imaging been done? If so, summarize results (including date)	
Is macroscopic appearance of the intestine on initial or subsequent colonoscopies more consistent with CD or UC? Summarize results	
Is pathology more consistent with UC or CD (aka are there granulomas)? Summarize results	
Surgery planned	Ileocecal/ileoascending resection Mid-small bowel resection Segmental colectomy with reanastomosis Diverting ileostomy Diverting colostomy Colectomy with ileostomy and Hartmann pouch Colectomy with ileostomy and J pouch
Indication for procedure	Medically refractory disease Abdominal or perirectal abscess Stricture Other
Current steroid dose	
Biologic treatment and last dose	
Has pre-surgical teaching been done?	
Other concerns/comorbidities	

Clinical Question

A 12-year-old male with a 3-year history of ulcerative colitis, previously maintained on mesalamine, presents with a 2-week history of worsening bloody diarrhea. His last colonoscopy 2 years ago demonstrated a Mayo score of 1 and chronic active colitis on biopsy, but he was maintained on mesalamine because he was asymptomatic. On examination, he is mildly dehydrated, afebrile, and has a soft nontender abdomen. Abdominal plain film does not demonstrate a dilated colon. He is rehydrated with intravenous fluids and admitted for further management. Pediatric ulcerative colitis activity index is 50. Hemoglobin is 10. Of the following, which is a medically appropriate next step in inpatient management (choose one).

A. Abdominal CT scan
B. Intravenous methylprednisolone
C. Oral tacrolimus
D. NPO (no oral intake of food)
E. Transfusion

Correct answer is B. Intravenous methylprednisolone

References

1. Turner D, et al. Management of paediatric ulcerative colitis, part 2: acute severe colitis-an evidence-based consensus guideline from the European Crohn's and Colitis Organization and the European Society of Paediatric Gastroenterology, Hepatology and Nutrition. J Pediatr Gastroenterol Nutr. 2018;67(2):292–310.
2. Turner D, et al. Consensus for managing acute severe ulcerative colitis in children: a systematic review and joint statement from ECCO, ESPGHAN, and the Porto IBD working group of ESPGHAN. Am J Gastroenterol. 2011;106(4):574–88.
3. Regan BP, Bousvaros A. Pediatric ulcerative colitis: a practical guide to management. Paediatr Drugs. 2014;16(3):189–98.
4. Birimberg-Schwartz L, et al. Development and validation of diagnostic criteria for IBD subtypes including IBD-unclassified in children: a multi-

centre study from the pediatric IBD Porto group of ESPGHAN. J Crohns Colitis. 2017;11(9):1078–84.

5. Bousvaros A, et al. Differentiating ulcerative colitis from Crohn disease in children and young adults: report of a working group of the North American Society for Pediatric Gastroenterology, Hepatology, and Nutrition and the Crohn's and Colitis Foundation of America. J Pediatr Gastroenterol Nutr. 2007;44(5):653–74.
6. Bressler B, et al. Clinical practice guidelines for the medical management of nonhospitalized ulcerative colitis: the Toronto consensus. Gastroenterology. 2015;148(5):1035–58.e3
7. Hyams JS, et al. Outcome following thiopurine use in children with ulcerative colitis: a prospective multicenter registry study. Am J Gastroenterol. 2011;106(5):981–7.
8. Kotlyar DS, et al. Risk of lymphoma in patients with inflammatory bowel disease treated with azathioprine and 6-mercaptopurine: a meta-analysis. Clin Gastroenterol Hepatol. 2015;13(5):847–58.e4; quiz e48–50
9. Joosse ME, et al. Malignancy and mortality in paediatric-onset inflammatory bowel disease: a 3-year prospective, multinational study from the paediatric IBD Porto group of ESPGHAN. Aliment Pharmacol Ther. 2018;48(5):523–37.
10. Novak G, et al. The safety of vedolizumab for the treatment of ulcerative colitis. Expert Opin Drug Saf. 2017;16(4):501–7.
11. Herfarth H, et al. Methotrexate is not superior to placebo in maintaining steroid-free response or remission in ulcerative colitis. Gastroenterology. 2018;155(4):1098–108.e9
12. Carbonnel F, et al. Methotrexate is not superior to placebo for inducing steroid-free remission, but induces steroid-free clinical remission in a larger proportion of patients with ulcerative colitis. Gastroenterology. 2016;150(2):380–8.e4
13. Turner D, et al. Appraisal of the pediatric ulcerative colitis activity index (PUCAI). Inflamm Bowel Dis. 2009;15(8):1218–23.
14. Turner D, et al. Development, validation, and evaluation of a pediatric ulcerative colitis activity index: a prospective multicenter study. Gastroenterology. 2007;133(2):423–32.
15. Dotson JL, et al. Feasibility and validity of the pediatric ulcerative colitis activity index in routine clinical practice. J Pediatr Gastroenterol Nutr. 2015;60(2):200–4.
16. Turner D, et al. Severe paediatric ulcerative colitis: incidence, outcomes and optimal timing for second-line therapy. Gut. 2008;57(3):331–8.
17. Feld LG, et al. Clinical practice guideline: maintenance intravenous fluids in children. Pediatrics. 2018;142(6):e20183083.
18. Livshits A, et al. Abdominal X-ray in pediatric acute severe colitis and radiographic predictors of response to intravenous steroids. J Pediatr Gastroenterol Nutr. 2016;62(2):259–63.

19. Kleer CG, Appelman HD. Ulcerative colitis: patterns of involvement in colorectal biopsies and changes with time. Am J Surg Pathol. 1998;22(8):983–9.
20. Mohammed Vashist N, et al. Endoscopic scoring indices for evaluation of disease activity in ulcerative colitis. Cochrane Database Syst Rev. 2018;1:CD011450.
21. Cohen S, et al. Cytomegalovirus infection in pediatric severe ulcerative colitis-a multicenter study from the pediatric inflammatory bowel disease Porto Group of the European Society of Pediatric Gastroenterology, Hepatology and Nutrition. Pediatr Infect Dis J. 2018;37(3):197–201.
22. Obih C, et al. Specific carbohydrate diet for pediatric inflammatory bowel disease in clinical practice within an academic IBD center. Nutrition. 2016;32(4):418–25.
23. Forbes A, et al. ESPEN guideline: clinical nutrition in inflammatory bowel disease. Clin Nutr. 2017;36(2):321–47.
24. Goel R, Cushing MM, Tobian AA. Pediatric patient blood management programs: not just transfusing little adults. Transfus Med Rev. 2016;30(4):235–41.
25. Dignass AU, et al. European consensus on the diagnosis and management of iron deficiency and anaemia in inflammatory bowel diseases. J Crohns Colitis. 2015;9(3):211–22.
26. Crowe EP, DeSimone RA. Transfusion support and alternatives for Jehovah's witness patients. Curr Opin Hematol. 2019;26(6):473–9.
27. Scott LJ. Ferric carboxymaltose: a review in iron deficiency. Drugs. 2018;78(4):479–93.
28. De Franceschi L, et al. Clinical management of iron deficiency anemia in adults: systemic review on advances in diagnosis and treatment. Eur J Intern Med. 2017;42:16–23.
29. Zitomersky NL, et al. Risk factors, morbidity, and treatment of thrombosis in children and young adults with active inflammatory bowel disease. J Pediatr Gastroenterol Nutr. 2013;57(3):343–7.
30. Zitomersky NL, Verhave M, Trenor CC 3rd. Thrombosis and inflammatory bowel disease: a call for improved awareness and prevention. Inflamm Bowel Dis. 2011;17(1):458–70.
31. Szigethy E, Knisely M, Drossman D. Opioid misuse in gastroenterology and non-opioid management of abdominal pain. Nat Rev Gastroenterol Hepatol. 2018;15(3):168–80.
32. Crandall WV, Halterman TE, Mackner LM. Anxiety and pain symptoms in children with inflammatory bowel disease and functional gastrointestinal disorders undergoing colonoscopy. J Pediatr Gastroenterol Nutr. 2007;44(1):63–7.
33. Mackner LM, et al. Psychosocial issues in pediatric inflammatory bowel disease: report of the North American Society for Pediatric Gastroenterology, Hepatology, and Nutrition. J Pediatr Gastroenterol Nutr. 2013;56(4):449–58.

34. Stapersma L, et al. Effectiveness of disease-specific cognitive behavioral therapy on anxiety, depression, and quality of life in youth with inflammatory bowel disease: a randomized controlled trial. J Pediatr Psychol. 2018;43(9):967–80.
35. Turner D, et al. Combination of oral antibiotics may be effective in severe pediatric ulcerative colitis: a preliminary report. J Crohns Colitis. 2014;8(11):1464–70.
36. Turner D, et al. Antibiotic cocktail for pediatric acute severe colitis and the microbiome: the PRASCO randomized controlled trial. Inflamm Bowel Dis. 2020;26(11):1733–42.
37. Turner D, et al. Severe pediatric ulcerative colitis: a prospective multicenter study of outcomes and predictors of response. Gastroenterology. 2010;138(7):2282–91.
38. Nalagatla N, et al. Effect of accelerated infliximab induction on short- and long-term outcomes of acute severe ulcerative colitis: a retrospective multicenter study and meta-analysis. Clin Gastroenterol Hepatol. 2019;17(3):502–9.e1
39. Church PC, et al. Intensified infliximab induction is associated with improved response and decreased colectomy in steroid-refractory paediatric ulcerative colitis. J Crohns Colitis. 2019;13(8):982–9.
40. Ogata H, et al. A randomised dose finding study of oral tacrolimus (FK506) therapy in refractory ulcerative colitis. Gut. 2006;55(9):1255–62.
41. Watson S, et al. Outcomes and adverse events in children and young adults undergoing tacrolimus therapy for steroid-refractory colitis. Inflamm Bowel Dis. 2011;17(1):22–9.
42. Williams JG, et al. Infliximab versus ciclosporin for steroid-resistant acute severe ulcerative colitis (CONSTRUCT): a mixed methods, open-label, pragmatic randomised trial. Lancet Gastroenterol Hepatol. 2016;1(1):15–24.
43. Lichtiger S, et al. Cyclosporine in severe ulcerative colitis refractory to steroid therapy. N Engl J Med. 1994;330(26):1841–5.
44. Christensen B, et al. Safety and efficacy of combination treatment with calcineurin inhibitors and vedolizumab in patients with refractory inflammatory bowel disease. Clin Gastroenterol Hepatol. 2019;17(3):486–93.
45. Barnes EL, et al. The burden of hospital readmissions among pediatric patients with inflammatory bowel disease. J Pediatr. 2017;191:184–9.e1
46. Singh N, et al. Multi-center experience of vedolizumab effectiveness in pediatric inflammatory bowel disease. Inflamm Bowel Dis. 2016;22(9):2121–6.
47. Ledder O, et al. Vedolizumab in paediatric inflammatory bowel disease: a retrospective multi-centre experience from the paediatric IBD Porto group of ESPGHAN. J Crohns Colitis. 2017;11(10):1230–7.

48. Dolinger MT, et al. Dual biologic and small molecule therapy for the treatment of refractory pediatric inflammatory bowel disease. Inflamm Bowel Dis. 2021;27(8):1210–4.
49. Rinawi F, et al. Risk of colectomy in patients with pediatric-onset ulcerative colitis. J Pediatr Gastroenterol Nutr. 2017;65(4):410–5.
50. Hyams JS, et al. Clinical and biological predictors of response to standardised paediatric colitis therapy (PROTECT): a multicentre inception cohort study. Lancet. 2019;393(10182):1708–20.
51. Ryan DP, Doody DP. Surgical options in the treatment of ulcerative colitis. Semin Pediatr Surg. 2017;26(6):379–83.
52. Hait EJ, et al. Pouch outcomes among children with ulcerative colitis treated with calcineurin inhibitors before ileal pouch anal anastomosis surgery. J Pediatr Surg. 2007;42(1):31–4; discussion 34–5

Management of Pediatric Patients Hospitalized with Crohn's Disease

12

Christopher J. Moran and Esther Israel

Case

A 17-year-old female with 2 years of ileocolonic Crohn's disease is admitted with 4 days of fevers and right lower quadrant pain. Labs demonstrate a leukocytosis of 17,500 and elevated inflammatory markers (c-reactive protein of 217 and erythrocyte sedimentation rate of 96). CT imaging demonstrates a 3 cm, rim-enhancing fluid collection anterior to the terminal ileum with a fistulous tract. The patient is admitted on intravenous antibiotics and ultimately has percutaneous drainage of the collection with a drain left in that has minimal drainage over the first 24 hours. The patient has the drain removed and is discharged home on 6 weeks of intravenous antibiotics and has infliximab therapy initiated 2 weeks following hospital discharge.

Crohn's disease (CD) is a chronic inflammatory condition that can affect any segment of the gastrointestinal tract. Symptoms

C. J. Moran
Pediatric Gastroenterology, MassGeneral Hospital for Children, Boston, MA, USA

E. Israel (✉)
Department of Pediatrics, Harvard Medical School, Boston, MA, USA
e-mail: eisrael1@partners.org

J. D. Feuerstein, A. S. Cheifetz (eds.), *Management of Inpatient Inflammatory Bowel Disease*,
https://doi.org/10.1007/978-1-0716-1987-2_12

typically include abdominal pain, diarrhea, and weight loss and frequently vary depending on location of involvement as well as the presence of complicating disease. Complicated subtypes include B2 (stricturing disease), B3 (internally penetrating disease), and B2B3 (involving both stricturing and internally penetrating disease) and carry different presentations compared to that of uncomplicated luminal disease (B1) [1]. While the presence of a complicated disease phenotype is rare (~4%) at the time of diagnosis in children, complicated disease increases up to 15% within the first 3 years of diagnosis [2]. Hospitalizations can occur with all of the subtypes.

Severe flares of CD often result in hospitalization which leads to both significant direct costs and indirect costs such as lost school for the child and lost work for the parent. Within the first 3 years after CD diagnosis, up to 35–43% of children require hospitalization, and that number rises to as high as 67% at 10 years following CD diagnosis [2, 3]. The overall population of children with very early-onset CD (diagnosed within the first 5 years of life) does not appear to have higher rates of hospitalization than their older counterparts although the severity of very early-onset inflammatory bowel disease (VEO-IBD) is often consolidated at specialized tertiary care hospitals and requires significant healthcare resources including frequent hospitalizations [3, 4]. Debruyn et al. demonstrated that the incidence of hospitalization in pediatric CD has increased from 1997 to 2009 [5]. Although many have hypothesized that more aggressive initial therapy with antitumor necrosis factor (anti-TNF) agents might reduce hospitalizations, studies have shown mixed results [6, 7]. Overall, hospitalization costs remain a significant driver of overall CD costs, behind only prescription drug costs [8].

Racial differences exist with regard to hospitalization rates in CD. Non-Hispanic Black adults have been shown to be hospitalized at higher rates compared to their Caucasian counterparts [9]. African-American children with CD had higher rates of perianal disease at diagnosis compared to Caucasian children (9% vs 5%), and they have been shown to develop perianal disease during their disease duration with higher frequency [10, 11]. In addition, African-American children with CD who are hospitalized are more likely than hospitalized Caucasian children with CD to be readmitted within 12 months [10]. It is not clear whether these differences represent racial disparities in the care of CD or differences in genetic factors leading to more complicated disease.

Luminal Crohn's Disease

Luminal CD makes up the vast majority of pediatric CD cases at diagnosis as well as over long-term follow-up [2]. Flares of luminal CD often involve abdominal pain and diarrhea and may result in excessive weight loss. They often incur high rates of outpatient office visits and oral steroid use prior to hospitalization.

Initial management of luminal CD flares begins with assessing hydration and the severity of the flare. Intravenous fluid resuscitation may be required. When children with CD present with abrupt changes in stool habits such as diarrhea, infectious etiologies should always be considered. *Clostridia difficile* (*C. difficile*) should be specifically evaluated especially in patients with risk factors for *C. difficile* (i.e., recent infection with *C. difficile*, recent hospitalization, emergency room evaluation, or antibiotic use) or risk factors for having severe flares of IBD due to *C. difficile* (i.e., hypoalbuminemia, anemia, or elevated creatinine) [12, 13]. Guidelines for pediatric ulcerative colitis (UC) recommend empiric treatment for *C. difficile* if there is high suspicion while waiting for definitive test results [14]. Consideration for this strategy in pediatric CD is also reasonable if there is moderate to high severity of the CD flare.

Consensus guidelines recommend that all children with CD have small bowel imaging to identify complicated disease at the time of diagnosis [15]. Further, evaluation for penetrating disease often is necessary in the setting of fever (especially if not done recently) as the presence of an abscess may preclude specific therapies. Decisions on the most appropriate imaging studies to perform commonly revolve around computerized axial tomography (CAT) scans and magnetic resonance imaging (MRI) scans. Ongoing concerns regarding the risk of accumulating burden of ionizing radiation in patients with CD often make MR imaging more desirable, but the need for urgent evaluation in the hospitalized patient may ultimately require CT imaging. There may be a role in the use of ultrasound to evaluate for intra-abdominal imaging, but this modality is quite dependent on skill and experience of the performing radiologist. The sensitivity of ultrasonography for intra-abdominal abscesses in adult CD can be as high as 90%, but it is dependent on both the depth of the abscess location and the radiologist's experience [16, 17].

Treatment of luminal CD may include either nutritional therapy or anti-inflammatory medications. In some severe cases, a decision to embark on a combined approach using both exclusive enteral nutrition (EEN) and medication is also reasonable.

EEN utilizing a liquid formula to provide > = 90% of calories has become a first-line therapy for CD whether the patient is in the hospital or in an outpatient setting for 8–12 weeks [18]. EEN has been demonstrated to be more effective than corticosteroids in attaining mucosal healing [19]. It appears that the protein source for EEN (polymeric vs elemental formula) does not affect efficacy but polymeric formulas are better tolerated by the patient drinking them [20].

In children with CD who have failed initial therapy with either EEN or outpatient oral corticosteroids (or potentially both), most experts would consider intravenous corticosteroids as a bridge to a maintenance therapy such as immunomodulatory therapy with thiopurines or methotrexate [18] or nutritional maintenance therapy. The immunomodulators are unlikely to play an immediate role in the treatment of children with CD who are hospitalized. The decision for starting intravenous corticosteroids while hospitalized should be balanced against the past history of other pulses of steroids and the degree of growth failure. Strong consideration should be given to initiation of anti-TNF therapy such as infliximab for such patients [18]. There are limited data on the use of other biologics or alternative immunosuppression in hospitalized pediatric CD. Vedolizumab offers a non-TNF-driven treatment modality in patients who have failed intravenous steroids and have previously been shown to be anti-TNF primary nonresponders [21]. Although the adult literature suggests that the response may be delayed, children with IBD may have a relatively faster response [22]. One specific concern for hospitalized patients with CD is that there appears to be an increased risk of postoperative complications in children and adults treated with vedolizumab who require surgery [23, 24]. Consideration for possible surgery in the near future should be balanced against the potential benefit of vedolizumab. However, the use of tacrolimus has been proposed as a bridge to vedolizumab maintenance therapy which may help navigate this risk [25]. Hamel et al. proposed concomitant initiation of tacrolimus and vedolizumab with initial goal tacrolimus troughs of 10–15 ng/dL and titration to 8–10 ng/dL once rectal bleeding has resolved [25]. The additive risk of multiple immunosuppressive effects must be evaluated in the context of the risk of severe CD flares not responding to first-line therapy. Future options for primary nonresponders to anti-TNF may also include ustekinumab although there are not any current data on its use in hospitalized CD.

Long-term outcomes demonstrate that hospitalizations for CD carry high risk for future need for surgery. *Falaiye* et al. reported that 42% of children hospitalized for Crohn's colitis who received infliximab during that admission ultimately required a surgical resection within 2 years [26].

Fistulizing Crohn's Disease

Fistulizing CD may present with more severe fevers and pain (compared to luminal CD) due to the presence of intra-abdominal abscesses. Fistulae may develop proximal to a fibrotic stricture or may develop in a severely inflamed segment of the bowel due to transmural involvement. Internally penetrating CD (B3) is only present in 2.6% of the RISK cohort of pediatric CD in the first few years of follow-up [27]. Older age at diagnosis (of pediatric CD), African-American ancestry, and the presence of antibodies directed against *Saccharomyces cerevisiae* (ASCA) and flagellin (CBir1) are associated with an increased risk of developing internally penetrating CD [27].

All patients with known internally penetrating disease who present with fevers and abdominal pain should be thoroughly evaluated for an intra-abdominal abscess. High fever or marked elevations in c-reactive protein (CRP) or erythrocyte sedimentation rate (ESR) should further prompt concern for an intra-abdominal abscess even for those without a history of internally penetrating CD. A diagnosis of an intra-abdominal abscess typically requires three-dimensional imaging either in the form of MR or CT imaging. CT scanning may be more readily accessible than MRI in a patient with the concern for an abscess given the need to make a relatively prompt diagnosis. Further delineation by ultrasonography of an abscess that may have a relatively superficial position may allow for subsequent follow-up by ultrasonography.

The presence of an intra-abdominal abscess requires immediate attention before proceeding to anti-inflammatory therapy for the underlying CD. Small abscesses may be amenable to intravenous antibiotics alone although larger or multifocal abscesses often will require either drainage via interventional radiology (IR) or a surgical procedure to remove the abscess pocket (and potentially the involved segment of the intestine). Traditionally, an abscess diameter of >2–3 cm prompts strong consideration for a drainage procedure combined with antibiotics over antibiotic-only approaches [17, 28]. Percutaneous drainage of an intra-abdominal abscess not only allows for control of the localized infection, but culture data may allow for optimization of antimicrobial therapy. Risk of percutaneous drainage includes the development of a persistent enterocutaneous fistula, but that risk appears to be relatively low (<3% of cases) [17]. It is generally assumed that microbes contained within the abscess pocket are derived from the local bowel microbiome with the relevant microbes in adult CD being specifically *E. coli* (most commonly), *Streptococcus*, *Enterococcus*, as well as *Candida* species [29]. It is not clear if the microbial spectrum of pediatric CD abscesses is similar as the long duration of some fistulizing CD in adults may modify the local microbiome. Growing literature describes increasing rates of pathogen resistance to fluoroquinolone and β-lactam antibiotics [29, 30]. Risk factors for antibiotic resistance include recent immunosuppression with corticosteroids and high blood leukocyte counts [29]. Empiric antibiotic coverage regimens for intra-abdominal abscesses typically include piperacillin-tazobactam, cefepime, or meropenam [28]. Given concerns about antibiotic resistance as well as the interest in tailoring therapy, acquisition of culture and antibiotic sensitivity data is ideal.

Ultimately, children admitted to the hospital for an intra-abdominal abscess need definitive therapy for their fistulizing disease. Following percutaneous drainage of an intra-abdominal abscess, it is typically recommended that antibiotics be continued for at least 7 days to await culture results and to monitor for both clinical improvement in pain and fever and serologic improvement of the CRP [28]. The majority of pediatric CD patients who are hospitalized for an intra-abdominal abscess eventually require a surgical resection [31]. A small study in adult CD with intra-abdominal abscesses suggested that early surgical resection may have long-term advantages over immediate percutaneous drainage in both early abscess control and prevention of abscess recurrence [32]. Given the limited research into the value of early surgery for all fistulizing CD complicated by abscess, the decision regarding surgery should be made on a case-by-case basis, but children with more extensive fistulae or large abscesses may be more likely to benefit from early surgery.

Long-term maintenance therapy in children with penetrating CD is frequently anti-TNF based whether it is as primary treatment for a diseased segment or as postoperative prophylaxis after resection. Strict guidelines on the timing of anti-TNF initiation are lacking. In patients undergoing surgical resection (with the majority of disease resected), one could consider initiating anti-TNF 4–6 weeks post-resection. In patients not undergoing a resection whose abscess has been either drained or for small abscesses that have fully responded to antibiotic therapy, earlier initiation (due to the likelihood of active intestinal disease) of biologic therapy should be considered along a timeline of 2–4 weeks following abscess resolution.

Stricturing Crohn's Disease

As CD progresses, it may be complicated by obstruction although obstruction can also be the initial presentation of the disease. Obstruction is the most common cause for surgery in patients with CD [33]. Obstruction can be related to one of three processes or a combination of them – acute inflammation, fibrostenotic disease, and postoperative adhesions. Bowel obstruction may be a result of significant edema of the mucosa from extensive inflammation and associated spasm of the bowel. It can be precipitated by dietary indiscretion with foods which are not easily digested (e.g., ingestion of nuts or corn). Obstruction in this setting may be intermittent and can often be reversed with conservative measures and anti-inflammatory agents. Ongoing transmural inflammation of the bowel can result in thickening of the bowel wall and narrowing of the lumen, hence the term stricturing or fibrostenotic disease (phenotype B2) which can also contribute to the acute onset of obstruction. Finally, patients who have had previous surgical procedures can present with obstructive symptoms secondary to adhesions.

Epidemiology of Stricturing Disease in Pediatrics

The development of stricturing disease is an important complication of CD managed in childhood and adolescence. The cumulative incidence of stricturing disease in a large pediatric cohort was 13.5% and 20.5% 5 and 10 years after diagnosis, respectively [34]. Patients with colonic disease are less likely to have stricturing disease complications compared with patients with ileocolonic or ileal disease [35]. Risk factors for stricturing disease which are relevant to pediatric patients include the presence of perianal disease and the need for steroids during the first flare [36]. A history of smoking is another risk factor for CD progressing to stricture. Deep mucosal ulcerations in the small bowel have also been identified as predictive of a patient's progression to stricturing disease, as has prior appendectomy [37].

Management

Patients who present acutely with clinically suspected bowel obstruction require hospitalization. This generally manifests with vomiting, often bilious, and severe abdominal pain. Initial management includes assessment for hydration and degree of discomfort, and serologic evaluation including electrolytes and markers of inflammation. Diagnostic imaging such as CT scanning or MRI is performed to confirm the site of the obstruction. The elements of fibrosis and inflammation may be distinguished to try to separate active inflammation from chronic fibrostenotic disease. No diagnostic imaging modality, however, is validated to absolutely differentiate between the two. Additionally, the presence of complications such as an abscess can be assessed. Radiologic testing shows dilated loops of proximal intestine terminating at the site of the obstruction. If the blockage is due to progressive inflammation, bowel wall thickening and inflammatory change are also noted. As the terminal ileum, cecum, and ascending colon are the most commonly affected parts of the bowel, it may be difficult to distinguish this from appendicitis with obstruction.

The approach to management of the patient with obstruction is at first conservative, if possible. Rehydration and electrolyte replacement with management of the symptoms of nausea and vomiting with antiemetics and pain with analgesics is primary. All enteral feeding and drinking is discontinued, and nasogastric intubation for bowel decompression is used for those with active ongoing emesis and for symptomatic relief. The patient is then observed for 2–3 days to monitor whether conservative management has been effective.

Steroids are given as an attempt to relieve the active component of the inflammation causing the obstruction as long as there is no evidence of an abscess. Other considerations if conservative medical intervention is not effective include active interventions to relieve the obstruction. If due to fibrostenotic narrowing, choices for intervention include endoscopic balloon dilatation, surgery with strictureplasty, surgical resection, or a combination of those therapies. Endoscopically accessible short-segment (<5 to 10 cm) stenosis is a good candidate for endoscopic dilatation though a stricture which is connected to a fistula or abscess is a contraindication for endoscopic dilatation. Since strictureplasty can preserve bowel length, it is preferred over bowel resection for nonphlegmonous strictures, and laparoscopy is preferable to open surgery with reduced postoperative pain and decreased lengths of stay [38]. There does not appear to be a significant difference between outcomes or complication rates between surgical resection and strictureplasty in pediatric CD though there is one pediatric study which found a higher risk to re-stricture following strictureplasty [33, 39]. For patients with previous surgeries, adhesions may be noted and might require lysis.

Simultaneous with the evaluation for the obstruction is an evaluation of the patient's nutritional status. Equally important is an evaluation of the patient's nutritional state. Patients who are nutritionally compromised should undergo nutritional repletion with parenteral nutrition to reverse their catabolic state, preferably prior to surgery.

Perianal Disease

Perianal involvement is a common potentially significant source of morbidity for patients with CD. Features of perianal disease include skin tags, fissures, fistulas, and abscesses. Hospitalization of patients with perianal disease occurs in the presence of a fistula resulting in an abscess.

Epidemiology

In the largest cohort yet examined, 4% of pediatric patients with CD disease had evidence of perianal disease at diagnosis with 30% developing perianal disease by 6 years after the initial diagnosis [11]. Although earlier studies suggested there was a significant association of perianal CD with younger age at diagnosis, complicated intestinal disease, and ileal disease location, this has not been substantiated in more recent studies [11].

Management

The presence of a perianal fistula with abscess is generally the precipitating event for a hospitalization in this group of patients.

Perianal pain, buttock pain, and purulent anal or vaginal discharge are generally the first signs that an abscess is present. An urgent pelvic MRI has become an essential tool for children to provide important information about the location and extent of the abscess and connection to a fistulous tract. Recently transperianal ultrasound has been shown to have good diagnostic accuracy for detection of perianal fistulae [40].

When an abscess is identified in the perianal area, antibiotics are generally started – metronidazole 20–30 mg/kg/day +/– ciprofloxacin10–20 mg/kg/day. In the event of a superficial abscess that can be seen in the perianal area, prompt surgical drainage is undertaken (typically during an exam under anesthesia). These are often extremely painful. If a fistula can be identified leading to a simple abscess, a fistulotomy is performed. More complicated abscesses arising from fistulas above the dentate line need to be drained and treated with placement of a noncutting seton.

Once the acute problem is managed surgically, anti-TNF agents would be used as the primary medical induction therapy for complex perianal CD. After successful induction, anti-TNF-alpha scheduled maintenance is necessary. There is some indication that there is a benefit to have a higher trough level of the anti-TNF-alpha [41] in the presence of perianal disease. Antibiotics are generally continued until drainage from the abscess or fistula has stopped.

Additional Considerations for Hospitalized Pediatric Crohn's Disease

Nutrition

While managing the inflammatory component of CD and its complications, clinicians must also pay attention to the nutritional consequences of inflammation. Nutritional consultation is a required part to every hospitalization for CD. In addition to developing a therapeutic strategy to reduce inflammatory burden, one must also develop a nutritional program that reverses the malnutrition that likely has developed during the CD flare. Clinicians must remain vigilant about nutritional complications such as refeeding syndrome and thromboembolic risk.

While there does not exist data describing the incidence of refeeding syndrome in hospitalized children with CD, it must remain a consideration. There are case reports describing the onset of refeeding syndrome in children hospitalized for CD flares. Risk factors for refeeding syndrome include undernutrition >10 days and acute weight loss which are both relevant in CD. In patients with large weight losses who are assumed to have absorbed poor calories recently, serial measurement of phosphorus, potassium, and magnesium should be performed, and repletion should occur when deficiencies occur [42]. When these deficiencies are detected, clinicians should focus on cautious advancement of caloric intake, and thiamine supplementation should occur.

IBD is often considered a pro-thrombotic condition, and there appears to be an increased risk of clotting in pediatric IBD patients. Zitomersky et al. reported an incidence of 1.9% of thromboembolism in hospitalized pediatric IBD patients [43]. Colonic IBD involvement (ulcerative colitis and CD) was the most significant risk factor, but also family history of thromboembolism, presence of a central line, and oral contraceptive use appeared to modify the risk of thromboembolism. Although thromboembolic risk is well-recognized in pediatric IBD, pediatric gastroenterologists do not frequently employ pharmacologic measures to reduce the risk [44]. Careful consideration of proactive measures to reduce thrombosis in these patients should be considered including pharmacologic prophylaxis.

Pain Management

Pain is likely to be one of the presenting complaints during most admissions for Crohn's disease, regardless of the specific precipitating event for the admission. Primary management of the pain, of course, is to relieve the specific complication resulting in the admission – relief of the obstruction, resolution of the abscess, or getting the disease activity under control. However, while supporting the patient in this, pain control needs to be addressed. Pharmacologic agents and nonpharmacologic approaches can work together to help with pain relief. Available agents for the acute management of pain include narcotics and nonsteroidal anti-inflammatory agents. Both of these classes of medications have challenges with patient with inflammatory bowel disease. There is a long history of concerns of worsening inflammatory bowel disease with NSAIDs. A recent review and analysis of published studies, however, did not reveal a consistent association between the use of NSAIDs and exacerbation of Crohn's disease [45]. Thus, there are little data in the literature to support the common recommendation to avoid all NSAIDs, and they can be used, in moderation, to alleviate pain. Along the same lines, concern regarding the use of narcotics and the risk of decreasing colonic motility and precipitating toxic megacolon may prevent adequate attempts at pain relief. If the inflammation is not pancolonic, narcotics should certainly be considered to ease pain. There are no specific data for children and adolescents in this regard. Additionally, nonpharmacologic approaches such as distraction techniques, especially with the help of child life services, can be helpful in the approach to pain management.

Mental Health

Flares of CD that require hospitalization have broad ranging effects. Beyond the obvious physical suffering of the patients, they are withdrawn from their routine daily activities while in the hospital and likely for days to weeks prior to the hospitalization. Special attention should be paid to the mental health of these hospitalized patients. It is well-known that children and adolescents with IBD are at higher risk for psychiatric disorders. Psychosocial support should be strongly considered for all hospitalized patients as well as identifying patients who might need further help once discharged.

References

1. Levine A, Griffiths A, Markowitz J, et al. Pediatric modification of the Montreal classification for inflammatory bowel disease: the Paris classification. Inflamm Bowel Dis. 2011;17:1314–21.
2. Lindoso L, Mondal K, Venkateswaran S, et al. The effect of early-life environmental exposures on disease phenotype and clinical course of Crohn's disease in children. Am J Gastroenterol. 2018;113:1524–9.

3. Benchimol EI, Mack DR, Nguyen GC, et al. Incidence, outcomes, and health services burden of very early onset inflammatory bowel disease. Gastroenterology. 2014;147:803–13. e7; quiz e14–5
4. Kelsen JR, Conrad MA, Dawany N, et al. The unique disease course of children with very early onset-inflammatory bowel disease. Inflamm Bowel Dis. 2020;26(6):909–18.
5. Debruyn JC, Soon IS, Hubbard J, et al. Nationwide temporal trends in incidence of hospitalization and surgical intestinal resection in pediatric inflammatory bowel diseases in the United States from 1997 to 2009. Inflamm Bowel Dis. 2013;19:2423–32.
6. Rahman A, Jairath V, Feagan BG, et al. Declining hospitalisation and surgical intervention rates in patients with Crohn's disease: a population-based cohort. Aliment Pharmacol Ther. 2019;50:1086–93.
7. Murthy SK, Begum J, Benchimol EI, et al. Introduction of anti-TNF therapy has not yielded expected declines in hospitalisation and intestinal resection rates in inflammatory bowel diseases: a population-based interrupted time series study. Gut. 2020;69(2):274–82.
8. Kuenzig ME, Benchimol EI, Lee L, et al. The impact of inflammatory bowel disease in Canada 2018: direct costs and health services utilization. J Can Assoc Gastroenterol. 2019;2:S17–33.
9. Nguyen GC, Chong CA, Chong RY. National estimates of the burden of inflammatory bowel disease among racial and ethnic groups in the United States. J Crohns Colitis. 2014;8:288–95.
10. Dotson JL, Kappelman MD, Chisolm DJ, et al. Racial disparities in readmission, complications, and procedures in children with Crohn's disease. Inflamm Bowel Dis. 2015;21:801–8.
11. Adler J, Dong S, Eder SJ, et al. Perianal Crohn disease in a large multicenter pediatric collaborative. J Pediatr Gastroenterol Nutr. 2017; 64:e117–24.
12. Micic D, Yarur A, Gonsalves A, et al. Risk factors for Clostridium difficile isolation in inflammatory bowel disease: a prospective study. Dig Dis Sci. 2018;63:1016–24.
13. Ananthakrishnan AN, Guzman-Perez R, Gainer V, et al. Predictors of severe outcomes associated with Clostridium difficile infection in patients with inflammatory bowel disease. Aliment Pharmacol Ther. 2012;35:789–95.
14. Turner D, Ruemmele FM, Orlanski-Meyer E, et al. Management of paediatric ulcerative colitis, part 2: acute severe colitis-an evidence-based consensus guideline from the European Crohn's and Colitis Organization and the European Society of Paediatric Gastroenterology, Hepatology and Nutrition. J Pediatr Gastroenterol Nutr. 2018;67:292–310.
15. Bruining DH, Zimmermann EM, Loftus EV Jr, et al. Consensus recommendations for evaluation, interpretation, and utilization of computed tomography and magnetic resonance enterography in patients with small bowel Crohn's disease. Radiology. 2018;286:776–99.
16. Maconi G, Sampietro GM, Parente F, et al. Contrast radiology, computed tomography and ultrasonography in detecting internal fistulas and intra-

abdominal abscesses in Crohn's disease: a prospective comparative study. Am J Gastroenterol. 2003;98:1545–55.
17. Feagins LA, Holubar SD, Kane SV, et al. Current strategies in the management of intra-abdominal abscesses in Crohn's disease. Clin Gastroenterol Hepatol. 2011;9:842–50.
18. Ruemmele FM, Veres G, Kolho KL, et al. Consensus guidelines of ECCO/ESPGHAN on the medical management of pediatric Crohn's disease. J Crohns Colitis. 2014;8:1179–207.
19. Borrelli O, Cordischi L, Cirulli M, et al. Polymeric diet alone versus corticosteroids in the treatment of active pediatric Crohn's disease: a randomized controlled open-label trial. Clin Gastroenterol Hepatol. 2006;4:744–53.
20. Zachos M, Tondeur M, Griffiths AM. Enteral nutritional therapy for induction of remission in Crohn's disease. Cochrane Database Syst Rev. 2007;4:CD000542.
21. Sandborn WJ, Feagan BG, Rutgeerts P, et al. Vedolizumab as induction and maintenance therapy for Crohn's disease. N Engl J Med. 2013;369:711–21.
22. Conrad MA, Stein RE, Maxwell EC, et al. Vedolizumab therapy in severe pediatric inflammatory bowel disease. Inflamm Bowel Dis. 2016;22:2425–31.
23. Zimmerman LA, Zalieckas JM, Shamberger RC, et al. Postoperative complications of pediatric patients with inflammatory bowel disease treated with vedolizumab. J Pediatr Surg. 2018;53:1330–3.
24. Lightner AL, Mathis KL, Tse CS, et al. Postoperative outcomes in vedolizumab-treated patients undergoing major abdominal operations for inflammatory bowel disease: retrospective multicenter cohort study. Inflamm Bowel Dis. 2018;24:871–6.
25. Hamel B, Wu M, Hamel EO, et al. Outcome of tacrolimus and vedolizumab after corticosteroid and anti-TNF failure in paediatric severe colitis. BMJ Open Gastroenterol. 2018;5:e000195.
26. Falaiye TO, Mitchell KR, Lu Z, et al. Outcomes following infliximab therapy for pediatric patients hospitalized with refractory colitis-predominant IBD. J Pediatr Gastroenterol Nutr. 2014;58:213–9.
27. Kugathasan S, Denson LA, Walters TD, et al. Prediction of complicated disease course for children newly diagnosed with Crohn's disease: a multicentre inception cohort study. Lancet. 2017;389:1710–8.
28. Pfefferkorn MD, Marshalleck FE, Saeed SA, et al. NASPGHAN clinical report on the evaluation and treatment of pediatric patients with internal penetrating Crohn disease: intraabdominal abscess with and without fistula. J Pediatr Gastroenterol Nutr. 2013;57:394–400.
29. Reuken PA, Kruis W, Maaser C, et al. Microbial spectrum of intra-abdominal abscesses in perforating Crohn's disease: results from a prospective German registry. J Crohns Colitis. 2018;12:695–701.
30. Park SK, Kim KJ, Lee SO, et al. Ciprofloxacin usage and bacterial resistance patterns in Crohn's disease patients with abscesses. J Clin Gastroenterol. 2014;48:703–7.

31. Rypens F, Dubois J, Garel L, et al. Percutaneous drainage of abdominal abscesses in pediatric Crohn's disease. AJR Am J Roentgenol. 2007;188:579–85.
32. Lobaton T, Guardiola J, Rodriguez-Moranta F, et al. Comparison of the long-term outcome of two therapeutic strategies for the management of abdominal abscess complicating Crohn's disease: percutaneous drainage or immediate surgical treatment. Color Dis. 2013;15:1267–72.
33. Romeo E, Jasonni V, Caldaro T, et al. Strictureplasty and intestinal resection: different options in complicated pediatric-onset Crohn disease. J Pediatr Surg. 2012;47:944–8.
34. Gupta N, Bostrom AG, Kirschner BS, et al. Incidence of stricturing and penetrating complications of Crohn's disease diagnosed in pediatric patients. Inflamm Bowel Dis. 2010;16:638–44.
35. Muller KE, Lakatos PL, Arato A, et al. Incidence, Paris classification, and follow-up in a nationwide incident cohort of pediatric patients with inflammatory bowel disease. J Pediatr Gastroenterol Nutr. 2013;57:576–82.
36. Herman Y, Rinawi F, Rothschild B, et al. The characteristics and long-term outcomes of pediatric Crohn's disease patients with perianal disease. Inflamm Bowel Dis. 2017;23:1659–65.
37. Andersson RE, Olaison G, Tysk C, et al. Appendectomy is followed by increased risk of Crohn's disease. Gastroenterology. 2003;124:40–6.
38. Page A, Sashittal S, Chatzizacharias N, et al. The Role of laparoscopic surgery in the management of children and adolescents in inflammatory bowel disease. Medicine 2015;94:e874.
39. Bamford R, Hay A, Kumar D. Resection leads to less recurrence than strictureplasty in a paediatric population with obstructive Crohn's disease. Surg Res Pract. 2014;2014:709045.
40. Lee EH, Yang HR, Kim JY. Comparison of transperianal ultrasound with colonoscopy and magnetic resonance imaging in perianal Crohn disease. J Pediatr Gastroenterol Nutr. 2018;66:614–9.
41. Yarur AJ, Kanagala V, Stein DJ, et al. Higher infliximab trough levels are associated with perianal fistula healing in patients with Crohn's disease. Aliment Pharmacol Ther. 2017;45:933–40.
42. Fuentebella J, Kerner JA. Refeeding syndrome. Pediatr Clin N Am. 2009;56:1201–10.
43. Zitomersky NL, Levine AE, Atkinson BJ, et al. Risk factors, morbidity, and treatment of thrombosis in children and young adults with active inflammatory bowel disease. J Pediatr Gastroenterol Nutr. 2013;57:343–7.
44. Chien KA, Hammad HT, Gerber L, et al. Pediatric gastroenterologists' approach to venous thromb oembolism prophylaxis in pediatric inflammatory bowel disease. J Pediatr Gastroenterol Nutr. 2018;66:286–8.
45. Moninuola OO, Milligan W, Lochhead P, et al. Systematic review with meta-analysis: association between acetaminophen and nonsteroidal anti-inflammatory drugs (NSAIDs) and risk of Crohn's disease and ulcerative colitis exacerbation. Aliment Pharmacol Ther. 2018;47:1428–39.

Management of Pregnant Women Hospitalized with a Flare of Inflammatory Bowel Disease

13

Punyanganie S. de Silva, Rahul S. Dalal, and Sonia Friedman

P. S. de Silva
Division of Gastroenterology, Hepatology, and Endoscopy, Department of Medicine, Brigham and Women's Hospital, Harvard Medical School, Boston, MA, USA

Harvard Medical School, Brigham and Women's Hospital, Center for Crohn's and Colitis, Chestnut Hill, MA, USA
e-mail: PDESILVA@BWH.HARVARD.EDU

R. S. Dalal
Division of Gastroenterology, Hepatology, and Endoscopy, Department of Medicine, Brigham and Women's Hospital, Harvard Medical School, Boston, MA, USA

S. Friedman (✉)
Division of Gastroenterology, Hepatology, and Endoscopy, Department of Medicine, Brigham and Women's Hospital, Harvard Medical School, Boston, MA, USA

Center for Clinical Epidemiology, Odense University Hospital, Odense, Denmark

Research Unit of Clinical Epidemiology, Department of Clinical Research, University of Southern Denmark, Odense, Denmark

Harvard Medical School, Brigham and Women's Hospital, Center for Crohn's and Colitis, Chestnut Hill, MA, USA
e-mail: sfriedman1@partners.org

J. D. Feuerstein, A. S. Cheifetz (eds.), *Management of Inpatient Inflammatory Bowel Disease*,
https://doi.org/10.1007/978-1-0716-1987-2_13

Epidemiology of and Risk Factors for Hospital Admissions of Pregnant Women with IBD

The majority of women with inflammatory bowel disease (IBD) have a normal pregnancy and deliver a healthy baby. Studies have demonstrated that approximately 80% of female patients conceive while their disease is in remission. In such cases, the IBD tends to remain in remission throughout the pregnancy and in the postpartum period [1]. However, active disease is a risk to a normal pregnancy and can on occasion lead to hospital admissions. In addition, a small minority of women may experience an initial flare of newly diagnosed IBD while pregnant, necessitating hospital admission.

Flares of Existing Diagnosis of IBD During Pregnancy

Of women with IBD who conceive while having active disease, 66% continue to have active disease or worsening IBD symptoms. Colitis symptoms can deteriorate in up to 45% of patients with ulcerative colitis (UC) and 33% of Crohn's disease (CD) patients who conceive while their disease is active, thereby increasing admission risk [2].

In a more recent study by de Lima-Karagiannis et al., out of a total of 298 pregnancies in 229 IBD patients (157 CD, 66 UC, and 6 IBD unclassified) resulting in 226 live births, active disease at conception was strongly associated with disease relapse during pregnancy (adjusted odds ratio (aOR) = 7.66; 95% confidence interval (CI), 3.77–15.54) [3]. This study also noted that pregnant women with UC did relapse more often than women with CD, independent of maternal age, smoking, periconceptional disease activity, previous IBD surgery, and the use of immunosuppressives or anti-tumor necrosis factor (anti-TNF) (aOR = 3.71; 95% CI, 1.86–7.40).

Of note, flares of UC during pregnancy are not limited to those with moderate to severe disease. A recent Japanese study of 68 women with UC recruited between 2013 and 2019 noted 15 adverse pregnancy outcomes which occurred in 13 patients [4]. Nonadherence to medication was a significant independent risk factor associated with relapse with a significantly higher proportion of women on mesalamine monotherapy relapsing due to nonadherence during the first trimester ($p = 0.002$).

Disease extent has also been recognized as a major outcome predictor in pregnant UC patients, with patients with pancolitis possibly at a higher risk of obstetric complications of ulcerative colitis vs. those with limited disease [5]. Patients with unstable UC are also more at risk of adverse fetal outcomes. A large population-based study from the USA revealed that pregnancy complicated by IBD was associated with increased incidence of small-for-gestational age birth (OR = 1.46, 95% confidence interval (CI) = 1.14–1.88), spontaneous preterm birth (OR = 1.32, 95% CI = 1.00–1.76), and preterm premature rupture of membranes (OR = 1.95, 95% CI = 1.26–3.02). Further stratifying by IBD subtypes, only UC was significantly associated with increased incidence of ischemic placental disease, spontaneous preterm birth, and preterm premature rupture of membranes [6]. A recent case-control study demonstrated that patients with UC in remission are less likely to flare during pregnancy than those who have active disease at the time of conception [7]. Of note, pregnancy itself does not influence the course of preexisting UC or the overall incidence of flare-ups during gestation (estimated to be between 14 and 34%) [8, 9]. Crohn's complications during pregnancy are less frequent than that of UC [9].

New-Onset Inflammatory Bowel Disease During Pregnancy

New-onset IBD is rare in pregnancy. Evidence for this is mostly based on case reports and small case series [7, 10–19]. It has however been associated with significantly poor outcomes including miscarriage, intrauterine death, abortion, Cesarean section, preterm delivery, fetal retinopathy, and toxic megacolon. Many of these reported cases are outdated, and one can presume that there are better outcomes due to improvements in IBD therapy and more coordination between multidisciplinary teams; however further studies in this regard are needed. As per Brunelli et al., it is felt that prevention of complications from new-onset IBD during pregnancy can be limited by early flexible sigmoidoscopy in patients with bloody diarrhea [19, 20], intense fetal monitoring, and an awareness that fever in pregnancy may be blunted due to decreased maternal core temperature [21], increased levels of placenta-derived anti-inflammatory factors, and altered brain sensitivity to fever inducing prostaglandins [22].

The need for colorectal surgical intervention is more common in de novo presentation of IBD. In a recent systematic review of 32 papers including 86 patients requiring surgery for IBD during pregnancy, 18% of cases were de novo presentations [23].

Stable Inflammatory Bowel Disease with Pregnancy Complication

While it is well documented that women who are in remission should remain on their current IBD therapy during pregnancy, there is still the risk of other pregnancy-related complications which could lead to inpatient admission [24]. Women with IBD often suffer from weight loss and malnutrition, both of which may be exacerbated due to hyperemesis gravidarum or even normal emesis during pregnancy [25]. Close monitoring of weight at routine antenatal and gastroenterology visits is necessary, and should there be any concern for failure to gain weight or weight loss, then prompt nutritional advice and therapy, preferably with dietician involvement, is recommended. Occasionally weight loss in itself may necessitate admission to the hospital; however it is more likely that hyperemesis gravidarum would be the main reason for admission. Crohn's disease especially is related to low birth weight and prematurity [26]. In a meta-analysis by Cornish et al., they found a 1.87-fold increase in prematurity (<37 weeks' gestation) and twice the normal amount of low birth weight (<2500 g) when compared with controls [27].

Corticosteroids are often necessary to control the symptoms of inflammatory bowel disease flares. While women with IBD often require corticosteroids for treatment of flares, they are also more susceptible to developing gestational diabetes [28]. This may prompt admission to hospital, or, alternatively, may be a consequence of recent inpatient admission for an IBD flare. Gastroenterological awareness of this complication, particularly in inpatients on high-dose corticosteroid therapy, is therefore important as gestational diabetes mellitus has been linked to significant short- and long-term outcomes in the baby. In the PIANO registry, corticosteroid use was associated with gestational diabetes (OR 2.8, 95% CI 1.3–6.0) [29]. Of note, in a separate retrospective study, this increased risk was not seen with budesonide; therefore, this may be a suitable option to use in women who have milder flares [30]. However, it is also important to note that inadequate control of a flare can lead to significant complications such as fetal distress, premature delivery, and miscarriage. Therefore, clinical judgment and close collaboration with obstetricians should be utilized with regard to deciding on an optimal corticosteroid dosage. This will depend on individual disease severity, trimester of pregnancy, and other comorbidities. Although it is considered optimal to use prednisone at less than 20 mg/day in pregnancy, it is generally accepted that higher doses are allowable for aggressive disease [31].

Consideration should also be made regarding the risk of venous thromboembolic events (VTE). Women with IBD, but particularly UC, are at increased risk of VTE during pregnancy [32]. Prophylactic low molecular weight heparin should therefore be considered in all hospitalized women with IBD. Of note, physicians should also be aware that women with Crohn's disease are also at a higher risk of antepartum hemorrhage. In a study by Broms et al., women with stable CD had a higher risk of antepartum hemorrhage (aOR, 1.66; 95% CI, 1.12–2.45) [32]. If thromboembolism is suspected, then per American Society of Hematology guidelines, in pregnant women with suspected pulmonary embolism, ventilation-perfusion (V/Q) lung scanning over computed tomography (CT) pulmonary angiography (conditional recommendation, low certainty in evidence about effect) is suggested [33]. Of note, in both established and *de novo* IBD, active disease increases the risk for thromboembolic events and emergency Cesarean delivery. Therefore, active disease should be treated aggressively [34].

A multidisciplinary team of obstetricians, gastroenterologists, midwives, clinical nurse specialists, the primary care practitioner, nutritionists, and if relevant, a colorectal surgeon is therefore needed during inpatient pregnancy care. This team approach is important in discussing and managing prenatal care, delivery, and postnatal care. In addition, treating gastroenterologists should also be aware that patients with IBD are also more susceptible to coronary artery disease [35]. Since pregnancy in itself is an acquired risk factor for thromboembolic events, often a cardiologist's input may be required in such high-risk patients.

Investigations in Inpatient IBD

An accurate assessment of disease activity among pregnant patients with IBD can be challenging, as common symptoms of pregnancy, such as changes in bowel habits, fatigue, and rectal bleeding due to hemorrhoids, may be similar to symptoms associated with worsening disease activity secondary to IBD. As with evaluating nonpregnant patients, providers can use a variety of tools to assess disease activity in the pregnant patient, though one must be aware that some tests, such as serum levels of inflammatory markers (including C-reactive protein), can increase in pregnancy [36]. Endoscopic procedures can be performed if necessary, but there are special considerations after 24 weeks when the fetus is viable. Fecal calprotectin, a stool marker of inflammation, has been shown to be a reliable marker of disease activity, as it is not affected by pregnancy [37–39]. Several studies have shown that fecal calprotectin levels in pregnancy significantly correlate with active disease in all trimesters of pregnancy [37, 39]. Hemoglobin and albumin have not been shown to be reliable markers of disease activity during pregnancy, and endoscopic scores, such as the Harvey-Bradshaw index, are not validated in pregnancy and may be challenging to interpret as the index includes assessment of abdominal mass, which is difficult to assess during pregnancy.

Endoscopy is generally safe during pregnancy for appropriate indications such as a flare of inflammatory bowel disease. A sigmoidoscopy can be performed without sedation to assess colitis activity. Sedation, if needed, should be performed by anesthesia with fetal monitoring after the first trimester. In a nationwide population-based cohort study from Sweden of endoscopy during pregnancy, exposure to any endoscopy during pregnancy was associated with an increased risk of preterm birth (adjusted relative risk (aRR), 1.54; 95% confidence interval [CI], 1.36–1.75) or small for gestational age (aRR, 1.30; 95% CI, 1.07–1.57) but not of congenital malformation (aRR, 1.00; 95% CI, 0.83–1.20) or stillbirth (aRR, 1.45; 95% CI, 0.87–2.40) [40]. The authors concluded that this risk was minimal and attributed it to "intrafamilial factors or disease activity."

Concern has been expressed about the safety of MRI exposure in the first trimester, due to the heating of sensitive tissues by radiofrequency fields and exposure to the loud acoustic environment. Administration of gadolinium in pregnancy is discouraged because of possible teratogenicity in the first trimester during organogenesis. Additionally, gadolinium may cross the placenta in the second or third trimester, where it may be excreted by the fetal kidneys into the amniotic fluid and then recirculated by the fetus. Theoretically, persistence of dissociated-free gadolinium could cause nephrogenic systemic fibrosis (NSF) in the child. In a large database study from Ontario, Canada, of 1,424,105 deliveries, the overall rate of MRI was 3.97 per 1000 pregnancies. Comparing gadolinium MRI (n = 397) with no MRI (n = 1,418,451), exposure to MRI during the first trimester of pregnancy compared with non-exposure was not associated with increased risk of harm to the fetus or in early childhood. Gadolinium MRI at any time during pregnancy was associated with an increased risk of a broad set of rheumatological, inflammatory, or infiltrative skin conditions (adjusted risk difference of 45.3 per 1000 person-years (95% CI, 11.3–86.8)) and for stillbirth or neonatal death (adjusted risk difference of 47.5 per 1000 pregnancies (95% CI, 9.7–138.2)) [41].

Medical Management of Complicated IBD During Pregnancy

Studies describing the medical treatment and colitis response rates among patients with a severe relapse of IBD during pregnancy necessitating hospital admission are very limited. Common medical reasons for admission involve the need for intravenous (IV) corticosteroid therapy, initiation of biologic therapy, optimization of malnutrition, and control of gastrointestinal blood loss.

A case-control study of 18 hospitalized pregnant patients with IBD flares (11 UC, 6 CD, 1 indeterminate colitis) at 2 large treatment centers between 1989 and 2001 revealed that the majority of hospitalizations were in the early second trimester (mean gestation 15.9 weeks (range 8–35)) [42]. Patients on average required a hospital stay of greater than 7 days (mean of 10.4 days (range 3–31)). As to be expected, all IBD patients in this study received IV hydrocortisone (mean dose 199 mg/day). In this study, which was undertaken in the prebiologic era, five patients were induced with cyclosporine. Nowadays, patients with a severe IBD flare during pregnancy may instead require initiation of a biologic. If patients are already established on biologics, as previously mentioned, they should continue. Additionally, it is acceptable to initiate new biologic therapy during pregnancy if clinically indicated. Post-authorization data published by the European Medicines Agency on the use of anti-TNF biologics during pregnancy have not demonstrated any increased risk of malformations; however infliximab was associated with an increased risk for secondary unfavorable outcomes such as Cesarean section, preterm birth, small for gestational age, and low birth weight [43], although these results may be due to increased IBD activity.

Unsurprisingly, most studies have noted that following inpatient treatment for a severe IBD flare during pregnancy, there is a higher risk of preterm delivery and low birth weight. It is more likely that these adverse outcomes are more due to the actual disease process rather than the treatment received. A Danish study of 219 women with IBD treated in the third trimester with anti-TNF therapy revealed no increased risk of low birth weight or preterm birth associated with the drug [44].

Data about outcomes of pregnancies with vedolizumab are limited. A review of pregnancies that occurred within the vedolizumab trials revealed 27 unintended pregnancies in female participants, and no significant safety concerns were identified [45]. More recently, the CONCEIVE study assessed 79 pregnancies of IBD patients and failed to identify any increased risk of miscarriage, prematurity, or low birth weight [46].

The data for ustekinumab in pregnancy are also limited to case studies and registry data. These data from the rheumatology literature suggest that ustekinumab is not associated with increased risk of miscarriage or congenital malformation [47]. Data in pregnancy in women with IBD are limited to case reports with variable outcome including miscarriage and healthy delivery [48, 49].

Data are also limited for tofacitinib in pregnancy associated with UC, where 11 cases of maternal exposure and 14 cases of paternal exposure have been identified across intervention studies. Outcomes include 15 healthy infants, with no neonatal or fetal deaths, no congenital malformations, two spontaneous abortions, and two medical terminations [50].

Clostridium difficile Infection and IBD

It is well recognized that patients with IBD have a higher incidence and prevalence of *Clostridium difficile* infection. Gastroenterologists should bear in mind that this pertains to the period during pregnancy as well, and prompt evaluation and treatment should be initiated should any suspicion arise. In addition, avoiding long-term antibiotics and ciprofloxacin is also recommended. In a large retrospective cohort study on women admitted for delivery using the Nationwide Inpatient Sample from the United States, both UC and CD were identified as significant risk factors for the diagnosis of *C. difficile* infection. Another independent risk factor was long-term antibiotic use [51]. The diagnosis of *C. difficile* infection in pregnancy was associated with a significant increase in poor outcomes such as maternal death (aOR 56.8, 95% CI 35.8–90.1), sepsis (aOR 59.1, 95% CI 48.8–71.6), paralytic ileus (aOR 33.1, 95% CI 27.5–39.8), venous thromboembolism (aOR 8.1, 95% CI 6.5–10.2), and hospital stays greater than 2 weeks (aOR 24.3, 95% CI 21.6–27.4) [51]. Therefore, while it is imperative that sick pregnant patients are treated appropriately, awareness of the adverse safety profile of these medications in pregnancy is necessary (Table 13.1).

Surgical Management of Complicated IBD During Pregnancy

Women who are pregnant should receive optimal medical and surgical care regardless of pregnancy status, and, if indicated, surgery should not be postponed until postpartum [52]. Women with obstruction, abscess, refractory colitis, hemorrhage, and appendicitis, among other medical conditions, may require more emergent surgery during pregnancy. A study using the Danish national registries of 1,202,870 pregnancies, including 4490 (0.4%) women who had non-obstetric abdominal surgery during pregnancy, showed increased risk of small for gestational age, very preterm births, preterm birth, and miscarriage among women who underwent surgery during pregnancy; the greatest risk for these outcomes occurred within 14 days after surgery [53]. The risk of miscarriage decreased with time after surgery and, after 2 weeks, approached that of pregnancies without surgery. Baseline characteristics showed that women who underwent non-obstetric abdominal surgery during pregnancy were more likely obese, smokers, diabetic, or diagnosed with rheumatoid arthritis or IBD. A systematic review of surgical management of complicated IBD in pregnant patients noted 86 cases over a 60-year period and noted that a free or contained small bowel perforation was the commonest reason for surgery in CD and medically refractory or fulminant UC or toxic megacolon was the main indication for surgery in UC [23]. Of note, of the 56 patients with UC who underwent surgery, 14 (25%) were newly diagnosed with UC during pregnancy [23]. In this review, several authors had recommended laparoscopy as the operative approach of choice in the first and second trimesters, due to its diagnostic and therapeutic role, smaller incision, likelihood of less adhesion formation, and

Table 13.1 Recommendations for medical therapy during pregnancy

Drug	Data source	Data in pregnancy	Recommendation
Aminosalicylates	2	All mesalamine preparations are now phthalate-free	Maintain prepregnancy dosage
Sulfasalazine	2	Azulfidine EN contains phthalates	Maintain prepregnancy dosage Consider adding 2 mg folate supplementation
Azathioprine/6-mercaptopurine	2	Possible increased risk of infant infection when used in combination with biologic	Continue as monotherapy. Consider withholding as combination therapy due to increased risk of infant infection Therapeutic drug monitoring recommended
Cyclosporine	2	Limited data in pregnancy Associated with hypertension, unfavorable outcomes[a]	Use as salvage therapy if appropriate
Methotrexate	1,2	Teratogenicity	Contraindicated in pregnancy
Corticosteroids	2,4	Cleft palate	For active flares, not maintenance therapy
Antibiotics	2,3	Reserved for perianal disease and pouchitis	Not recommended for planned maintenance therapy (amoxicillin/metronidazole (2nd and 3rd trimester) preferred over ciprofloxacin)
Adalimumab	1,2	No increased rate of malformations or other unfavorable outcomes[a]	Plan final pregnancy injection 2–3 weeks before EDD[c], and resume postpartum (1–2 weeks if weekly dosing)
Certolizumab pegol	1,2	No increased rate of malformations or other unfavorable outcomes[a]	May continue scheduled dosing throughout pregnancy

(continued)

Table 13.1 (continued)

Drug	Data source	Data in pregnancy	Recommendation
Infliximab	1,2	No increased rate of malformations Increased risk for adverse secondary outcomes but may be due to increased disease activity[b]	Plan final pregnancy infusion 6–10 weeks before EDD and resume postpartum. (If every 4-wk dosing, then 4–5 wk before EDD). Base dosing on prepregnancy weight during pregnancy and immediate postpartum. Can check level at 28 weeks to see if additional dose needed as levels increase in third trimester
Vedolizumab	1,2	Limited human data	Plan final pregnancy dose 6–10 weeks before EDD and resume postpartum. (If every-4-week dosing, then 4–5 wk before EDD).
Tofacitinib	2	Limited human data	Consider other options, particularly in first trimester
Ustekinumab	2	Limited human data	Plan final pregnancy dose 6–10 weeks before EDD and resume postpartum. (If every-4-week dosing, then 4–5 wk before EDD).

1. Br J Clin Pharmacol. 2020 Mar;86(3):580–590. doi: https://doi.org/10.1111/bcp.14145
2. Gastroenterology. 2019 Apr;156(5):1508–1524. doi: https://doi.org/10.1053/j.gastro.2018.12.022. PubMed PMID: 30658060
3. Nat Rev Gastroenterol Hepatol. 2014 Feb;11(2):116–27. doi: https://doi.org/10.1038/nrgastro.2013.135. PubMed PMID: 23897285
4. Birth Defects Res A Clin Mol Teratol. 2016 Jun;106(6):494–9. doi:https://doi.org/10.1002/bdra.23509. PubMed PMID: 27301563

[a]Unfavorable outcomes in this regard include spontaneous abortions, minor birth defects, preterm delivery, birth size, and serious or opportunistic infections and no stillbirths or malignancies

[b]Including Cesarean section, preterm birth, small for gestational age, and low birth weight

[c]Expected date of delivery

quicker recovery. Surgery in pregnancy requires a multidisciplinary management involving gastroenterologists, obstetricians, neonatologists, surgeons, and nutritionists.

Delivery in IBD

In pregnancy complicated by IBD – be it CD or UC – the mode of delivery is usually planned based on obstetric indications. This is applicable even in severe flares of IBD. Most women can undergo vaginal delivery unless there is active perianal disease present at time of delivery [52]. In addition, women with previous ileal pouch-anal anastomosis (IPAA) may be advised to undergo Cesarean section as it is thought to prevent anal sphincter injury [52]. Cesarean section should also be considered here to avoid future pouch dysfunction in IPAA patients and maintain sphincter functionality. The integrity of the anal sphincter can be disturbed by mechanical pressure during vaginal birth. Episiotomy has a risk of causing rectovaginal fistulas and nonhealing wounds during periods of active perianal disease; therefore it is not recommended [54, 55]. In general, it is best to avoid an operative vaginal delivery (i.e., forceps or vacuum delivery) as these patients may have increased long-term complications [52].

In a retrospective study of 61 patients with perianal CD, 11 were delivered vaginally, and 50 underwent delivery by Cesarean section. No difference was noted in the rates of postpartum perianal surgical intervention or luminal disease flares based on mode of delivery [56]. However if perianal disease is active, there can be up to a tenfold increased risk for fourth-degree laceration [56, 57]. As per AGA guidelines, group B streptococcus screening culture collection from perineal area at 35–37 weeks' gestation and inspection enable physicians to decide on a suitable mode of delivery and revise if appropriate based on the presence of infection or active perianal disease [52].

In pregnant patients with either new or established ostomies, mode of delivery is again largely dictated by obstetric indication. Stomal problems, such as displacement, enlargement, retraction, stenosis, and prolapse, may occur with stretching of the abdominal wall. Postpartum care may require coordination with a colorectal surgeon and an ostomy/wound nurse. If a Cesarean section is required, simply covering the ostomy with gauze is adequate to protect the operative field [52].

Details of mode of delivery are summarized in Fig. 13.1.

Pregnancy Outcomes in IBD

Adverse pregnancy outcomes occur more frequently in women with inflammatory bowel diseases (IBD) compared to the general population [58, 59]. IBD has been shown to increase the risk of spontaneous preterm birth as well as indicated preterm delivery secondary to maternal and fetal complications [60]. Adverse maternal outcomes in IBD include C-section, gestational diabetes, and preeclampsia. A recent meta-analysis by Tandon and colleagues has identified a pooled odds ratio (OR) of 1.79 (95% CI 1.16–2.77) for C-section among patients with IBD compared to controls [61]. After stratifying by IBD type, the higher odds of C-section remained for those with UC, but not those with CD. While higher rates of C-section may be due to current guidelines recommending planned C-section for patients with active perianal disease or ileal pouch-anal anastomosis [52, 62], the majority of C-section deliveries among IBD patients occur for emergent indications [63, 64]. Patients receiving combination therapy with anti-TNFs and immunomodulators are also more likely to require C-section [7]. Regardless of corticosteroid use during pregnancy, patients with IBD are more likely to develop gestational diabetes (OR 2.96, 95% CI 1.47–5.98) compared to healthy controls [61]. The etiology of this risk is unknown, but a link with vitamin D deficiency is suspected [65]. There is no increased risk for pre-eclampsia among patients with IBD compared to healthy controls, and there is no increased incidence of preeclampsia among patients exposed to anti-TNFs, immunomodulators, or budesonide compared to those not exposed to these therapies [61].

Placental complications including chorioamnionitis, placental abruption, and placenta previa do not appear to be significantly

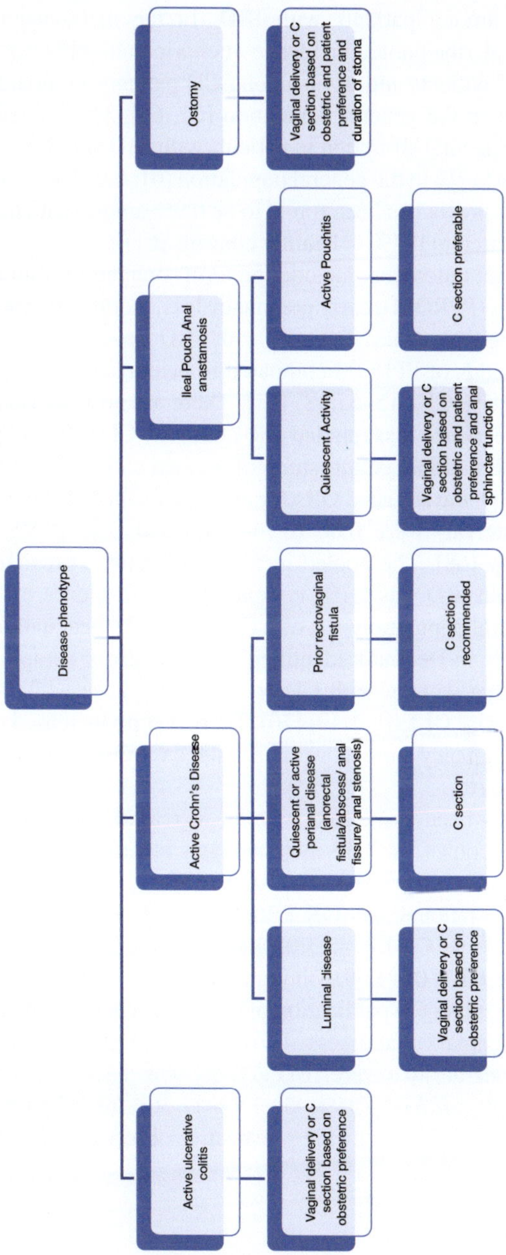

Fig. 13.1 Mode of delivery

increased among patients with IBD. In the meta-analysis by Tandon et al., the pooled incidence of chorioamnionitis was 0.3% among UC patients and 0.2% among CD patients, compared to a rate of 4% in the general population [61, 66]. The pooled incidence of placental abruption in patients with IBD was 3.3%, compared to up to 1% in the general population [61, 67]. The incidence of placenta previa has been found to be 0.9% among patients with IBD compared to 0.7% in healthy controls [61].

Obstetric outcomes include preterm premature rupture of membranes (PPROM), early pregnancy loss, therapeutic abortion, and ectopic pregnancy. Patients with IBD have a significantly increased odds of PPROM compared to healthy controls (pooled OR 12.1, 95% CI 2.15–67.98) [61]. There are no increased odds of early pregnancy loss (pooled OR 1.63, 95% CI 0.49–5.43) [61]. In a Danish national cohort study of women with UC and CD or without IBD, the adjusted ORs for an elective abortion (95% confidence interval) were 0.80 (0.74–0.86) and 0.96 (0.89–1.04), respectively [68]. The pooled incidence of ectopic pregnancy in patients with IBD was 1.1%, compared to a prevalence of 0.64% in the general population [61, 69]. However, a 22-year nationwide cohort study in Denmark identified a higher risk of ectopic pregnancy among women with CD compared to those without IBD (OR 1.23, 95% CI 1.01–1.49) [70]. There was no increased risk of ectopic pregnancy among women with UC (OR 0.98, 95% CI 0.80–120) [70].

IBD has been associated with an increased risk of neonatal adverse outcomes. A 2015 meta-analysis identified significantly increased odds of preterm birth (OR 1.85, 95% CI 1.67–2.05), small for gestational age (OR 1.36, 95% CI 1.16–1.60), stillbirth (OR 1.57, 95% CI 1.03–2.38), and congenital anomalies (OR 1.29, 95% CI 1.05–1.58), though the authors concluded that the latter is subject to publication bias [59]. In a nationwide cohort study in Denmark that assessed IBD activity and pregnancy outcomes, moderate to severe IBD activity was associated with an adjusted OR of 3.60 (95% CI 1.14–11.36) for preterm birth [71]. A recent US nationwide prospective observational study of

1,490 completed pregnancies in women with IBD resulting in 1431 live births with follow up of 1010 infants to one year, found that the use of biologics (anti-TNF, anti-integrin, and anti-interleukin-12/23), thiopurines, or combination therapy was not associated with an increased risk of spontaneous abortion, congenital malformations, preterm birth, low birth weight, or infant infections through the first year of life [72]. However, more active disease was associated with an increased risk of spontaneous abortion (HR 3.41, 95% CI 1.51–7.69) and preterm birth with increased infant infections (OR 1.73, 95% CI 1.19–2.51). Therefore, it is recommended that these therapies should be continued during pregnancy to reduce the risk of adverse pregnancy and neonatal outcomes.

Conclusion

Despite advances in IBD medical therapy, IBD appears to be associated with increased rates of adverse pregnancy outcomes including C-section, gestational diabetes, PPROM, preterm birth, stillbirth, and small for gestational age. However, many adverse outcomes appear to be related to IBD activity rather than biologic or thiopurine therapy, which are felt to be safe during pregnancy. Additional large, prospective studies are needed to identify IBD-specific predictors for pregnancy complications. Validated prediction models with the ability to risk-stratify individual IBD patients prior to conception would greatly facilitate prenatal counseling in this high-risk population.

It is imperative that in order to minimize inpatient admission, gastroenterology providers counsel female patients with IBD that if they are planning for pregnancy, potential risks of IBD and pregnancy be discussed first. Regular medical visits and the importance of following a set treatment plan should be discussed. The importance of not only regular obstetric but also gastroenterology monitoring (usually in each trimester) should also be discussed.

Clinical Vignette

A 32-year-old G1P0 female at 12 weeks' gestation presents with 1 week of progressive lower abdominal pain and frequent bloody diarrhea. She was diagnosed with ulcerative pancolitis 2 years ago and, after an initial course of corticosteroids, has been in remission on vedolizumab monotherapy every 8 weeks. Her last infusion was 2 weeks prior to presentation. On day 1 of hospital admission, a flexible sigmoidoscopy was performed and notable for Mayo grade 3 inflammation continuously to the hepatic flexure. Pathology was negative for viral inclusions. CRP was 33 and she was started on IV methylprednisolone. On day 3 of hospitalization, her CRP is 110 and there has been no improvement in her bowel frequency. What is the next best step in management?

Best Answer

Infliximab TNF-alpha antagonists have been shown to be safe in pregnancy [73]. Infliximab can be administered at an intravenous induction dose of 5 mg/kg. A second dose at 10 mg/kg can be given if there is insufficient clinical response within 5 days. Live vaccines should be delayed for 6 months for infants exposed to TNF-alpha antagonists as serum levels may be detectable for several months.

Alternative Approaches

Cyclosporine Cyclosporine is also an effective induction agent for acute severe ulcerative colitis during pregnancy [42]. Its use has not been associated with congenital malformations, but there may be an increased risk of premature delivery [74]. A maintenance agent will have to be chosen after induction.

Surgery Medical therapy should be optimized prior to consideration of surgery. Colectomy has been associated with spontaneous abortion or fetal death in up to 50% of cases [75].

Would Avoid

Dose Interval Reduction of Vedolizumab to Every 4 Weeks While dose intensification has been shown to recapture response in about half of IBD patients who lose response to vedolizumab, the acuity of this patient's symptoms and need for a timely clinical response indicate a more aggressive approach [76].

Tofacitinib Tofacitinib should be avoided in pregnancy, as it has been associated with congenital malformations in animals.

References

1. Mogadam M, Korelitz BI, Ahmed SW, et al. The course of inflammatory bowel disease during pregnancy and postpartum. Am J Gastroenterol. 1981;75(4):265–9.
2. Miller JP. Inflammatory bowel disease in pregnancy: a review. J R Soc Med. 1986;79(4):221–5.
3. de Lima-Karagiannis A, Zelinkova-Detkova Z, van der Woude CJ. The effects of active IBD during pregnancy in the era of novel IBD therapies. Am J Gastroenterol. 2016;111(9):1305–12.
4. Watanabe C, Nagahori M, Fujii T, Yokoyama K, et al. Non-adherence to medications in pregnant ulcerative colitis patients contributes to disease flares and adverse pregnancy outcomes. Dig Dis Sci. 2020; https://doi.org/10.1007/s10620-020-06221-6. [Epub ahead of print] PubMed PMID: 32249373
5. Puri A, Bharadwaj V, Sachdeva S. Extent of disease is a major outcome predictor in patients with ulcerative colitis and pregnancy. Indian J Gastroenterol. 2015;34(2):108–11.
6. Getahun D, Fassett MJ, Longstreth G, et al. Association between maternal inflammatory bowel disease and adverse perinatal outcomes. J Perinatol. 2014;34(6):435–40.
7. Bortoli A, Pedersen N, Duricova D, European Crohn-Colitis Organisation (ECCO) Study Group of Epidemiologic Committee (EpiCom), et al.

Pregnancy outcome in inflammatory bowel disease: prospective European case-control ECCO- EpiCom study 2003–2006. Aliment Pharmacol Ther. 2011;34:724–34.
8. Riis L, Vind I, Politi P, et al. Does pregnancy change the disease course? A study in a European cohort of patients with inflammatory bowel disease. Am J Gastroenterol. 2006;101:1539–45.
9. Dubinsky M, Abraham B, Mahadevan U. Management of the pregnant IBD patient. Inflamm Bowel Dis. 2008;14:1736–50.
10. Abramson D, Jankelson IR, Milner LR. Pregnancy in idiopathic ulcerative colitis. Am J Obstet Gynecol. 1951;61:121–9.
11. Willoughby CP, Truelove SC. Ulcerative colitis and pregnancy. Gut. 1980;21:469–74.
12. Greenfield C, Pounder RE, Craft IL, et al. Severe ulcerative colitis during successful pregnancy. Postgrad Med J. 1983;59:459–61.
13. Bohe MG, Ekelund GR, Genell SN, et al. Surgery for ulcerative colitis during pregnancy. Dis Colon Rectum. 1983;26:119–122.
14. Anderson JB, Turner GM, Williamson RC. Fulminant ulcerative colitis in late pregnancy and the puerperium. J R Soc Med. 1987;80:492–4.
15. Beniada A, Benoist G, Maurel J, Dreyfus M. Inflammatory bowel disease and pregnancy: report of 76 cases and review of the literature. J Gynecol Obstet Biol Reprod. 2005;34:581–8.
16. Haq AI, Sahai A, Hallwoth S, et al. Synchronous colectomy and cesarean section for fulminant ulcerative colitis: case report and review of the literature. Int J Color Dis. 2006;21:465–9.
17. Orabona R, Valcamonico A, Salemme M, et al. Fulminant ulcerative colitis in a healthy pregnant woman. World J Gastroenterol. 2015;21:6060–4.
18. Uchino M, Ikeuchi H, Matsuoka H, et al. Surgery for severe ulcerative colitis during pregnancy: report of two cases. Case Rep Gastroenterol. 2015;9:74–80.
19. Brunelli R, Perrone S, Perrone G, et al. New-onset ulcerative colitis in pregnancy associated to toxic megacolon and sudden fetal decompensation: case report and literature review. J Obstet Gynaecol Res. 2019;45(7):1215–21.
20. Cappell MS, Colon VJ, Sidhom OA. A study at 10 medical centers of the safety and efficacy of 48 flexible sigmoidoscopies and 8 colonoscopies during pregnancy with follow-up of fetal outcome and with comparison to control groups. Dig Dis Sci. 1996;41:2353–61.
21. Hartgill TW, Bergersen TK, Pirhonen J. Core body temperature and the thermoneutral zone: a longitudinal study of normal human pregnancy. Acta Physiol. 2011;201:467–74.
22. Pillay V, Savage N, Laburn H. Interleukin-1 receptor antagonist in newborn babies and pregnant women. Pflugers Arch. 1993;424:549–55.
23. Killeen S, Gunn J, Hartley J. Surgical management of complicated and medically refractory inflammatory bowel disease during pregnancy. Color Dis. 2017;19(2):123–38.

24. Winter R, Nørgård BM, Friedman S. Treatment of the pregnant patient with inflammatory bowel disease. Inflamm Bowel Dis. 2016;22(3):733–44.
25. Friedman S. Gestational weight gain: a new factor influencing pregnancy outcomes in women with inflammatory bowel disease. Dig Dis Sci. 2017;62(8):2070–1.
26. Beaulieu DB, Kane S. Inflammatory bowel disease in pregnancy. Gastroenterol Clin N Am. 2011;40(2):399–413.
27. Cornish J, Tan E, Teare J, et al. A meta-analysis on the influence of inflammatory bowel disease on pregnancy. Gut. 2007;56(6):830–7.
28. Leung YP, Kaplan GG, Coward S, et al. Intrapartum corticosteroid use significantly increases the risk of gestational diabetes in women with inflammatory bowel disease. J Crohns Colitis. 2015;9:223–30.
29. Lin K, Martin CF, Dassopoulos T, et al. Pregnancy outcomes amongst mothers with inflammatory bowel disease exposed to systemic corticosteroids: results of the PIANO registry. Gastroenterology. 2014;146:S-1.
30. Truta B. Potential risks of immunosuppressant drugs to the pregnant patient. American College of Gastroenterology: Honolulu; 2015.
31. Mitchell K, Kaul M, Clowse M. The management of rheumatic diseases in pregnancy. Scand J Rheumatol. 2010;39(2):99–108.
32. Broms G, Granath F, Linder M, et al. Complications from inflammatory bowel disease during pregnancy and delivery. Clin Gastroenterol Hepatol. 2012;10:1246–52.
33. Bates SM, Rajasekhar A, Middeldorp S, et al. American Society of Hematology 2018 guidelines for management of venous thromboembolism: venous thromboembolism in the context of pregnancy. Blood Adv. 2018;2(22):3317–59.
34. van der Woude CJ, Ardizzone S, Bengtson MB, et al. European Crohn's and Colitis Organization. The second European evidenced-based consensus on reproduction and pregnancy in inflammatory bowel disease. J Crohns Colitis. 2015;9(2):107–24.
35. Tsigkas G, Davlouros P, Despotopoulos S, et al. Inflammatory bowel disease: a potential risk factor for coronary artery disease. Angiology. 2017;68(10):845–9.
36. Tandon P, Leung K, Yusuf A, Huang VW. Noninvasive methods for assessing inflammatory bowel disease activity in pregnancy: a systematic review. J Clin Gastroenterol. 2019;53(8):574–81.
37. Julsgaard M, Hvas CL, Gearry RB, et al. Fecal calprotectin is not affected by pregnancy: clinical implications for the management of pregnant patients with inflammatory bowel disease. Inflamm Bowel Dis. 2017;23(7):1240–6.
38. Bálint A, Berényi A, Farkas K, et al. Pregnancy does not affect fecal calprotectin concentration in healthy women. Turk J Gastroenterol. 2017;28(3):171–5.
39. Kammerlander H, Nielsen J, Kjeldsen J, et al. Fecal calprotectin during pregnancy in women with moderate-severe inflammatory bowel disease. Inflamm Bowel Dis. 2018;24(4):839–48.

40. Ludvigsson JF, Lebwohl B, Ekbom A, et al. Outcomes of pregnancies for women undergoing endoscopy while they were pregnant: a nationwide cohort study. Gastroenterology. 2017;152(3):554–63.
41. Ray JG, Vermeulen MJ, Aditya Bharatha A, et al. Association between MRI exposure during pregnancy and fetal and childhood outcomes. JAMA. 2016;316(9):952–61.
42. Reddy D, Murphy SJ, Kane SV, et al. Relapses of inflammatory bowel disease during pregnancy: in-hospital management and birth outcomes. Am J Gastroenterol. 2008;103(5):1203–9.
43. Ghalandari N, Dolhain RJEM, Hazes JMW, et al. The pre- and post-authorisation data published by the European medicines agency on the use of biologics during pregnancy and lactation. Br J Clin Pharmacol. 2020;86(3):580–90.
44. Kammerlander H, Nielsen J, Knudsen T, Kjeldsen J, Friedman S, Nørgård BM. Anti-TNF-α use during the third trimester of pregnancy in women with moderate-severe inflammatory bowel disease and the risk of preterm birth and low birth weight. Inflamm Bowel Dis. 2017;23(11):1916–23.
45. Mahadevan U, Vermeire S, Lasch K, et al. Vedolizumab exposure in pregnancy: outcomes from clinical studies in inflammatory bowel disease. Aliment Pharmacol Ther. 2017;45(7):941–50.
46. Moens A, van der Woude CJ, Julsgaard M, et al. Pregnancy outcomes in inflammatory bowel disease patients treated with vedolizumab, anti-TNF or conventional therapy: results of the European CONCEIVE study. Aliment Pharmacol Ther. 2020;51(1):129–38.
47. Götestam Skorpen C, Hoeltzenbein M, Tincani A, et al. The EULAR points to consider for use of antirheumatic drugs before pregnancy, and during pregnancy and lactation. Ann Rheum Dis. 2016;75:795–810.
48. Venturin C, Nancey S, Danion P, et al. Fetal death in utero and miscarriage in a patient with Crohn's disease under therapy with ustekinumab: case-report and review of the literature. BMC Gastroenterol. 2017;17:80.
49. Klenske E, Osaba L, Nagore D, et al. Drug levels in the maternal serum, cord blood and breast milk of a ustekinumab-treated patient with Crohn's disease. J Crohns Colitis. 2019;13(2):267–9.
50. Mahadevan U, Dubinsky MC, Su C, et al. Outcomes of pregnancies with maternal/paternal exposure in the tofacitinib safety databases for ulcerative colitis. Inflamm Bowel Dis. 2018;24:2494–500.
51. Ruiter-Ligeti J, Vincent S, Czuzoj-Shulman N, Abenhaim HA. Risk factors, incidence, and morbidity associated with obstetric clostridium difficile infection. Obstet Gynecol. 2018;131(2):387–91.
52. Mahadevan U, Robinson C, Bernasko N, et al. Inflammatory bowel disease in pregnancy clinical care pathway: a report from the American Gastroenterological Association IBD parenthood project working group. Am J Obstet Gynecol. 2019;220(4):308–23.
53. Rasmussen AS, Christiansen CF, Ulrichsen SP, et al. Non-obstetric abdominal surgery during pregnancy and birth outcomes: a Danish registry-based cohort study. Acta Obstet Gynecol Scand. 2019;epub only.

54. Brandt LJ, Estabrook SG, Reinus JF. Results of a survey to evaluate whether vaginal delivery and episiotomy lead to perineal involvement in women with Crohn's disease. Am J Gastroenterol. 1995;90:1918–22.
55. Poturoglu S, Ormeci AC, Duman AE. Treatment of pregnant women with a diagnosis of inflammatory bowel disease. World J Gastrointest Pharmacol Ther. 2016;7(4):490–502.
56. Cheng AG, Oxford EC, Sauk J, et al. Impact of mode of delivery on outcomes in patients with perianal Crohn's disease. Inflamm Bowel Dis. 2014;20(8):1391–8.
57. Hatch Q, Champagne BJ, Maykel JA, et al. Crohn's disease and pregnancy: the impact of perianal disease on delivery methods and complications. Dis Colon Rectum. 2014;57(2):174–8.
58. Nguyen GC, Boudreau H, Harris ML, et al. Outcomes of obstetric hospitalizations among women with inflammatory bowel disease in the United States. Clin Gastroenterol Hepatol. 2009;7:329–34.
59. O'Toole A, Nwanne O, Tomlinson T. Inflammatory bowel disease increases risk of adverse pregnancy outcomes: a meta-analysis. Dig Dis Sci. 2015;60:2750–61.
60. Mountifield R, Bampton P, Prosser R, et al. Fear and fertility in inflammatory bowel disease: a mismatch of perception and reality affects family planning decisions. Inflamm Bowel Dis. 2009;15:720–5.
61. Tandon P, Govardhanam V, Leung K, et al. Systematic review with meta-analysis: risk of adverse pregnancy-related outcomes in inflammatory bowel disease. Aliment Pharmacol Ther. 2020;51:320–33.
62. Nguyen GC, Seow CH, Maxwell C, et al. The Toronto consensus statements for the management of inflammatory bowel disease in pregnancy. Gastroenterology. 2016;150:734–57.
63. Burke KE, Haviland MJ, Hacker MR, et al. Indications for mode of delivery in pregnant women with inflammatory bowel disease. Inflamm Bowel Dis. 2017;23:721–6.
64. Sharaf AA, Nguyen GC. Predictors of cesarean delivery in pregnant women with inflammatory bowel disease. J Can Assoc Gastroenterol. 2018;1:76–81.
65. Aghajafari F, Nagulesapillai T, Ronksley PE, et al. Association between maternal serum 25-hydroxyvitamin D level and pregnancy and neonatal outcomes: systematic review and meta-analysis of observational studies. BMJ. 2013;346:f1169.
66. Fowler JR, Simon LV. Chorioamnionitis. StatPearls. Treasure Island: StatPearls Publishing; 2019. https://www.ncbi.nlm.nih.gov/books/NBK532251/
67. Tikkanen M. Placental abruption: epidemiology, risk factors and consequences. Acta Obstet Gynecol Scand. 2011;90:140–9.
68. Nørgård BM, Magnussen B, Fedder J, et al. The risk of elective abortion in women with Crohn's disease and ulcerative colitis: a nationwide cohort study. Inflamm Bowel Dis. 2019;25(3):561–7.

69. Hoover KW, Tao G, Kent CK. Trends in the diagnosis and treatment of ectopic pregnancy in the United States. Obstet Gynecol. 2010;115:495–502.
70. de Silva PS, Hansen HH, Wehberg S, et al. Risk of ectopic pregnancy in women with inflammatory bowel disease: a 22-year nationwide cohort study. Clin Gastroenterol Hepatol. 2018;16:83–9.
71. Kammerlander H, Nielsen J, Kjeldsen J, et al. The effect of disease activity on birth outcomes in a nationwide cohort of women with moderate to severe inflammatory bowel disease. Inflamm Bowel Dis. 2017;23:1011–8.
72. Mahadevan U, Long MD, Kane SV et al. Crohn's Colitis Foundation Clinical Research Alliance. Pregnancy and Neonatal Outcomes After Fetal Exposure to Biologics and Thiopurines Among Women With Inflammatory Bowel Disease. Gastroenterology. 2021 Mar;160(4):1131-1139. https://doi.org/10.1053/j.gastro.2020.11.038. Epub 2020 Nov 21. PMID: 33227283; PMCID: PMC7956164.
73. M, Chaparro A, Verreth T, Lobaton E et al. (2018) Long-Term Safety of In Utero Exposure to Anti-TNFα Drugs for the Treatment of Inflammatory Bowel Disease: Results from the Multicenter European TEDDY Study. American Journal of Gastroenterology 113(3) 396–403. https://doi.org/10.1038/ajg.2017.501.
74. Benjamin B O, Hackman T, Einarson G et al. Pregnancy outcome after cyclosporine therapy during pregnancy: A meta-analysis. Transplantation 2001; 71(8) 1051–55 https://doi.org/10.1097/00007890-200104270-00006.
75. Dozois EJ, Wolff BJ, Tremaine WJ e al. Maternal and Fetal Outcome After Colectomy for Fulminant Ulcerative Colitis During Pregnancy: Case Series and Literature Review. Diseases of the Colon & Rectum 2006; 49(1) 64–73. https://doi.org/10.1007/s10350-005-0210-x.
76. Laurent PB, Silvio DM, Lieven A et al. Loss of Response to Vedolizumab and Ability of Dose Intensification to Restore Response in Patients With Crohn's Disease or Ulcerative Colitis: A Systematic Review and Meta-analysis. Clinical Gastroenterology and Hepatology 2019;17(5)838–46.e2 https://doi.org/10.1016/j.cgh.2018.06.026.

Index

J. D. Feuerstein, A. S. Cheifetz (eds.), *Management of Inpatient Inflammatory Bowel Disease*,
https://doi.org/10.1007/978-1-0716-1987-2

V

W

MIX
Papier aus verantwortungsvollen Quellen
Paper from responsible sources
FSC® C105338
FSC
www.fsc.org

If you have any concerns about our products,
you can contact us on
ProductSafety@springernature.com

In case Publisher is established outside the EU,
the EU authorized representative is:
Springer Nature Customer Service Center GmbH
Europaplatz 3, 69115 Heidelberg, Germany

Printed by Libri Plureos GmbH
in Hamburg, Germany